T0322986

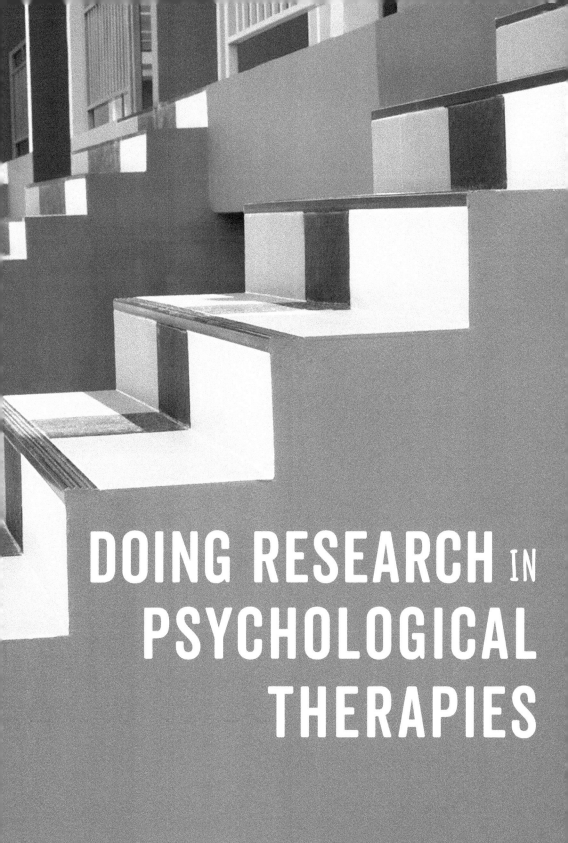

DOING RESEARCH IN PSYCHOLOGICAL THERAPIES

JOEL VOS

DOING RESEARCH IN PSYCHOLOGICAL THERAPIES

A STEP-BY-STEP GUIDE

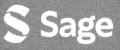
Sage

S Sage

1 Oliver's Yard
55 City Road
London EC1Y 1SP

2455 Teller Road
Thousand Oaks, California 91320

Unit No 323-333, Third Floor, F-Block
International Trade Tower Nehru Place
New Delhi – 110 019

8 Marina View Suite 43-053
Asia Square Tower 1
Singapore 018960

Library of Congress Control Number: 2023931168

British Library Cataloguing in Publication data

A catalogue record for this book is available from the British Library

Editor: Susannah Trefgarne
Editorial Assistant: Esmé Sawyer
Production Editor: Gourav Kumar
Copyeditor: Tom Bedford
Proofreader: Larry Baker
Indexer: KnowledgeWorks Global Ltd
Marketing Manager: Ruslana Khatagova
Cover Design: Naomi Robinson
Typeset by KnowledgeWorks Global Ltd

ISBN 978-1-5297-3374-7
ISBN 978-1-5297-3373-0 (pbk)

'Unless we get the practice of research right, we will not provide the right research to underpin and inform practice'.

(Barkham & Lambert, 2021, p174)

CONTENTS

ONLINE RESOURCES

Visit the author's website **https://joelvos.com/doingresearch** to access the following resources:

Downloadable templates A–I

Student resources

- Recommended reading
- Online tables (extra; downloadable)
- Downloadable figures

Lecturer resources

- Teaching plan for research modules
- Pedagogical tips and tricks

Other resources

- Research proposal checklist
- Thesis checklist
- Research proposal PowerPoint presentation
- Thesis PowerPoint presentation

ABOUT THE AUTHOR

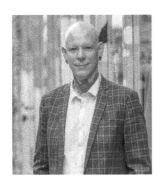

Joel Vos, PhD, MSc, MA, CPsychol, FHEA, is a psychologist, philosopher, and psychological therapist. He works as a Senior Researcher and Senior Lecturer at the Metanoia Institute in London. He is Director of IMEC International Meaning Events and Community, and is a consultant and board member to several mental health services. In the past he has worked at the University of Roehampton and the New School of Psychotherapy and Counselling in the United Kingdom, and at Leiden University in the Netherlands. He has extensive experience in helping students doing research in psychological therapies. For example, he has been teaching research methods and design for almost two decades, and has redesigned the research programmes at several universities. He has supervised and examined hundreds of master and doctorate students. Joel has published over 160 articles and chapters. His recent books with Sage include *The Psychology of COVID-19* in 2021 and *Mental Health in Crisis* together with Ron Roberts and James Davies in 2019. Other books include *Meaning in Life: An Evidence-Based Handbook for Practitioners* (Bloomsbury, 2019) and *The Economics of Meaning in Life* (University Professors Press, 2020). His recent research focuses on mixed methods studies, systematic reviews, and meta-analyses of psychological therapies, humanistic and existential therapies, meaning in life, social movements, critical psychology, and social justice.

Read more on his personal website: https://joelvos.com.

PART I
BASIC SKILLS

1

How to Become a Researcher on Psychological Therapies

Chapter aims

This chapter introduces how you can use practical steps to become a motivated, self-critical, scholarly, and realistic researcher on psychological therapies. This chapter also explains how to use this book.

Steps in chapter

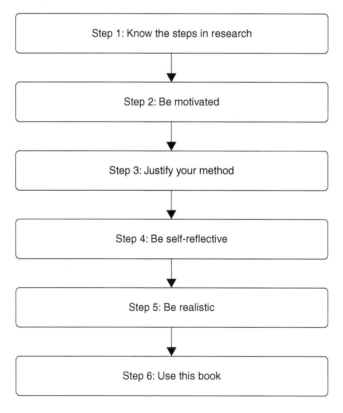

Step 1: Know the steps in research

Definition

This section explains how a step-by-step approach can help you develop your research project, and how this differs from other books.

Explanation

I remember starting my first research project. I was sitting behind my computer in my student room, surrounded by piles of books and syllabi. I told myself: 'I must know what to do because I have all the knowledge in these key texts!' But I did not know what steps to take. I felt overwhelmed. Many landmark books gave brilliant theoretical introductions to research but they did not give the practical guidance I needed. Other books were too detailed about specific methods. I needed someone guiding me around these landmark publications, telling me which book to pick up and which step to take, and when. Someone needed to break down the overwhelming research process into small steps; as Henry Ford said, 'nothing is particularly hard if you divide it into small jobs'. As nobody at that time had developed a step-by-step guide to doing research, I created my own, and have developed it during the approximately 170 research projects I have conducted and supervised since then, with helpful input from students and colleagues. Over the years, I have written many texts to guide my students and colleagues, which have organically evolved into the publication of this book.

This book is for anyone doing research in psychological therapies. I use 'psychological therapies' as an umbrella term for any treatment offered by a professional ('therapist') to an individual ('client') to reduce their psychological problems and/or improve their psychological well-being. Under this umbrella, you can find fields such as psychotherapy, counselling, clinical and community psychology, psychiatry, mental health nursing, social work, and coaching. Undoubtedly you will know your field's unique history, philosophy, and traditions. This book focuses on the generic principles of therapy research, as there is often much overlap between their research aims, methods, and findings (Grawe, 1997; Orlinsky, 2009).

This book guides beginning and experienced researchers in simple steps to develop their research, from developing a research idea to conducting literature reviews, designing research, analysing data, and writing theses and articles. This book provides a comprehensive overview of all steps in research, based on the 29 consecutive conceptual steps found in the 200 most frequently cited articles on psychological therapies (see Chapter 3; Vos, 2014). If you systematically follow these steps, you will develop a coherent and logical framework for your research, and use the best practices and latest research trends. This book provides a rich compendium of resources for each step of research, including explanatory tables, reflective questions, and references. The step-by-step approach ensures that you do not forget crucial steps, know which decisions to make at each stage of the research process, and get going again when you feel lost. These steps also fulfil the research requirements from the main psychology bodies, such as the American Psychological Association (APA) and British Psychological Society (BPS).

This book does not aim to make you an expert in each research method, but provides an overview of the most frequently used research methods, explains how to select the best method for your research, and gives recommendations for further reading. This book is like a hiking map where you can see all possible roads, and you may subsequently decide to further examine particular landmarks in the landscape yourself.

Step 2: Be motivated

Definition

The more meaningful a research project is, the more motivated and dedicated researchers are, and the more likely they will persevere and succeed (Vos, 2017). Therefore, this section describes the motivations that I have observed in my research students over decades of research teaching.

Improving the field

Many students want to improve the field, such as making therapy more effective and helping therapists understand their clients better. A survey of 384 therapists showed that therapists prefer research that does justice to the complexities of therapy and that has potentially practical implications, such as emphasising how therapy is done, moments of change, processes, development of the therapeutic relationship, comparison with other therapies, and connection between theory and practice (Morrow-Bradley & Elliott, 1986).

To impact your field, your research must be innovative and relevant. Therefore, this book will guide you to start your research project with a literature review, to know which studies have already been done and how you could make a unique contribution. You also need to select a strong research methodology to ensure that your findings can be trusted and are worthy of sharing with colleagues. Furthermore, it is insufficient to write a thesis that ends up in a drawer collecting dust: the findings must be transferred for example via presentations and articles in academic journals. Therefore, to optimise your potential impact, this book explains how to conduct a literature review, identify your potential contributions, and develop a robust research proposal and dissemination plan.

Developing a professional identity

Our research expertise gives us a distinctive professional status from pop-scientists and quack-practitioners: research findings can offer key justifications for therapeutic practices. This gives us a more authoritative voice (and possibly better positions and salaries). Many professional bodies and health insurance providers require practitioners to have research expertise.

Becoming a better therapist

Many professional bodies expect trainees to become scientist-practitioners, integrating research and practitioner skills (Lane & Corrie, 2007), as doing research can teach crucial skills for therapeutic practices, such as understanding which interventions are effective, and becoming more critical about the empirical foundations and limitations of practices. Doing research may socialise practitioners with values such as subjectivity, inter-subjectivity, reflexivity, pluralism, empowerment, ethical commitment, and valuing diversity. Furthermore, since the 1990s there has been a global trend towards evidence-based practice, as Chapter 3 will explain.

Institutional needs

Research can help mental health services evaluate the coverage of their target population, the quality of their services, and identify opportunities for improvement with more reliable information than therapists' subjective self-reflection.

Giving voice to individuals

A growing number of researchers argue that all research should lead to practical knowledge that can make a difference to people. Research can give a voice to people whose experiences have rarely been heard, do justice to their subjective experiences, and follow a social justice agenda. Of course, it seems unlikely that one research project will solve all problems, but it may contribute to developing a body of research that can make a difference in the long term. Research can inform stakeholders, such as clients, therapists, researchers, and policy-makers, in academic and public debates. If done ethically, participating in research can also be an empowering experience for participants. This means that researchers do not merely follow ethical guidelines as a tick-box exercise but value the unique experiences of the participants and the possible impact of research.

Enjoying research

Many trainees enjoy doing research they are passionate about and do something different than their university modules and clinical work.

Step 3: Justify your method

Definition

Consider a broad range of research methods. Even though you may not use some methods, you need to justify why your method seems better than others for your project.

Components

Everybody does research, but not everybody is a researcher. If you want to buy a TV, you may examine its specs and read some reviews. However, you will not systematically compare all reviews and conduct tests of its technical standards, as in daily life, you do not need this methodological rigour.

This is where academic research differs from our naive daily life enquiries. According to the Oxford Dictionary, research is 'the careful study of a subject, to discover new facts or information about it'. This definition highlights that research does not merely focus on regurgitating our existing knowledge but on collecting 'facts or information'. A research project could explore a new topic, e.g., 'how do clients experience cognitive behaviour therapy (CBT) for dog phobia?' (explorative aim), or test a hypothesis, e.g., 'CBT for dog phobia reduces anxiety' (hypothesis-testing aim). Our aims need to be modest, as we cannot answer all questions in one project. Consequently, research is often circular: you explore or test a topic/hypothesis (aim), collect new facts/information (method), interpret the results (analysis), and compare them with your original ideas (discussion). New questions may arise, which may be answered in a new round of information collection. Therefore, research is often an accumulative process whereby researchers build on each others' work.

As this definition indicates, research also uses a 'careful' method to achieve its aims. Different methods exist to explore or test our topics/hypotheses, which may lead to different facts/information. Whatever method we choose, we need to justify that this method provides reliable, valid, or trustworthy findings.

Quantitative methods

Many studies on psychological therapies use quantitative methods, which focus on numbers, such as questionnaires. In line with the popularity of quantitative methods in medicine, experiments like Randomised Controlled Trials (RCTs) often rank highest in the subjective knowledge hierarchy in psychology. For example, a researcher may use a depression questionnaire to test their hypothesis that clients are depressed ('hypothetical-deductive research'). This seems to assume that a questionnaire can directly measure the client's reality, like medical doctors directly test body temperatures with a thermometer. The quantitative world seems directly measurable and quantifiable, and results can (usually) be generalised between clients because universal laws determine it. Furthermore, quantitative researchers assume that the totality of the client's lived experiences can be reduced, albeit with inevitable errors, to a pre-selected number of 'variables' or 'factors'.

Qualitative methods

Although quantitative methods cast valuable light on general trends and mechanisms across individuals, and test hypotheses, they may not do full justice to the richness and uniqueness of how individuals make sense of their world and experiences. Therefore, qualitative researchers explore the rich, unique experiences of individuals, which may reach beyond the stereotypical rigid answer options in questionnaires/experiments. Qualitative research, such as using interviews, may help to build ideas from individual experiences about the therapy process ('explorative-inductive research') or from a critical-theoretical lens ('critical-deductive research'). Since the turn of the millennium, increasing numbers of qualitative studies have been published on psychological therapies.

Methodological pluralism

The previous paragraphs sketched a stereotypic distinction between quantitative and qualitative research paradigms. Some authors have argued that quantitative and qualitative methods are incommensurable or that there is a hierarchy of true objective science versus the subjective research of arts/philosophy. However, there seems to be an increasing consensus about needing a plurality of research perspectives to understand the dynamic complexities of psychological therapies. Psychological therapies seem to have many facets like a diamond: you need to cast light from different angles to see as many facets as possible (Vos, 2021a). Different angles show various aspects of people's experiences, and all are part of the complex totality of psychological therapies. Innovation often happens in the collaboration and confrontation between different research paradigms (Kuhn, 1970; Popper, 2005). Therefore, this book follows methodological pluralism, the idea that we can attain reliable, valid, and trustworthy data in many different ways; there is no knowledge hierarchy with one best type of research. Pluralism does not mean that all researchers combine quantitative and qualitative methods ('mixed methods'), but that researchers know when to use which method, and they justify their methods while recognising their limitations and valuing alternatives.

Step 4: Be self-reflective

Definition

A critical difference between quack and science is the self-reflective attitude that researchers show throughout the research.

Explanation

Luborsky and colleagues (1999) showed why it is important to reflect critically on your biases and influences on the research process. In their systematic review of clinical trials, they found that the theoretical background of the lead researcher predicts the study out-comes, called researcher-allegiance effects, i.e., the belief in the superiority of a specific treatment. Researchers tend to focus on findings supporting their beliefs, expectations, or preferences. This is one of the greatest threats to the validity of studies (Munder, 2013). For example, a cognitive behavioural therapist lead researcher is more likely conclude that CBT is effective. Cuijpers and Cristea (2016) also found that therapists are less effective when giving interventions they do not fully believe or are not trained in. Therefore, this book invites researchers to critically reflect on their beliefs, justify their decisions, and honestly examine the strengths and weaknesses of their research.

Step 5: Be realistic

Definition

Develop realistic expectations about your research and research process.

Explanation

Research is often not as perfect and streamlined as journals and books may suggest: research is often messy, changing, non-linear, and frustrating. Novice researchers often start with high ideals about research, but quickly learn they need to adjust their expectations. For example, they do not have enough time, money, research skills, or interested participants. Research can be an emotional roller-coaster, starting with beginner's enthusiasm and leading to inevitable disappointments and challenges. Doing your first research project may also feel like entering a dark forest, without your usual routines and confronted with unfamiliar procedures, which may trigger unsettling emotions or even existential anxieties. Thus, doing research involves facing our emotions and constructively coping with them. Developing yourself as a researcher is like being a journeyman learning a craft from master-craftsmen, where you learn the finer points of the research craft from other researchers, lecturers, and supervisors. Therefore, it is important to develop realistic expectations of research (Duffy & Dik, 2013). Chapter 2 explains how to cope with the emotional and relational sides of research. Other handbooks may introduce the specific expectations about research in specific fields (e.g. Barker, Pistrang & Elliott, 2015; McLeod, 2022; Vossler & Moller, 2014).

Step 6: Use this book

Definition

This section explains how to use this book.

Overview of chapters

Part I offers an introduction to research. Chapter 2 explains basic academic skills which students with prior academic learning can skip (although this may be a good refresher for them). Part II guides in developing essential skills relevant for all researchers. Chapter 3 gives an overview of the main trends in research, which can inspire readers to become aware of possible research topics and methods. Following these general trends, Chapter 4 guides the reader in finding a research topic. At this stage, researchers may only have a general direction for their research because they may not know their field in-depth yet. Therefore, Chapter 5 helps readers to plan and conduct literature reviews. Following the gap identified in the literature, Chapter 6 explains how to formulate the research aims, questions, and/or objectives. Chapter 7 helps to find the best study design to achieve the research aims. Whereas Part II was relevant for all types of methods and topics, Part III of the book gives detailed information for developing and conducting quantitative research (Chapter 8), qualitative research (Chapter 9), and mixed methods research (Chapter 10). Chapter 11 is again relevant for all researchers, explaining how to apply the chosen research methods ethically and how to develop ethics proposals. Chapter 12 describes how to write the discussion of research papers, write a thesis, and disseminate findings.

Steps within each chapter

Each chapter is structured in multiple steps, starting with an overview of all steps. Each step starts with a definition, followed with an explanation of specific components, procedures, and examples. Each chapter ends with exercises for self-reflection, homework, or classroom discussion.

Templates in the Appendix

Researchers can use and adjust the templates in the Appendix as the basis of their research texts: research interest statement, literature review plan, literature review, methodology essay, essay on critical self-reflection and reflexivity, research proposal, ethics proposal, thesis, article. These templates guide researchers in doing their research via clear structures of headings/sub-headings and checklists so they do not forget any important steps. The chapters explain how to use the templates.

Online resources

Additional resources can be found on https://joelvos.com/doingresearch. This includes all templates and figures in downloadable and editable Word files. The website offers checklists and PowerPoint presentations for the research proposal and thesis. The website also provides extra resources for each chapter, referred to as 'online tables', with extra explanations, exercises, and examples. Lecturers can find a template design of research modules and lecture topics, and pedagogical tips and tricks.

■■■■■■ Reflective questions ■■■■■■

- What are your motivations, expectations, and emotions about doing research?
- Select a topic you are interested in, and search for and read three relevant 'literature reviews', 'meta-analyses', or 'handbooks' (e.g., use these search terms in scholar.google.com).

2

How to Develop Basic Academic Skills

Chapter aims

All researchers should have mastered basic skills in academic reasoning and writing. Students may want to train these skills by using them like muscles in academic exercises such as writing essays and conducting feasibility studies. The next chapters assume readers have mastered these basic academic skills. (Recommended reading includes: the APA *Publication Manual*, 2020); Birkenstein & Graff, 2018; and Swales & Feak, 2019.

Steps in chapter

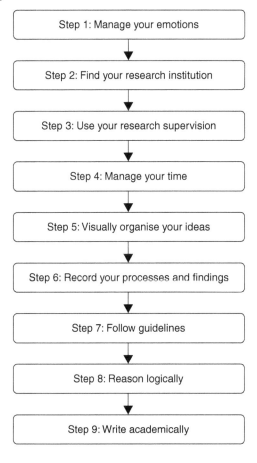

Step 1: Manage your emotions

Step 2: Find your research institution

Step 3: Use your research supervision

Step 4: Manage your time

Step 5: Visually organise your ideas

Step 6: Record your processes and findings

Step 7: Follow guidelines

Step 8: Reason logically

Step 9: Write academically

Step 1: Manage your emotions

Definition

Many researchers experience research as a roller-coaster of positive and negative emotions. Learning to identify and cope effectively with disruptive research-related emotions is essential.

Explanation

Researchers have identified many emotions during research: unrealistic optimism, beginner's despair, urgency, anxiety, frustration, second-year exhaustion, perfectionism, helplessness, magical thinking, being over-relaxed, lack of motivation, arrogance, self-confirmation bias, good-cop/bad-cop supervisors, imposter syndrome, and taking feedback personally. Common traps are not giving complete arguments, not justifying all research decisions, cherry-picking literature, insufficient critical self-reflection, and forgetting to ask for key information from research participants (Kasket & Gil-Rodriguez, 2011). These emotions and traps are normal and will not cause problems, as long as they are identified and managed effectively. Use your psychological skills to identify your feelings, and check with others how realistic and helpful your thoughts are about the research process. You may want to share your research-related emotions and thoughts with your therapist (Online Table 2.1 offers emotional self-help resources).

Step 2: Find your research institution

Definition

Find the appropriate research institution.

Components

You may want to select a research institute with a good research culture (Duffy et al., 2013; Gelso et al., 2013), with features such as:

- Role models with good research knowledge and behaviour
- Positive reinforcement of research activities
- Students participate in research
- Research is explained as an interpersonal experience
- The limitations of research are underlined
- Multiple research approaches are taught
- Importance is put on following your research interests
- Connections between research and practice are shown
- Statistics are explained via applications and research designs
- Students are taught how research can be done in practice settings
- Research supervisors offer rapport and role modelling
- Encouragement and opportunities to work with peers/fellow students

Step 3: Use your research supervision

Definition

Find the appropriate research supervisor, discuss expectations, and use their feedback.

Components

Appropriate supervisor

Brilliant researchers are not automatically competent supervisors. The main tasks of a supervisor are to help you develop your research skills, improve your research project, achieve the goals of your program, and follow ethical guidelines. The supervisor will not take over your research or writing, but give feedback to stimulate the development of your academic skills. Often, the feedback and the working relationship change over time, as supervisors become less proactive and less detailed in their feedback when students become more skilled and independent. A good supervisor fosters a constructive supervisor–supervisee relationship in which it feels safe to share uncertainties, anxieties, and frustrations. Vital relational processes in supervision include containment/safety, clarity/rigour, and compassion/empathy; therefore, the ideal supervisor has the following characteristics (Bager-Charleson & McBeath, 2021):

- Formal allowance to give research supervision
- Research experience/publications, preferably with publications in peer-reviewed journals
- Expertise on topic/methodology
- Supervision experience
- Self-reflective, knowing their limitations, open-minded
- Showing empathy, trust, openness
- Able to contain complex issues
- Sensitive to diversity
- Feedback and explaining its rationale
- Feedback on research progress and details
- Feedback on good aspects and aspects that could be improved
- Feedback on research products and skills, not on the person
- Attention to emotions and relational ruptures

Discuss expectations

To facilitate a good supervisory relationship, discuss your expectations in the first meeting and reflect on this regularly, such as:

- How often and where will you meet
- How many hours are available, holidays, etc.
- Who will take the initiative and plan meetings
- How much time does the supervisor need to respond to emails and read documents
- What type of feedback does the student want at which stage
- What are key goals/deadlines
- Will the research be published, and if so, will the supervisor co-author
- Use questionnaires (e.g., Mutual Expectations Regarding Supervision Questionnaire)
- Summarise your agreements via a letter-of-understanding
- Evaluate progress, e.g., in annual progress reports

Use feedback

A difficult skill to learn is using feedback constructively. The following reflections may help:

- Research is like chiselling – you create the final form after many rounds of improvement, conversations, and feedback. Research involves much rewriting. Let a text rest for some time to look at it again with fresh eyes. Envisage rewriting not as a vicious circle but a virtuous spiral where you return to the text at a better level.
- Supervisors help you improve your research project and skills; their feedback is not about you personally.
- Ask for feedback in multiple rounds, e.g., first generic, then detailed.
- Examination boards, reviewers, and journal editors consist of multiple experts; together, they have more expertise and see blind spots you and your supervisor may have overlooked. Their input can improve your skills and research project.
- Remind yourself that supervisors, reviewers, and examiners are fallible humans: even Einstein's thesis was initially rejected. Unfortunately, sometimes feedback says more about their research paradigm or ideological/political/financial agenda. Reflect on how realistic their feedback is.
- Kill your darlings, e.g., ideas and texts you like that are unnecessary/problematic. Not everything fits in one project: a good project is a feasible project. Researchers call this parsimony or Ockham's Razor: choose the simplest research opportunity, idea, or interpretation. You may not want to kill your darlings permanently but save them for later, e.g., keep a working document, a deleted-texts document, and a research logbook.
- Do not rigidly stick to your hypotheses, but seriously consider plausible rival hypotheses.
- Actively ask for academic support from supervisors, mentors, lecturers, and fellow researchers/students. Share emotions and ask for emotional support.

Step 4: Manage your time

Definition

Research is time-intensive and often competes with other activities. Therefore, develop good time management skills.

Suggestions

- Pencil-in research timeslots in your calendar (better too many and too long)
- Tell others not to disturb you
- Get into the habit of sitting down for research, even if you are not effective
- Identify and stop procrastination
- Use time-management tools, e.g., diaries, to-do list apps.
- Use good equipment, e.g., multiple screens for simultaneously open files/datasets.
- Save your files in multiple places, e.g., computer/laptop, external drives/USB sticks, email them to yourself, preferably use data-protected cloud storage.
- Use good software, e.g., text editors, data-analysis software.
- Look after yourself: enough sleep, relaxation, physical exercise, mindfulness are all important. The best ideas often pop up outside of work.

Step 5: Visually organise your ideas

Definition

Visualisation may help to quickly and creatively convey complex ideas.

Suggestions

- Flowcharts: e.g., LucidChart, SmartDraw, PowerPoint/Word.
- Post-its: e.g., write one idea per post-it and move post-its to create groups/patterns (see exercise in Online Table 2.2).
- Mind-mapping: e.g., tree-structures, spider-diagrams, sociograms, enterprise architecture (e.g., LucidChart, Canva, Matchware), statistical structures (e.g., Bayesian networks, structural equation modelling).

Step 6: Record your processes and findings

Definition

Research can quickly become complicated, and you may forget why you made certain decisions and how you conducted parts of your research. Supervisors and journal editors may ask you to show and justify your procedures and findings. Like Hansel and Gretel, leave a trail of pebbels. Use a systematic method to record both your findings and processes/decisions.

Suggestions

Organise all research material in a computer/laptop folder or physical binder. Consider the following tabs/sub-folders:

- **Document-versions:** standardise file titles and save frequently, e.g., 'Doing Research JV18062021 ST22062021' refers to this book's title, initials, date of writing, date that ST edited this. The editor will use 'comments' and 'track changes' to differentiate between their and my edits.
- **Reflective research journal:** Chapter 4 explains that most qualitative researchers reflect in research journals.
- **Process logbook:** write for each research step what you did and why, e.g., save codes, search terms, SPSS-syntax; if needed, later copy-paste these codes/search terms and reuse them.
- **Literature process logbook:** record how you did each round of your literature search, e.g., search terms, search engines, number of references (Table 2.1).
- **Literature content logbook:** summarise findings from relevant literature; you may use this when writing your literature review (Table 2.2).
- **Recording references:** keep a record of relevant references (e.g., write or copy-paste references in a separate Excel/Word file). Referencing software can save time: you can insert references manually or import these from search engines into a database, which you can later use to cite-while-you-write and automatically print a reference list (e.g., Mendeley, Zotero, RefWorks, EndNote, or Reference Manager; check YouTube tutorials).
- **Publications:** e.g., literature review.

- **Inspiration:** e.g., texts, ideas, discussions.
- **Guidelines:** e.g., professional bodies, university forms.
- **Minutes of research/supervision meetings.**
- **Data-collection instruments:** e.g., questionnaires, interview schedule.
- **Research and ethics proposals.**
- **Raw data:** e.g., initial interview transcripts, SPSS data file.
- **Transformed data:** e.g., transformed SPSS data file, syntax.
- **Findings:** e.g., NVivo/SPSS output.
- **Draft thesis.**

Table 2.1 Literature process logbook example (explained in Chapter 5)

Date	27/08/22 17:00
Database	Web-of-Science
Keywords	Topic = (depress* OR bipolar) AND (cognitive behaviour therapy)
Type of study	Review OR meta-analysis OR overview
Limitations	Publication year > 2000 Author = James
Results	6
Comments	Results limited because only showing recent studies from James on CBT for depression.

Table 2.2 Literature content logbook example (explained in Chapter 5)

Content logbook reference	27/08/22 17:00
Referencing software number	1
Article reference	James, 2018
Problem/population	Depression in children 8–15 years
Intervention	Cognitive behaviour therapy (CBT)
Comparison group	Meaning centred psychotherapy (MCP)
Outcome measure	Patient Health Questionnaire (PHQ-9)
Study type	Randomised controlled trial
Study quality (1–7)	2 Low quality due to small sample size (N CBT=6, N MCP=5)
Findings	Small effect size (Cohen's D=0.1)
Relevance	Relevant to answer my research question into MCP effects.

Step 7: Follow guidelines

Definition

All research steps should follow academic, ethical, and legal guidelines (see Online Table 2.3.).

Suggestions

Search for research and ethics guidelines from the following groups:

- **Your research institute/university:** e.g., guidelines, handbooks
- **National:** e.g., UK Research Integrity Body
- Professional bodies: e.g., APA, BPS
- **Publication manuals and referencing guidelines:** e.g., APA, Harvard, author instructions from journals (tip: buy the APA *Publication Manual* for academic writing, referencing, and layout; search for APA Word templates online)
- **Authorship guidelines:** e.g., International Committee of Medical Journal Editors, Committee on Publication Ethics

Step 8: Reason logically

Definition

Academic texts should use logical arguments. Logical reasoning may not come naturally and may need training.

Suggestions

Check whether your arguments have a logical structure

An argument is a train of thought, e.g., with a premise and conclusion. You can often quickly identify the different components of an argument as they are marked or can be marked with words such as 'therefore', 'but', 'and'. Explicate the logic behind your text by using such words (Online Tables 2.4–2.5).

Prevent logical fallacies and cognitive biases

Logical fallacies seem persuasive but weaken an argument. You may want to look up common fallacies to identify and prevent these in your texts, e.g., straw man, correlation/causation conflation, appeal to authority, false dilemma, hasty generalisation, anecdotal evidence, bandwagon, slippery slope, red herring, *ad hominem* and *tu quoque*. Closely related are cognitive biases, which are ways of thinking usually regarded as irrational or due to poor judgment, e.g., confirmation bias and black-or-white thinking.

Give evidence for your arguments

Each part of an argument should be supported by solid evidence. For example, in a deductive argument, justify that a general principle applies to a situation. In an inductive argument, justify that the situation can be generalised.

Step 9: Write academically

Definition

Academic texts differ from non-academic ones. Learn writing with an academic tone, clear structure, accurate strength-of-claim and referencing, and critical self-reflection.

Components

Academic tone

Academic tone can, for example, be found in the following:

- **Audience:** researchers, academically trained therapists
- **Purpose:** specific topic
- **Organisation:** systematic, logical structure
- **Fundaments:** trustworthy evidence instead of subjective opinion
- **Formal style:** Latinisation (e.g., cf., i.e.); no 'we'/'I', contractions (don't), and street language ('stuff', 'things')
- **Presentation:** no linguistic errors, neutrality (e.g., gender, sexual orientation, religion)
- **Concise sentences:** short sentences, where possible combined sentences (e.g., -ing clauses), no unnecessary clauses/circumlocutions (e.g., 'this study' replaces '*the present* study'), no redundant formulations (e.g., they were *both* alike; a *total* of 68 participants), few passive sentences
- **Clear terminology:** key concepts/words are defined and operationalised
- **Academic terminology:** use correct words (check dictionary, thesaurus), specific (e.g., 'individuals who...' instead of 'people'), no clichés/empty phrases (e.g., 'needle in a haystack'), avoid labelling (e.g., 'older homosexual individuals' rather than 'elderly gays'), no colloquial expressions (e.g., 'report' instead of 'write-up'), no unnecessary jargon, limited use of easily confused words such as 'this'/'it', no anthropomorphisms (e.g., 'this article examines...'), use synonyms instead of repeating words, accurate collocation (check collocation-dictionaries), quotation marks are only used for citations.

Clear structure

Academic texts have a clear structure (Swales & Feak, 2019):

- **Division in parts:** a text consists of multiple parts, such as head, body, and lower part. Each part may have various sub-parts. For example, most articles/theses have an introduction (e.g., background, rationale, aims), methodology, findings, and discussion (e.g., conclusions, strengths, limitations, explanations, implications).
- **Appropriate lengths:** each part of a text has an appropriate size relative to other parts, e.g., no disproportionally lengthy introductions or discussions.
- **Parts are logically connected:** there is coherence and flow between text parts. The author tells why each part is needed and how each part connects with other parts. Many texts follow a funnel model: the introduction describes the broad field, followed by specific methods and findings, which the discussion may interpret considering broad literature and implications.
- **Explicate structure:** the author's first task is to handle reader expectations; be clear what your text is about, do what you promise, and have a strong ending in which you show how you have lived up to your promises. Psychologists call this the

'tell-tell-and-tell principle': first, tell what you will tell (introduction), tell it (body), and tell what you have told (end). The explication and justification of the textual structure handle readers' expectations and pre-empt possible criticisms.

- **Introduction structure:** you may want to include the following in the introduction of a part/chapter/section: explicit aim or main message; how this builds on previous parts/chapters/sections (e.g., summarise main findings so far and tell the remaining problem this part/chapter/section aims to solve); how this section fits in the broader text and may help achieve overall research aims; the method in the section; justify aim and method (e.g., why discuss these topics and exclude others). The author continuously explains and justifies the structure, making the author's logical reasoning transparent (Table 2.3).
- **End structure:** a part/chapter/section usually finishes with some sentences with a brief conclusion/synthesis ('In sum', 'Thus'), followed by a reminder of how this main message fits in the broader text/helps to answer the research aim/objective/question, and reflections on remaining issues/problems discussed in the next section ('However'; 'Therefore') (Table 2.4).
- **Create tree-structure before writing:** Before writing, decide the key message, aim, and structure of each part/chapter/section. Many authors write these decisions as a tree-structure with numbered first-order and second-order headings (Table 2.5; Online Table 2.6 explains how to develop tree-structures).

Linking-phrases and linking-words

An explicit structure in a text can handle readers' expectations and explicate the logical reasoning and arguments. The textual structure can be explicated via linking phrases, e.g., 'This section aims to…', 'As discussed previously', 'Thus, we have discussed that… therefore, now…'. Linking words are, for example, 'but' 'however', 'therefore', 'thus', 'in sum', 'concluding'. Use structuring elements, e.g., 'first… second…', 'on the one hand, on the other hand' (more examples in Online Table 2.6).

Accurate strength-of-claim

Use formulations reflecting the strength of your evidence for the claim. Each field has its own subjective hierarchy of weak/strong evidence. Table 2.6 gives a hierarchy often seen in psychological therapies.

Accurate referencing

Each statement requires a reference: who said what? Explicate if something is your own opinion. Use formal referencing guidelines, e.g., the APA *Publication Manual*. Furthermore, plagiarism is a cardinal sin which could lead to failing assignments and getting expelled. Plagiarism means presenting another person's work as your own, e.g., paragraphs, sentences, arguments, ideas, or theories. Plagiarism can occur intentionally (deliberately copying texts) or unintentionally (forgetting references). Self-plagiarism means using your own texts/essays/ideas. Prevent plagiarism by including references. Most universities and journals use plagiarism software to detect direct and slightly adjusted copies.

Table 2.3 Example introduction structure

This part/chapter/section answers question B. That is, the previous part/chapter/section answered question A but not B. However, question B is also important for the following reasons (describe reasons that justify why you need to write this part/chapter/section). Therefore, this part/chapter/section aims to answer B. This helps achieve the overarching research aim/objective/question (explain how answering B may serve the overall research aims). This part/chapter/section answers B with the following method (explain and justify how this method helps answer B). B can be separated into sub-themes B1, B2, and B3. Therefore, this part/chapter/section is structured with sections B1, B2, and B3. This part/chapter/section ends with a discussion of the findings, which will show the key findings of B (mention key message/conclusion from this part/chapter/section). This will show that this part/chapter/section could only answer B, but due to the limits of the method, could not answer C, which will therefore be discussed in the next part/chapter/section.

Table 2.4 Example end structure

In sum, this part/chapter/section answered question B by discussing B1, B2, and B3. The key message/findings/conclusion is 1/2/3. However, the findings 4/5/6 seemed to be exceptions/surprising, which may be explained with arguments/research from others 7/8/9. To remind the reader, this part/chapter/section followed previous parts/chapters/sections answering question A but not B. Therefore, this part/chapter/section discussed B, which has helped further to answer the research aim/objective/question. However, the method used in this part/chapter/sectionwas limited for the following reasons (describe limitations of the method) and this part/chapter/section could therefore could not answer question C. Furthermore, the findings raised new questions about C. Therefore, the next part/chapter/section discusses C.

Table 2.5 Example textual tree-structure

Chapter 5. Title

5.1. First order heading 1

    5.1.1. Second order heading 1

    5.1.2. Second order heading 2

      -*Third order heading 1*

      -*Third order heading 2*

5.2. First order heading 2

Etc.

Table 2.6 Example strength-of-claim

Very strong evidence → very strong formulation
Evidence:

- Common fact (e.g., the sun rises in the east)
- Published systematic literature review with meta-analyses according to formal guidelines

Example-formulation:

- It is common knowledge…
- Overall, research shows…
- Researchers agree…
- It is very likely…

Table 2.6 Example strength-of-claim (Continued)

Strong evidence → strong formulation
Evidence:

- Three/more quantitative studies in a peer-reviewed high-impact journal with good study validity and reliability
- A published systematic literature review

Example formulation:

- It is very probable/highly likely…
- It seems almost certain…
- Several studies show…

Relatively strong evidence → relatively strong formulation
Evidence:

- One quantitative study in a peer-reviewed high-impact journal with good validity/reliability
- Other good systematic literature reviews, e.g., meta-ethnography, narrative-reviews
- A literature review/chapter in an authoritative handbook by authoritative researchers

Example formulation:

- This study indicates…
- Author X argues…

Relatively weak evidence → relatively weak formulation
Evidence:

- One trustworthy published qualitative study
- Trustworthy book/chapter
- Trustworthy expert opinion/conference keynote

Example-formulation:

- It is probable/possible/likely…
- It seems/maybe…
- Expert X suggests…

Weak evidence → weak formulation
Evidence:

- Article in non-peer-reviewed journal
- Unpublished thesis
- Own clinical experience
- Non-systematic case study

Example formulation:

- It might/appears/could possibly…
- There is a slight possibility…
- Based on limited data/small study…
- In the opinion of some authors…
- This seems to suggest…

Very weak evidence → very weak formulation
(Rarely used in research publications)
Evidence:

- Own opinion
- Popular media, newspapers, magazines, pop-science books

Example formulation:

- This opinion maker suggests it might be…
- In my opinion…

Self-reflection

All humans are fallible. Reflect on your text's limitations, such as: 'This study showed B but not C, possibly due to the limitations of the method', 'Findings are restricted to…', 'The findings cannot be taken as evidence for…', 'Unfortunately, we are unable to conclude from this data…'

━━━━━ **Reflective questions** ━━━━━

- Examine your emotions and thoughts about research, examine how realistic and helpful they are, and formulate alternatives (use Online Table 2.1).
- Examine your strengths and weaknesses, and how these may aid or hinder in research: e.g., writing, logical reasoning, listening, being systematic, personality characteristics, independence, flexibility, openness, analytical and self-reflective skills.
- Examine how appropriate your institution and supervisor are for your research.
- Examine how you cope with feedback, manage time, organise ideas, record research processes and findings, and how you could improve these (organise folders like Step 6).
- Identify relevant guidelines/handbooks/forms (Step 7).
- Select three frequently cited articles in your field. Examine their academic tone, structure, visual organisation, strength-of-claim, referencing, critical self-reflection, logical structure, and logical fallacies. What are the strengths and weaknesses? What lessons can you learn?
- Develop your skills to identify logical fallacies and cognitive biases. Search for instructions, lectures, and examples of fallacies and biases. Select a speech by an influential politician/scientist and identify logical fallacies and cognitive biases.
- Develop your writing skills. Select two pages you have written. With the help of this chapter and proofreading checklists (Online Table 2.5), identify weaknesses in logical reasoning and academic writing. Rewrite accordingly. Alternative exercise: give mutual feedback to texts of peers.
- Take control of your academic self-development. Identify which academic skills need improvement, and make an improvement plan (e.g., do extra reading, ask for advice, follow workshops).

PART II
ESSENTIAL SKILLS

3

How to Develop a Conceptual Overview of Your Research Area

Chapter aims

This chapter gives an overview of the broad landscape of research on psychological therapies. This overview may help readers become aware of general research trends, identify topics they are interested in and position their research project. Like a large-scale map of the surroundings, this chapter describes the main highlights: the ten most cited groups of concepts in therapy research. The final section explains how researchers can develop the overall conceptual framework of their research. Chapters 4–5 will further guide readers in specifying their area of interest.

Steps in chapter

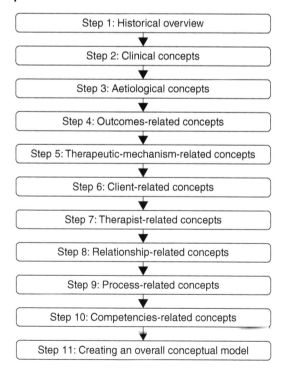

Step 1: Historical overview

Step 2: Clinical concepts

Step 3: Aetiological concepts

Step 4: Outcomes-related concepts

Step 5: Therapeutic-mechanism-related concepts

Step 6: Client-related concepts

Step 7: Therapist-related concepts

Step 8: Relationship-related concepts

Step 9: Process-related concepts

Step 10: Competencies-related concepts

Step 11: Creating an overall conceptual model

Step 1: Historical overview

Before you start a hiking trip, you buy a map to decide where you will be walking. Similarly, before you start your research project, you create an overview, mapping the broader research landscape in which your specific research project is embedded. A large-scale map shows you the highlights (e.g., villages, mountains) and roads connecting them. In research, a conceptual framework shows the main concepts and their coherent, logical relationships. It provides a tentative framework of the phenomena you are studying, which may guide the development of innovative research aims and appropriate methodologies (Maxwell, 2012).

For example, a conceptual framework of dog phobia may consist, amongst others, of clinical concepts defining the criteria of dog phobia ('clinical conceptual model') and aetiological concepts describing how dog phobia develops ('aetiological conceptual model'). A concept is an idea of what something is or how it works, and usually consists of multiple components (Jabareen, 2009). A conceptual model is a combination of concepts about a specific topic, such as the aetiology of dog phobia. A conceptual framework is a logical combination of multiple conceptual models, such as models about aetiology, clinical problem, therapeutic mechanisms, and outcomes. Thus, a conceptual framework may consist of multiple models, which may consist of multiple concepts, which may consist of multiple components (read more: Imenda, 2014; Ravitch & Riggan, 2016; Smyth, 2004).

Hikers know they should not conflate the map with the landscape (map/landscape fallacy). The map is just a representation of the landscape and they may discover mapping errors and landscape changes. Therefore, hikers prefer recently updated maps, and check their accuracy. Similarly, a bona fide research project is based on a coherent, logical conceptual framework supported by the latest research evidence (Kazdin, 2015; Vos, 2014). For example, researchers usually start by reviewing the most important concepts in the field, examining how strongly the main concepts are supported by research evidence, and how the concepts are coherently and logically connected. Thus, a conceptual framework enables researchers to say, 'Here's how I am positioning my problem within an established arena of ideas and here's why it matters... [Building a conceptual framework means] uncovering what is relevant and what is problematic among the ideas circulating around your problem, making new connections, and then formulating an argument that positions you to address that problem' (Schram, 2006, p.62).

What should be included in a conceptual framework about psychological therapies? This chapter explains the ten conceptual models found in the introductions/literature review sections of the 100 most cited qualitative and the 100 most cited quantitative therapy research publications (Online Tables 3.1–3.2 show all 29 conceptual models and how these are integrated in later chapters). Most publications mention clinical, aetiological, outcomes-oriented and therapeutic-mechanism-related models; some add client-related, therapist-related, relationship-related, process-related and competences-related models.

In different periods, therapy researchers seem to have focused on other concepts with different methods. The following is an evolution of conceptual frameworks in therapy research (Barkham, Lutz, & Castonguay, 2021; Strupp & Howard, 1992):

- **Pre-1950:** Research mainly aimed to demonstrate the legitimacy of psychological therapies in competition with other professions. For example, publications focused on case studies, proving clinical and aetiological models and explaining therapeutic mechanisms. The first rating scales were developed, particularly to rate session recordings. Many studies focused on client-centred and psychoanalytic therapies (Miller et al., 1993).
- **1950–1980:** Experimental study designs emerged, treatment manuals were used, and quantitative measurement instruments such as questionnaires were developed.

Research started to focus on outcomes and comparisons. Eysenck (1952) claimed that therapies are no better than spontaneous recovery, which triggered researchers to conduct controlled trials to prove therapy is more effective.

- **1980–1990:** Research focused on making therapy more cost-effective, such as the relationship between the length and effects of therapy ('dose-effect studies'). Studies also examined how therapeutic change occurs, for example by examining differences in effects for different treatments and their underlying therapeutic mechanisms. Meta-analyses became popular. Qualitative methods emerged to examine the therapeutic process and its relationship with therapeutic outcomes, including criteria for trustworthiness. Theoretical and political battles emerged over the definition of 'empirical evidence'.
- **1990–present:** Widely diverse topics are studied with a broad range of methods. More attention is given to qualitative research, clinically significant outcomes, therapeutic mechanisms, client-centred experiences, therapeutic relationships, processes, and competencies. Guidelines, checklists, and internal methods of rigour emerged were developed for qualitative research.

Step 2: Clinical concepts

Definition

The clinical model answers the question: what is the central clinical concept or psychological or experiential phenomenon that this study focuses on? Most research publications start with definitions of key clinical concepts and diagnostic criteria. The clinical model is particularly elaborated in quantitative, symptom-focused, and action-oriented studies.

Coherent, logical connections

The clinical conceptual model often stands in the centre of the overall conceptual framework, like all fibres lead to the spider in a web. For example, the aetiological model explains how the clinical phenomenon develops, and outcomes concern the impact of psychological therapies on this phenomenon. Some clinical concepts, such as psychiatric diagnoses, have been criticised for being too generic and insufficiently sensitive to diverse and minority groups (Vos, Roberts, & Davies, 2019).

Components

- Formal diagnosis and criteria from psychiatric manuals (e.g., DSM, ICD)
- Evidence for the diagnosis and criteria. Critical psychologists have questioned the evidence basis of some diagnoses (Vos, Roberts, & Davies, 2019)
- Historical change, controversies and socio-cultural differences of diagnoses and criteria, e.g., DSM diagnosis of homosexuality until the 1970s
- Prevalence and incidence of this phenomenon in the population
- Subjective experience of this phenomenon (e.g., qualitative studies about what it is like to live with these clinical problems and/or be diagnosed)
- Similarities, dissimilarities, and comorbidities with other clinical phenomena
- Neuropsychological processes associated with the phenomenon, such as the involvement of neurotransmitters, brain structures, and (stress) hormones

Cynophobia example

Dog phobia, cynophobia, is a specific phobia disorder defined by extreme fear triggered by seeing, encountering or thinking about dogs considered harmless by most people. Nine per-cent of the population suffers from cynophobia.

Step 3: Aetiological concepts

Definition

The aetiological conceptual model answers the question: how did the central clinical prob-lem originally develop, and which mechanisms influenced its continuation, aggravation, or extinction? Clinical problems may be caused directly or indirectly by disease-specific and generic aetiological factors, and their dynamic interaction (Garber & Hollon, 1991).

Coherent, logical connections

The aetiological concepts describe how the clinical phenomenon has evolved. The thera-peutic mechanisms often intervene in the aetiological causes to create positive outcomes. For example, if a clinical problem has developed due to avoidance of traumatic memories, the treatment could focus on processing the memory. Despite many studies on aetiologi-cal mechanisms and risk factors for developing psychopathology, our knowledge is limited regarding the aetiology of many psychological problems (Kazdin, 2007, 2009; Kraemer et al., 2001). Researchers have called for more aetiological research, particularly in minority groups and in relationship to other conceptual models.

Components

- Events initially causing the phenomenon: e.g., life-events, traumatic experiences, attachment style, style of upbringing, parental/intergenerational messages.
- Internal reinforcement: unhelpful or self-reinforcing coping mechanisms, behavioural responses, emotions, and thoughts reinforcing the phenomenon, e.g., avoidance, denial, withdrawal, rumination, hyper-reflection, misinterpretations.
- Social influences reinforcing the phenomenon: e.g., reward and punishment by others, role-models, cultural/social narratives/discourses.
- Neurobiological influences: e.g., genetics, temperament, physical diseases.
- Socio-economic factors: e.g., the following groups are at larger risk of developing mental health problems: women, individuals with low socio-economic status, individuals from Black, Asian, and minority ethnicities (BAME), lesbian, gay, bisexual, transgender, queer, and intersex (LGBTQI+) persons, and individuals with chronic or life-threatening physical disease (Vos, Roberts & Davies, 2019). Consequently, particular clinical problems may develop differently for these groups.
- Nature–nurture interaction: the pendulum in the nature–nurture debate has swung between the two sides over time (ibidem). Whereas medical doctors focused mainly on the biological origins of mental health disorders until the 19th century (nature), Sigmund Freud introduced some psychological origins (nurture). By the end of the 20th century, more attention was given to the neurocognitive origins of psychological problems (nature). Many contemporary researchers recognise the

aetiology of most psychological problems as a complex, dynamic, contextualised interaction between nature and nurture. For example, neurocognitive research shows that early-life adversity is associated with neurological and cognitive changes due to which individuals remember and interpret situations differently (Donohoe, 2022). Research has for example identified adversity/trauma as aetiological causes in many psychological disorders, inspiring the development of new holistic, multidisciplinary, trauma-focused treatments (McKay et al., 2021).

Cynophobia example

Most cynophobic individuals have had a traumatic experience with dogs, such as having been bitten. However, not all victims of dog attacks develop cynophobia. The anxiety is also reinforced by the client's avoidance of dogs, e.g., walking away when seeing a dog. That is, escape and avoidance reduce short-term anxiety but keep anxiety high long term, because the client learns that avoidance reduces anxiety ('avoidance learning'). Other factors may influence the development of cynophobia, such as the context and experiences with other dogs, and cognitive appraisal of the threat and resources to cope with the threat, as well as an anxious genetic predisposition and other traumatic and stressful life events.

Step 4: Outcomes-related concepts

Definition

The outcomes-related conceptual model answers the question: what are the outcomes of psychological therapies for the central clinical problem? Thousands of studies unequivocally tell that, in general, clients are better off after therapy than before therapy, often with large effect sizes. The question 'what are the outcomes of therapy' can be answered in many ways. This section introduces key concepts and findings in outcomes-related research. Recommended overviews include Cooper (2013), Kazdin (2011), Midgley, Hayes and Cooper (2017), Wampold and Imel (2015).

Coherent, logical connections

The outcomes-related conceptual model describes the effects of psychological therapies in which therapists use therapeutic mechanisms to change the experience of the clinical problem and/or prevent its aetiological causes. However, outcomes on their own do not explain why change happens (e.g., therapeutic mechanisms) and do not explain client-oriented, therapist-oriented, process-oriented, relationship-oriented, and competencies-oriented factors in therapy. As will be explained in later chapters, outcome studies may require complex study designs and may not be feasible for smaller student projects.

Components
Qualitative research

The first therapy research studies were case studies. A case study may give an in-depth and detailed examination of the history of a client's psychological phenomenon, therapeutic mechanisms, and outcomes from a subjective perspective which may not be found by merely using questionnaires/observations. A case study may help develop theories, understand client experiences, and create hypotheses about the therapeutic helpfulness and mechanisms (see Chapter 9). Subjective perceptions are at best modestly associated with quantitative therapy outcomes (Lambert, 2011; Lauer, 1999).

Quantitative research

The first case studies were often aggregated ideal-cases researched and written by the therapist, with a large risk of self-confirmation bias. It was sometimes also challenging to interpret the findings: without objective criteria or benchmarks, clients may say they have improved, but how big, reliable, and valid are their improvements?

To solve some of these problems, quantitative researchers developed standardised outcome measures such as questionnaires, as Chapter 8 will elaborate. To measure the standardised effects of therapy, researchers often give questionnaires before the first therapy session and after the last session, and they calculate the change in scores. Imagine Mary started with a score of 23 on the Patient Health Questionnaire (PHQ-9), indicating severe depression according to studies in norm groups (a norm group is a comparison group). After the last session, Mary had a score lower than 4, indicating minimal depression. However, these improved scores still need to be interpreted, as we do not know yet, for example, whether the changes were caused by the treatment, as Mary could have naturally improved without treatment.

Efficacy versus effectiveness

Psychological therapy is a complex process, often with multiple sessions and an accumulation of countless tiny interventions by a therapist. In medicine, a single intervention could be the administration of a surgery or giving a psychopharmaceutical drug, which can be one step of a longer treatment plan. A psychological intervention may be narrowly defined as a single action, strategy, or step by a therapist, usually as part of a larger treatment plan, intended to directly foster change in the client; an intervention may also indirectly facilitate change, for example by improving the therapeutic mechanisms, processes or relationships. For example, an empathic smile may help clients feel understood. Some interventions may be standardised and prescribed by a therapeutic school, such as creating a scale of subjective units of distress in CBT; other interventions may be non-specific and may be a spontaneous response by the therapists, such as paraphrasing or showing empathy. Therapists use the words 'intervention' and 'techniques' in various ways, and some schools do not prescribe specific interventions or techniques but describe 'principles' or 'attitudes'.

To understand which therapeutic intervention fosters client improvement, researchers have studied psychological therapies under ideal and controlled circumstances, such as research laboratories. In such labs, a standardised situation is created to minimise the influence of extra-therapeutic influences, ensuring that client changes can be attributed to the interventions. Many laboratory studies standardise the treatment to pre-determine which interventions clients will receive, for example via a structured treatment manual, explaining all therapeutic steps within and across sessions (Miller & Binder, 2002).

Laboratory studies may indicate efficacy but not effectiveness. Efficacy describes the performance of an intervention (e.g., treatment manual), under ideal and controlled circumstances (e.g., perfectly selected clients in whom you expect the largest change, without comorbid problems like clients in real-world situations often have). In contrast, effectiveness refers to performance under real-world conditions, for example in the daily life practice of a psychotherapist (also called 'ecologically valid', i.e., the study seems valid in real-world contexts). Research conducted in controlled laboratory situations show larger changes in clients than ecologically valid research in clinical practice (Barkham et al., 2008; Cahill, Barkham,

& Stiles, 2010; Nathan, Stuart, & Dolan, 2000). To know which therapeutic treatments work best in real-world conditions, focus on effectiveness studies.

Complexity of change

Researchers should not merely report positive pre-/post-treatment changes (Cuijpers et al., 2017). For example, the APA requires researchers also to report adverse/negative effects: how many individuals deteriorate, to what extent, and for how long? (Chan et al., 2013; Ioannidis et al., 2004). Not reporting potential harm can worsen therapy outcomes and lead to biased mental health care policies. Adverse events regard negative changes in physical and/or mental health in social or professional life relevant to the client, therapist, or others, such as new, recurrent or worsening symptoms, suicidality, aggression, drugs use, or medication. Therapeutic treatments fail in 5–20% of clients (Linden & Schermuly-Haput, 2014), 3–15% worsen (Lambert, 2007; Lilienfeld, 2007), 50% do not experience significant positive change or drop out (Westen & Morrison, 2001). Due to various factors, misunderstandings may remain unresolved and lead to clients quitting therapy (Rhodes et al., 1994).

An increase in reported symptoms may not necessarily be negative. For example, anxiety may rise when clients start facing their feelings after the first sessions; as clients learn to tolerate and cope with their emotions, their anxiety levels may decrease later. Nearing the end of therapy, symptoms may increase again, for example due to fear of having to manage emotions without the therapist, missing the therapeutic bond, or struggling with saying goodbye.

Whereas meta-analyses indicate that even though most clients report a reduction in mental health problems and few adverse effects, this does not automatically mean that they also experience more positive emotions and improved quality of life, including happiness, positive relationships, and meaning in life. Therefore, some researchers include quality-of-life and positive-psychological outcome measures as secondary outcomes next to primary outcomes such as symptoms of psychopathology (e.g., WHOQOL, SF-6D, Scales of Wellbeing, Meaning in Life Questionnaire, Positive Affects Negative Affects Scale). A reduction in psychiatric diagnoses such as depression may also not be the therapy goal for clients; studies on client needs and client goals indicate that many clients want to live a more meaningful life and work on life goals (e.g., measurable via Goal Attainment Form) (Andresen, Oades, & Caputi, 2011).

Therapeutic success may also be evaluated by looking at the number of people completing treatment and not prematurely dropping out. Researchers may examine the number and causes of dropout; for example younger, male, or emotion-suppressing clients are more likely to drop out.

Therapy may also be beneficial for sub-clinical symptoms and prevent mental health problems (Cuijpers et al., 2008).

In sum, change and dropout can be examined in many ways, and researchers should consider measuring multiple outcomes at multiple measurement-moments.

Research samples

Quantitative researchers are not merely interested in one client's experience but try to develop ideas about how clients generally experience therapy. What works for one individual may not work for other individuals. Therefore, researchers conduct studies in larger samples to identify what interventions help the most people. Researchers will try to argue that their sample represents the general population: what works for the clients in this study may work for most individuals.

Therapists hope to hear the following conclusions from a study. 'This intervention can help everyone with this type of problem, and therefore, health insurance providers or national health services should pay therapists to give this to all clients'. This type of reasoning is called induction, bearing the risk of the induction fallacy: what is good for the participants in this sample may not be good for the average person in the general population (e.g., the research sample may not be representative). There is also the risk of the deduction fallacy: what works in the general population may not work for a particular client. For example, research indicates that CBT has a significant effect with most cynophobic clients, but it may not with Mary. The conclusions and implications of clinical trials depend on the representativity, size, and inclusion/exclusion criteria of the research sample (Dechartres et al., 2014).

Clinical trial

Would Mary have spontaneously recovered from her psychological problems without therapy? Eysenck (1952) observed that psychological problems tend to decrease over time, regardless of treatment, which he called 'spontaneous remission'. Hypothetical reasons for natural improvement are countless, such as individuals trying to find their own solutions to problems, new life experiences, and 'corrective experiences'. Therefore, individuals may even improve while on waiting lists, although they may deteriorate if they expect a negative effect without treatment ('nocebo effect': Furukawa et al., 2014).

Therapists want to know that their therapeutic activities are an efficient use of their time and energy and that their clients' improvement is larger than spontaneous remission. Therefore, researchers design clinical trials in which the experimental group (clients receiving treatment) is compared with a control group, such as those on waiting lists or a no-intervention group. They statistically compare the extent of change in the experimental condition with the control group. Therapists of new interventions also want to know their therapy is not inferior to what is considered the gold standard in the field, and therefore researchers often give the gold standard treatment to the control group.

Therapists hope that their clients remain better for longer than they would have done with spontaneous remission. In the short term, most therapies are more effective than spontaneous remission. After the final therapy session, some clients continue to improve, for example because they apply the learned lessons in daily life. However, therapeutic effects often become smaller in the long term, and some clients may deteriorate/relapse. Despite the fading effectiveness of most therapies, fewer clients relapse in the long term after most psychological therapies than spontaneous remission or alternative interventions (Spielmans, Berman, & Usitalo, 2011; Steinert et al., 2014).

Therapists also want to know that their clients' improvements are real, and not artificially caused by the research process. For example, the Hawthorne effect happens when individuals know they are part of an experiment, so they work harder and improve more (e.g., individuals may respond either more affirmatively or more negatively, give socially desirable answers or avoid extreme answers). The placebo effect describes the outcomes of getting treatment without therapeutic effects, such as a pill without active ingredients. Researchers often add a placebo control group to a clinical trial to measure the extent to which individuals recover due to the artificial research experience, including spontaneous remission and the Hawthorne effect: the placebo-effect is strong (Wampold et al., 2005). To remove the Hawthorne effect altogether, participants and sometimes researchers do not know whether a participant is receiving the placebo or experimental intervention (blinded/double-blinded trials).

Research participants may be randomly allocated to the experimental condition or the control group, in what is called a randomised controlled trial (RCT), regarded as the gold standard in medical study designs. In psychological therapies, it is often impossible to create a blinded group who are offered placebo treatment, because it is difficult to design a treatment which feels like a treatment (like a blank white pill in medical trials) but which is not a real treatment (a pill without active ingredients). An option is to give the experimental groups and control groups treatments with relatively similar structures but without the key therapeutic mechanisms expected to be the main reason for change. Placebo-psychological therapies create some effects, but most bona fide psychological treatments are more effective than placebo (Nathan, Stuart, & Dolan, 2000). In sum, clinical trials should be designed and interpreted carefully (see Chapter 8).

Cynophobia example

Wolitzky-Taylor and colleagues (2008) conducted a systematic literature review and meta-analysis of 33 clinical trials on CBT for specific phobias, including cynophobia. All treatments were more effective than placebo-control groups. The effects remained long term, with few clients relapsing. Wolitzky-Taylor et al. also examined which therapeutic mechanisms could explain the effects and found that exposure and a larger number of sessions improved the outcomes. These findings imply that therapists may want to multi-session in-vivo exposure therapy for clients with cynophobia.

Step 5: Therapeutic-mechanisms-related concepts

Definition

Concepts related to therapeutic mechanisms answer the question: 'what is the basis for the effect', such as the processes or events responsible for change, the reasons why change has occurred, or how change came about (Kazdin, 2021). This includes information about the therapeutic mechanisms leading to the client's change, such as all steps between a therapeutic intervention and client outcomes (for an overview, see: Castonguay & Beutler, 2005).

Coherent, logical connections

As is common in the literature, this book uses the term 'mechanisms of change' as a broad umbrella term for all changes during therapy, and does not restrict this term to neurobiological mechanisms (Kazdin, 2007). This broad definition follows non-reductionist and pluralistic trends (Goss & Mearns, 1997) and interactional complex-systems approaches (Pennington, 2002). Effective therapeutic mechanisms may target the aetiological mechanisms causing the clinical problem, and subsequently lead to positive outcomes. Therapeutic mechanisms are not applied in a vacuum, and thus researchers may also want to describe the role of clients, therapists, relationships, processes, and competencies, as will be explained in this chapter's next steps. Some qualitative researchers have contested the simplism of linear cause-effect relationships (see Chapter 9).

Components

Biopharmaceutical versus psychological mechanisms: Overall, psychological therapies have relatively similar effects to pharmaceutical drugs (Spielmans, Berman, & Usitalo, 2011). Some studies indicate larger short-term effects for drugs, but psychological therapies may have longer-lasting effects. However, these generalising statements oversimplify the situation, that certain psychological disorders and symptoms, such as acute anxiety or acute psychoses, may benefit slightly more from pharmacological treatment (at least in the short term); pills may for example stabilise psychological stress, which may help clients become more open to change in psychological therapies (Bandelow et al., 2015; Cuijpers et al., 2008; Cuijpers et al., 2013). It is also important to consider the larger negative side effects, drug dependency, and dropout rates of psychopharmacological treatment.

The great psychotherapy debate: Wampold and Imel (2015) asked which therapies are relatively more effective than others. Systematic literature reviews and meta-analyses suggest that some psychological therapies for some psychological problems are supported by more evidence than others. Note the nuanced formulation: a lack of studies does not necessarily mean that a therapy cannot be effective, as future research may prove its effectiveness. Therefore, conclusions about which therapeutic interventions work best for whom should be interpreted in light of available studies. (Those wanting to know which therapeutic orientation works best for which client can read about this elsewhere: Cooper, 2013; Norcross, Beutler, & Levant, 2006; Wampold & Imel, 2015.)

The evidence-based therapies controversy: The interest in the relative effectiveness of therapies is related to what is known as 'evidence-based psychological therapies': therapists treat clients with the best available empirical research with clinical expertise in the context of the client's characteristics, culture, and preferences (see key texts on evidence-based therapies: Barkham, Hardy, & Mellor-Clark, 2010; Fisher & O'Donohue, 2006; Goodheart, Kazdin, & Sternberg, 2006; Nathan & Gorman, 2015; Norcross, Beutler, & Levant, 2006; Roth & Fonagy, 2006; Weisz & Kazdin, 2010). The idea that therapists need to justify their interventions with evidence follows from evidence-based medicine and has been promoted by many professional bodies.

The APA Division of Clinical Psychology used the following definition (Chambless & Ollendick, 2001; APA Presidential Task Force on Evidence-Based Practice, 2006). A therapy may be regarded empirically validated if it has at least two sufficiently powered experimental studies in which the treatment is superior to a pill/placebo/treatment and/or equivalent to an already established treatment, and/or more than nine single-case experimental designs compared with a control condition; furthermore, the experiments must be conducted with treatment manuals, clearly described samples, and examined by two independent research teams. Treatments may probably be efficacious if two experiments show that the treatment is more effective than a waiting-list control group, or a series of three experimental single-case studies.

Evidence-based therapies may improve health-care, policies, training, research, collaboration, and guideline development (Elliott, 1998). Evidence-based therapy guidelines often determine which treatments are funded by national health services and insurance providers. For example, 60% to 90% of supported treatments in mental health care are brief CBT for specific disorders (O'Donohue, Buchanan, & Fisher, 2000). However, evidence-based guidelines have also been criticised. For example, not all psychological problems, clients, and therapeutic approaches have been studied as extensively as CBT for specific disorders, and a lack of research does not mean that other therapies do not work (Vos, Roberts, & Davies, 2019). Furthermore, what researchers count as 'evidence' may depend on their research preferences and paradigms, which may change over time. Critics have also argued that evidence-based therapies may not include all relevant outcomes, focus too much on RCTs and on statistical significance instead of clinical significance and ecological validity, and may stimulate a dehumanised/technical approach to therapeutic practice (Elliott, 1998).

In response to these limitations, the APA Division of Psychotherapy developed different criteria, and instead focused on empirically supported therapy relationships (Norcross & Lambert, 2019; see Step 7). Furthermore, the APA Division of Counselling Psychology defined principles of empirically supported interventions in counselling psychology underlining the holistic understanding of psychological problems and the complexity of therapeutic practices

(Wampold, Lichtenberg, & Waehler, 2002). This included: measuring outcomes at different levels of specificity (e.g., general therapeutic effects, and specific effects for the approach, specific disorder, and specific client), not merely measuring a diagnosis, examining all scientific evidence (more than RCTs), absolute and relative efficacy (e.g., acceptability, cost-effectiveness), persuasive causal relationships, appropriate and broad outcome measures, and outcome measures should be tailored locally including the therapists' and clients' voices. A new APA Task Force of Empirically Based Principles of Therapeutic Change also examined client-related, therapist-related, relationship-related, and mechanism-related factors, as will be explained in the next steps.

In sum, there seems an ongoing debate over what is the best research evidence for psychological therapies, and some practitioners seem resistant to follow evidence-based practice (Lilienfeld et al., 2013). Professional bodies in different countries also seem to follow their own definitions of 'evidence' and 'evidence-based practice', such as the UK's NICE guidelines.

Equivalent therapies effect/dodo bird effect: A key criticism to the evidence-based movement is that differences between therapeutic schools are overemphasised (Wampold & Bhati, 2004). Most bona fide therapies seem to have relatively similar effects for most clients (Cuijpers et al., 2008; Luborsky et al., 2002; Wampold et al., 1997; Wampold & Imel, 2015). Bona fide therapies are therapeutic practices delivered in good faith, such as therapists trained in and committed to the therapy and being based on a sound conceptual framework (Wampold & Imel, 2015) consequently, this excludes for example guided self-help, which is usually non-effective (Cuijpers et al., 2010). Studies in ecologically valid clinical settings often show few differences in effectiveness between therapy orientations (e.g., Seligman, 1995). This finding of equivalent effects of bona fide therapies has been called the dodo bird effect (Wampold et al., 1997). This is named after the dodo bird in *Alice in Wonderland* who judged a race in which 'everyone has won and must have prizes'. For example, CBT may not be superior to other therapies in outcomes for depression, although it sometimes is for anxiety (Bandelow et al., 2015; Cuijpers et al., 2008; Wampold, Minami et al., 2005). However, the rule of thumb that 'all bona fide therapies are similarly effective' does not imply that therapists can give any therapy to any particular client, as therapies are often need to be tailored to unique clients (Chambless, 2002).

Specific factors: What matters may not be the generic therapeutic orientation, such as 'CBT' or 'humanistic therapy', but the specific interventions used by the therapist. The effects of specific interventions may be studied in laboratory experiments and clinical trials. Based on many reviews and meta-analyses, the following evidence-based mechanisms may be identified (e.g., Cooper, 2013). Evidence-based CBT techniques include exposure (in-vivo, imaginal, virtual reality, interoceptive exposure, with/without response prevention), cue exposure, systematic desensitisation, paradoxical intention, activity scheduling, and several cognitive techniques such as reframing. Evidence-based humanistic interventions include sensitive interpretations, non-directivity, deepening levels of experiencing and emotional processing, chair dialogues, and focusing – and recently mindfulness-based interventions (Goldberg et al., 2018). Other evidence-based techniques include therapeutic agreements/contracts, listening, paraphrasing, encouragement, questioning, advice, sensitively used touch, homework, feedback on client progress, and manualisation. Some studies examined the role of psychological and existential defence mechanisms in therapy which may impact the therapy process, therapeutic relationship, and outcomes. Furthermore, clients seem to benefit from therapists making and sharing systematic assessments and case formulations (Van Rijn, 2014).

Mechanisms of common factors: Thus, differences between therapeutic orientations do not seem to predict differences in therapeutic effects. This widespread conclusion has led researchers in recent years to shift their focus from examining differences between therapeutic orientations to their similarities. Their research has focused on common factors, a set of non-specific factors common to all therapies (Ahn & Wampold, 2001; Wampold & Imel, 2015). Examples include the role of the therapeutic relationship and instilling positive expectations/hope in therapy. This chapter's next steps zoom into several common factors. Lambert offered a resolution to the debate over whether therapy is effective thanks to specific factors unique to therapeutic orientations or thanks to common factors. Based on years of clinical and research experience, he suggested that specific factors cause 15% of the improvement in therapy, and 85% is caused by common factors such as expectancy/hope and placebo effects (15%), therapeutic relationship (30%), and client-variables (40%). Although the common factors theory seems supported across various outcomes (Stevens, Hynan, & Allen, 2000), some have argued that the design and quality of studies on common factors are insufficient to derive definite conclusions (Cuijpers, Reijnders, & Huibers, 2019).

Organisational factors: The effects and processes of therapy may depend on the organisation of the mental health service, at least in the self-report from clients and therapists (Vos, Roberts, & Davies, 2019). For example, although the National Health Service in the UK and similar organisations in other countries are based on stepped care, in which all clients start with the least-intensive treatment, little evidence exists that stepped care is superior to matched care (Firth, Barkham, & Kellett, 2015; Vos, Roberts, & Davies, 2019).

Neurocognitive and biophysical mechanisms: Since the end of the 20th century, many studies have described neuropsychological and biophysical mechanisms in psychological therapies (Naji & Ekhtiari, 2016). Most studies have examined the neurological basis of clinical and aetiological phenomena. Some studies explain therapeutic changes in neurocognitive terms, such as psychological stress measured via cortisol in saliva, baseline heart rate, and skin conductance. For example, the neurocognitive understanding of traumatic memory has inspired the development of EMDR (Eye Movement Desensitisation and Reprocessing). Recent themes in neurocognitive paradigms include neurodevelopmental disorders and neurodiversity, neuroplasticity (i.e., the ability to experience neurocognitive changes across the lifespan), and treatment of acquired brain injury and neurodevelopmental disabilities. Research into the contribution of genetics and gene-treatment is in its infancy. Increasing numbers of studies describe the role of psychedelics in treating psychological disorders such as PTSD and depression. Neurocognitive/biophysical studies have been criticised for their often small samples, simplistic models, rigid materialistic reductionism and a conflation of correlations and causes (i.e., the observation that certain subjective experiences correlate with certain brain patterns does not imply that these neurological processes *caused* subjective experiences, or that the treatment *should* focus on these neurological mechanisms). Recent neurocognitive and biophysical studies have more complex, multidisciplinary study designs. (See for an introduction: Mohlman, Deckersbach, & Weissman, 2015.)

Cynophobia example

Treatments in which phobic clients are directly exposed to the feared object (in-vivo) are more effective than those with imaginal or virtual exposure (in-vitro) (Wolitzky-Taylor et al., 2008). However, these effects only exist immediately post-therapy and not in the long term. Studies indicate that exposure is an effective mechanism because it addresses its specific aetiology. Exposure therapy prevents avoidance of the feared situation, and reduces anxiety via experiential habituation, self-efficacy, and weakening the learned associations between stimuli/dogs and responses/fear (e.g., although one dog bit in the past, not all dogs bite; Milosevic & McCabe, 2015).

Step 6: Client-related concepts

Definition

Client-related concepts answer the question what works best for which client and which characteristics help them in their therapeutic process.

Coherent, logical connections

Client-related factors can improve therapy outcomes, for example by helping clients benefit more from therapeutic mechanisms, relationships, and processes. The outcomes and experiences of therapy also seem to be influenced by the client's unique clinical and aetiological histories. Recent years have seen more research on the unique experiences, processes, and outcomes of minority groups such as BAME and LGBTQI+.

Components

One size of therapy does not fit all clients, as ultimately clients are responsible for making therapy work, not therapists (Duncan, Miller, & Sparks, 2011). The following is an incomplete overview of client factors in improving outcomes (Bohart & Tallman, 1998; Cooper, 2013; Xiao et al., 2017).

Clients improve more in therapy if they are more motivated and committed, have positive expectations, hope, faith, and realistic treatment expectations. Clients may have different preferences in therapy than therapists, for example they may want more directiveness and emotional intensity (Cooper et al., 2019). When therapy accommodates clients' preferences for therapy type and therapist, clients are less likely to drop out and the therapy effects are slightly better (Swift et al., 2018). Clients with manifest/observed mental health problems have larger effects than those with latent/underlying problems. Clients particularly benefit from therapy and are less likely to drop out if they are not diagnosed with a personality disorder, are securely attached, function psychologically and interpersonally well, are not perfectionistic, have social support, are psychologically minded, willing to confront emotions, ready to change, do not skip/non-attend sessions, and have confidence in the therapy and therapist. Socio-demographic characteristics such as gender and age have only small effects. However, some young people, men, and individuals with a minority ethnic background or lower socio-economic status may have more difficulties accessing therapy and are more likely to drop out, particularly if therapy is offered online, or if the type of therapy is not matched with the client's preferences; reasons not to access therapy seem diverse, including stigma (Cooper & Conklin, 2015; Swift, Callaghan, Cooper & Parkin, 2018; Swift & Greenberg, 2012).

Cynophobia example

Client characteristics do not seem to explain treatment effects for phobias (Wolitzky-Taylor et al., 2008).

Step 7: Therapist-related concepts

Definition

Therapist-related concepts answer the question how clients can benefit from particular therapist characteristics. These characteristics may be defined as a therapist's enduring and relatively stable traits that apply to the therapist in general, including outside the therapeutic relationship (Norcross, Beutler, & Levant, 2006). Orlinsky (2022) gives a good overview.

Coherent, logical connections

The therapist's characteristics explain 5.8% of the variability of therapy outcomes (Saxon, Firth, & Barkham, 2017), although some therapists are significantly more effective than others (Castonguay & Hill, 2017).

Components

Clients seem to improve more in therapy if their therapists have a higher level of psychological well-being, and sometimes if they have similar values, gender, and socio-economic status (Cooper, 2013; Norcross, Beutler, & Levant, 2006). Some personality characteristics, attachment style, mindfulness, meta-cognition, and theory of mind of therapists may improve the therapeutic relationship and outcomes. The therapists' multicultural competencies often improve the therapy process and outcomes (Tao et al., 2015). Many surveys have described the training, development and practices of therapists, showing large diversity (Orlinsky & Rønnestad, 2005). The therapist's professional training, supervision, and professional experience seem to have small effects on therapy outcomes, although they may influence the therapeutic processes, and the lack of effects may be due to poor study designs (Atkins & Christensen, 2001; Kühne et al., 2019; Murphy et al., 2018). For example, trainee therapists have relatively equivalent effects as experienced therapists (Vos et al., 2022). Better-designed studies are needed to understand why therapist factors only have small effects.

Cynophobia example

No studies can be found on therapist characteristics in phobia treatment.

Step 8: Relationship-related concepts

Definition

Relationship-related concepts answer the question of how clients may benefit from their relationship with the therapist.

Coherent, logical connections

Clients improve more if they have a positive relationship with the therapist, confirming the effectiveness of the relational focus in psychodynamic, person-centred, and other humanistic therapeutic approaches (Norcross & Lambert, 2019). More research is needed to understand the precise mechanisms and processes explaining the effects of relationship-related concepts, as well as research on which relational factors work best in which clients and therapists.

Components

Evidence-based relational factors

There is a myriad of concepts and terms for therapeutic relationships. This diversity of concepts and terms seems caused by the complex and multifaceted nature of relationships, and by paradigmatic/political differences between researchers. The research field was summarised in the landmark publication *Psychotherapy Relationships that Work* edited by Norcross and Lambert in 2019. Mearns and Cooper (2017) give a good introduction for practitioners in *Working at Relational Depth*. The meta-analyses included in their books showed that therapy is more effective if there is:

- a positive working alliance, i.e., therapists and clients have a strong collaborative relationship
- experiences of relational depth
- consensus about therapy goals and processes
- an empathic therapist, offering unconditional positive regard and validating the client's experiences
- an authentic and deep relationship, genuine and congruent therapist, fostering a sense of genuineness and congruence in the client
- stimulation of clients to express their emotions freely
- therapeutic work with transference (i.e., transferring early-life patterns of behaviour to the current relationship) and counter-transference (i.e., therapist responses to clients based on their life experiences)
- multiple strategies to repair ruptures in the working-alliance
- feedback-informed treatment – therapists collect real-time input from clients, for example via session-by-session routine outcome monitoring, to identify what is and what is not working in therapy, and subsequently adjust to meet their client's needs better (e.g., using the Session Rating Scale, Outcome Rating Scale)
- cohesion in therapy groups (see research overview on www.agpa.com).

Therapeutic responsiveness

A related concept is therapeutic responsiveness, which has also been formulated as attunement and personalising, tailoring, or matching therapies. Responsiveness can be defined as moment-to-moment behaviour influenced by emerging events, such as therapists being influenced by and responding to what clients do (Castonguay & Hill, 2017; Watson & Wiseman, 2021). This means that therapists try to understand the client's experiences and needs in their context and translate this awareness into appropriate responses and dynamic social interactions. Understandably, appropriate responsiveness seems to correlate with other relationship-related concepts, such as the working alliance. In other words, appropriate responsiveness involves personalising therapy to the unique client: what treatment by whom is the most effective for this individual with that specific problem and under which circumstances? Therapists can for example be responsive-to (i.e., give-attention-to) and responsive-with (give-intention-towards) the therapeutic relationship, technique, or specific client characteristic (Stiles, in Watson & Wiseman, 2021). Therapeutic responsiveness may for example be improved by training, clinical supervision, critical self-reflection, and reflexivity.

A researcher may merely measure the direct effects of a therapeutic intervention on clients. However, also with standardised treatment manuals, therapists will make at least some small adjustments to tailor interventions to clients; consequently, the effects may not merely be caused by the interventions but also by therapeutic-responsiveness. Therefore, instead of ignoring these effects of tailoring the treatment to clients, researchers may want to examine how therapists personalise the intervention and appropriately respond to the client's experiences and processes as they evolve moment-to-moment. For example, clients may be matched with particular treatment arms in a clinical trial, treatments may include systematic case formulations and plan analysis, treatments may be adjusted with the input of session-by-session routine outcome monitoring, and therapeutic techniques and competencies may be tailored to them. Researchers may also include questionnaires about the therapeutic relationship and interview therapists and clients about their experiences, conduct theory-building case studies and observe how therapists tailor therapy to clients in recordings of therapy sessions. Several studies indicate that subjective evaluations of responsiveness predict dropout and outcomes. Therefore, some researchers consider appropriate responsiveness as a common factor in therapies.

Other interpersonal research methods

Transference-related methods (also named 'central relationship pattern methodologies') focus on identifying repeated patterns in the therapeutic relationship and relationships outside the therapy room. This includes Luborsky's Core Conflictual Relationship Theme method, the Consensual Response Method, Plan Formulation Method, and Fundamental Repetitive and Maladaptive Emotional Structures. There is a long research history into interpersonal processes, following Sullivan's work, such as Leary's Interpersonal Diagnosis of Personality, Interpersonal Circle, Interpersonal Octagon, and Structural Analysis of Social Behaviour. In couples and family therapy, researchers may use dyadic measures (Sexton et al., 2004). In group therapy, researchers may use methods adjusted from individual therapy, but also analyse group processes such as group cohesion, interactions, roles, and phases (see agpa.org; Beck & Lewis, 2000).

Cynophobia example

No studies can be found on therapeutic relationships in cynophobia treatments. It may be hypothesised that therapists need to create a safe, empathic atmosphere for clients to face their fears.

Step 9: Process-related concepts

Definition

Process-related concepts regard the question of how clients and therapists experience the processes of change in therapy.

Coherent, logical connections

Many authors seem to divide all therapy research into two broad categories: outcome research and process research. In this broad definition, the therapy process also includes therapeutic mechanisms, the therapeutic relationship, and client and therapist characteristics. However, in the analysis of the 200 most cited articles on psychological therapies, many authors seemed to describe these as separate steps in their logical reasoning; for example, they separately discussed client-related and therapist-related concepts, before moving to relationship-related concepts. The separation of these steps also seems justified by the fact that the research into each of these steps has exponentially grown. Furthermore, this process-oriented step regards research into qualitative aspects of the processes of therapeutic change that have not been discussed yet. Process research is sometimes criticised for simplifying processes, limited generalisability, non-linearity (Timulak, 2008), and the impossibility getting insight into client experiences (Farber, 2003). (See the following overviews of process research: Elliott, 2010; Greenberg & Pinsof, 1986; Lambert & Hill, 1994; Riding & Lepper, 2005, Toukmanian & Rennie, 1992; Tryon, 2002.)

Components

Client helpfulness studies (CHS): Clients describe what they found helpful and unhelpful in therapy, and their perceptions of the processes of change, based on the phenomenological principle that clients' accounts of their experiences are a valid source of data (Cooper, McLeod, & Ogden, 2015). Although the self-report method limits the generalisability, these studies can deepen insights into therapeutic mechanisms, relationships, and processes. Most published CHS studies have used an interview schedule developed for that particular study, although some use standardised interview schedules such as the Client Change Interview (Elliott & Rodgers, 2008) or questionnaires such as Helpful Aspects of Therapy. A review of 18 qualitative studies showed that many clients report common helpful aspects (e.g., gaining new perspectives, feeling heard/understood/accepted, feeling engaged in the therapeutic process) and eight common hindering aspects (e.g., lacking guidance from therapists, feeling emotionally overwhelmed; Ladmanová, Řiháček, & Timulak, 2022).

Attribution of change: Therapists do not only want to know that clients change but also that this change can be attributed to therapy and not to extra-therapeutic factors such as life events outside therapy. Therefore, an interviewer may ask a client: 'In general, what do you think has caused these various changes? In other words, what do you think might have brought them about (outside of therapy and in therapy)?'; 'How likely would the change have been if you had not been in therapy?' (Elliot & Rodgers, 2008).

Sudden and gradual change: Some clients experience 'sudden gains' (Shalom & Aderka, 2020). However, therapeutic change is usually gradual, and clients experience different motivations, resistances, explicit ambivalences, and implicit internal (cognitive) conflicts towards change at different stages of therapy (Boswell, Bentley, & Barlow, 2015). Clients may go through 'stages of change': pre-contemplation (not recognising the problem), contemplation (recognising the problem but unsure about change), preparation/determination (preparing to change), action/willpower (changing) and maintaining the changes (i.e., the Transtheoretical Model of Behaviour Change; Prochaska & Norcross, 2001). Similarly, the Health Action Process Approach (Schwarzer & Luszczynska, 2015) describes motivational conditions of change. Several therapeutic interventions, such as motivational interviewing, focus on improving the client's expectations and motivations, preventing relapse and bridging therapeutic change to daily life.

Significant moments and sequences of moments: Increasing numbers of studies have investigated which specific moments/events/sequences in therapy are significant to the client and lead to change (Timulak, 2010). Researchers have for example investigated moment-by-moment change processes and interactions with sequential analytical methods, e.g., task analysis indicates clients resolve conflicts by softening a harsh critical voice into one of compassion (Greenberg, 2007).

Assimilation analysis: Assimilation analysis describes, interprets, or tests hypotheses about the client's progress within problematic themes across treatment, as problematic experiences often pass through a sequence of stages. Psychotherapy outcomes are understood as change in relation to particular problematic experiences, such as painful memories, threatening feelings, or destructive relationships. In successful psychotherapy, clients follow a regular developmental sequence of recognising, reformulating, understanding, and resolving the problematic experiences that brought them into treatment (Stiles, 2001).

Expert ratings: Chapter 9 exemplifies how researchers can use conversation and discourse analysis to examine any texts, transcripts of therapy sessions, language in audio recordings, non-verbal communication, etc. Raters may also use coding schemes to rate audio/video recordings of sessions, such as the Client Vocal Quality Scale, the Experiencing Scale (measuring the depth of a client's experiences), and Client Verbal Response Category System (categorising content). The therapist may be rated via the Accurate Empathy Scale, Therapist Experiencing Scale, therapeutic competencies scales, and the Structural Analysis of Social Behaviour.

Comprehensive process analysis: In comprehensive process analysis, researchers create pathways in which contributing factors and impacts relate to a particular target event and identify patterns repeated across events (Watson & Rennie, 1994). For example, clients need to avoid painful awareness at certain times, as avoidance can facilitate successful change later (Elliott, 1989).

Interpersonal process recall: Clients and/or therapists may use session recordings to rate each therapeutic intervention regarding its helpfulness (Elliott, 1986; Elliott & Shapiro, 1988).

Narrative analysis of change: Narrative analysis can help identify and analyse narratives in psychotherapy in line with social constructionism (Avdi & Georgaca, 2007). Example narrative data-collection tools include Multiple Code Theory and Adult Attachment Interviews. For example, McLeod (1997) has described the role of meta-narratives in different therapy orientations and therapeutic interactions, such as how clients and therapists make sense of the therapy process and clinical problems. Cognitive narrative analysis focuses on how individuals make sense of their experiences for example via talking, writing, and autobiographies. Grounded theory has also been used to develop theories about the therapeutic process, for example via systematic steps of conceptualisation and focused interviewing and data analysis (Toukmanian & Rennie, 1992). The Therapeutic Cycles Model offers a quantitative analysis of meaning in texts via computerised analysis of transcripts of therapy sessions.

Process-outcome research: Although rarely routinely administered, several questionnaires measure therapeutic processes. For example, clinical trials may include the Session Impact Scale (measuring positive and negative impact of therapy), Session Evaluation Scale (measuring depth, smoothness, positivity, and arousal after the session), Session Reactions Scale, Experiencing Scale, or Therapeutic Gains. Processes predict therapy outcomes (Norcross, Beutler, & Levant, 2006), and most therapeutic approaches share many common processes (Orlinsky, Grawe, & Parks, 1994; Prochaska & Norcross, 2018).

Cynophobia example

Some small studies exist on the therapeutic process of exposure therapy for animal phobias. Future studies may ask clients what they see as helpful and unhelpful, significant moments, and attribution of change.

Step 10: Competencies-related concepts

Definition

Competence frameworks answer the question which competencies therapists have and which skills they use in therapy. A competence describes what a therapist can do, as measurable semi-standardised skills, whereas competencies describe how individual therapists could achieve these standards, as specific behaviour (Vos, 2021b).

Coherent, logical connections

Competencies are examples of therapeutic mechanisms that therapists may use, such as relational skills. Therapeutic competencies have shown to improve therapy outcomes. More research is needed in the evidence and helpfulness of competence frameworks, which therapeutic competencies work best for which clients, and how this relates to other processes.

Components

To guarantee the competencies of psychologists, the APA called in 2006 to establish and implement competency standards throughout the field of psychology across all levels of applied training and professional practice. These benchmarks guide trainers and supervisors to assess their trainees' progress and ensure the highest quality of care. National health-care services and insurance providers often only fund therapists who can prove these competencies, for example by having graduated from an institute/university using a validated competence framework. Competence frameworks are often based on the best research evidence, similar to evidence-based medicine. However, some competence frameworks have been criticised for reflecting more the opinions of influential therapists than systematic reviews of evidence-based research (Roth, 2015).

Beutler listed five generic therapeutic competencies, later validated by others (Norcross & Karpiak, 2017): facilitating a positive therapeutic relationship, therapeutic knowledge of therapeutic mechanisms of change, therapeutic skills to implement effective techniques, being sensitive to the demands and uses of time in selecting interventions, and being creative and flexible when needed. Competence frameworks have also been developed for specific therapies and psychopathologies, such as clinical-psychology, cognitive behaviour therapy, psychoanalytic/psychodynamic therapy, humanistic psychotherapy (UCL Competence Frameworks), and existential psychotherapy (Vos, 2021b).

Cynophobia example

The UCL CBT-frameworks include competencies that therapists may use in exposure therapy, e.g., explaining the rationale, stopping avoidance, planning interventions, involving others, doing hierarchical exposure, and offering follow-up.

Step 11: Creating an overall conceptual framework

Definition

The conceptual framework of a research project gives a coherent overview of the main conceptual models and concepts, their logical connections, and research evidence.

Procedures

This chapter has given an overview of the therapy field. Like a hiker may briefly describe the landmarks and roads on a hiking map, researchers may start their research project by briefly describing the main concepts, relationships, and research evidence in their research area. For example, researchers may conduct non-systematic scoping mini-reviews for each of the nine conceptual models: clinical, aetiological, outcomes-related, therapeutic-mechanism-related, client-related, therapist-related, relationship-related, process-related, and competencies-related concepts. For example, researchers may provide clear, operational definitions of key concepts and describe what handbooks, key authors, systematic literature reviews, and meta-analyses say about these. They may also describe how the concepts are logically connected, for instance how therapeutic mechanisms may target the aetiological causes of dog phobia (the researcher may for instance visualise the findings in an overarching visual figure such as a mind-map). Elaborated examples of conceptual frameworks can for instance be found for existential therapies (Vos, 2017, 2019) and transactional analysis psychotherapy (Vos & van Rijn, 2021).

The conceptual framework may be used as a background section in a research proposal/thesis/article, which may help to identify a problem in the field or a gap in the literature that the research project aims to solve. Usually, the broad non-systematic background review of the conceptual framework is followed by a narrow systematic literature review on the specific problem/gap of the research project, to find all studies on similar topics (see Chapter 5).

The conceptual framework forms the foundations of the methodology, as Chapter 7 will explain. For example, a researcher may base a clinical trial on three conceptual hypotheses: behavioural avoidance reinforces cynophobia (aetiological hypothesis), exposure therapy prevents behavioural avoidance (therapeutic mechanism hypothesis), and exposure therapy reduces cynophobia (outcomes hypothesis). Whereas the clinical trial may only test hypotheses about outcomes, researchers need to justify the intervention by citing other research studies showing how its therapeutic mechanisms may address the aetiological causes of cynophobia.

Researchers may decide to look at the concepts through a specific lens. This is sometimes called a 'theoretical framework' which guides the researcher in their discussion of concepts, such as exploring the conceptual models of cynophobia predominantly through the theoretical lens of 'attachment theory'. Whereas a conceptual framework often consists of mostly empirical and some theoretical concepts, a theoretical framework seems to be more skewed towards describing theories, philosophy, values, and norms. The theoretical framework influences how researchers develop their conceptual framework via their literature reviews and subsequent research steps. If researchers decide to use a theoretical lens in their literature review and research project, they need to describe and justify this and critically reflect on how their theoretical position may limit their research. Researchers usually explicitly describe their theoretical lens at the start of their research proposal/thesis/article. For example, therapy researchers may start their research proposal, thesis or article with sketching the key theories in their field, and how this will influence their literature review and research project in general, such as theories about attachment, psychoanalysis, object-relations, stress-coping model, psychotrauma, congruence, emotion-focused theory, existentialism, postmodernism, structuralism, narratives, etc.

Some researchers use a critical-theoretical lens in their conceptualisation of their research project (Denzin & Lincoln, 2021). In recent years, increasing numbers of qualitative researchers seem to be using a critical-theoretical lens in their literature reviews, their formulation of research aims, and their methodological decisions. They argue that it is impossible to be systematic and neutral in research, and this illusion can limit our attention for important topics and silence oppressed and marginalised voices. Instead, they carefully look at the concepts and the dominant research paradigms through a critical-theoretical lens, and for example examine how processes of power/oppression have influenced the field. They highlight particular underexposed concepts or research methods and critique common research paradigms. Common critical-theoretical frameworks include critical theory, cultural studies, critical ethnography/discourse/grounded theory, Marxist theory, critical race theory, and feminist, post-colonial, LGBTQI+/queer/quare, indigenous/ethnic, critical pedagogy, and criticaltechnology theories; often, researchers focus on the intersection between critical theories

(Denzin & Lincoln, 2021). These researchers take up moral projects that decolonise, honour, and reclaim individual, counter-cultural, and indigenous cultural practices, and mobilise collective actions that may lead to radical politics of possibility, hope, love, care, and equality; therefore, they may focus their literature reviews and research aims on topics such as racism, sexism, homophobia/heterosexism, xenophobia, linguistic oppression, ableism, ageism, classism, elitism, economic inequality, religious oppression, Islamophobia, and anti-Semitism (Marshall, Gerstl-Pepin, & Johnson, 2020). Chapter 4 will describe how researchers may use critical self-reflection and reflexivity to become aware of their position and select or develop a critical-theoretical framework.

Cynophobia example

Exposure therapy for cynophobia seems based on an evidence-based, coherent, and logical conceptual framework. An individual could develop a phobia of dogs (clinical concept) after having been bitten by a dog with subsequent reinforcing avoidance behaviour (aetiology). This phobia could be treated by exposure to stop avoidance, create experiential habituation and extinction, and improve self-efficacy (therapeutic mechanism). This treatment is further supported by outcome research. More research is needed for client-oriented, therapist-oriented, and relationship-oriented factors. Future process-oriented research, such as client interviews about helpful/unhelpful factors, significant moments and attribution of change, may deepen our understanding of how clients experience exposure therapy for cynophobia.

━━━━ Reflective questions ━━━━

- Select three frequently cited articles in your field. Examine their conceptual steps. What are their strengths and weaknesses? What lessons can you learn?
- Examine the literature you have collected for your research project. Examine how many studies you have for each conceptual step and find extra studies for under-represented steps. Reflect: how strong is the evidence for each conceptual step, how coherent and logical are the relationships between studies; is there an unresolved gap/problem in the literature?

4

How to Find a Research Topic and Use Self-Reflection

Chapter aims

The first aim of this chapter is to help researchers find a researchable topic that interests them, leading to the formulation of a preliminary interest statement in the final step. At this stage, researchers may not be able to develop a specific research proposal yet, which they will further refine via a subsequent literature review, as the next chapter will explain. The second aim is to explain how researchers can use self-reflection, for example to find their research topic. The self-reflective skills can be used in all types and stages of research. (Recommended texts on reflexivity include Finlay & Gough, 2008; Willig, 2019.)

Steps in chapter

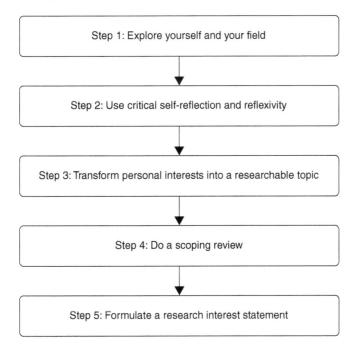

Step 1: Explore yourself and your field

Step 2: Use critical self-reflection and reflexivity

Step 3: Transform personal interests into a researchable topic

Step 4: Do a scoping review

Step 5: Formulate a research interest statement

Templates (see appendices in the back of the book)

A. Preliminary interest statement

E. Essay on critical self-reflection and reflexivity

Step 1: Explore yourself and your field

Definition

Research projects seem to sit at the intersection between personal interests, general research trends, and the needs in a specific field. To find a research topic, you may want to examine all three of these.

Components

Explore yourself

Whereas the feminist movement used the slogan 'the personal is political', this chapter's motto could be 'the personal is researchable'. You may find meaningful research topics and inspiration in your life experiences. Connecting your research with your personal life can make the research personally meaningful; we need to feel motivated to commit to a large research project.

People often already have an intuitive understanding of what is meaningful (Heidegger, 1927). For example, practitioners often use their clinical intuition and crystallised expertise about what may be meaningful for their clients without requiring conscious reflection and verbalisation. Similarly, many researchers use their life history, experiences, and intuitions. Everyday knowledge can yield powerful knowledge: for example, Morrow-Bradley and Elliott (1986) found that therapists learn the most from their client work, theoretical writings, being a client, supervision, and hands-on workshops; only 10% of the respondents reported research publications. See Table 4.1 with reflective prompts to explore your interests (expanded in Online Table 4.1).

There are pros and cons to researching a topic that is closely related to your personal experiences. The advantages of insider research is that researchers may generate more relevant ideas and innovative hypotheses, are not seen as strangers but as group members, understand the culture and jargon beyond stereotypes, and require less preparation time. Insider researchers may be criticised for being biased and insufficiently independent, 'forgetting' research competences, unconsciously selecting participants and routines, and experiencing role conflicts. Instead, outsider researchers seem more neutral and objective, and may stimulate participants sharing more sensitive information because of their temporary stay, but outsider researchers may experience a culture shock, need time to establish trust and understand the culture and jargon, and suffer from ingroup/outgroup bias (Abbas, 2022).

Explore your field

The classic advice at the start of a research project is to read as broadly as possible to identify possible research needs in the field. Some needs may seem important due to popular trends, education, and the media, whereas others may be underexposed (Stevens & Gabbay, 1991). Some topics may also have more momentum or seem more controversial or inert than others due to public and political pressure. Do not focus only on trends, but also on special populations, sub-types, exceptions, extensions of prior research to other populations, problems, outcomes, or theories. You may want to check whether a topic applies to new populations or contexts. You may for example look at relationships/correlations between phenomena, risk factors, protective factors, or causes of phenomena. You may want to describe, explore, or explain a little-understood phenomenon, or understand it in more depth. You may want to give voice to oppressed and marginalised voices, and contribute to social justice. You may also consider developing or evaluating new measurement instruments for a specific topic. While reading, write your thoughts and feelings in a reflective research journal (see Step 2). Table 4.2 offers possible ways to explore your research field.

Table 4.1 Reflective prompts about personal research interests

- Motivation to study psychological therapies
- General interests in life
- Meaning in life
- Topics that enthuse or frustrate you
- Societal trends
- Consider experiences of those with muted voices and injustices in society
- Therapeutic or professional experiences, e.g. case studies, difficult or positive moments
- Personal emotional struggles and development
- Ask friends and peers
- Do not only use your analytical-rational mindset but also use your intuition, unconscious processes, dreams, metaphors, and analogies (Bargar & Duncan, 1982)
- Write in a reflective research journal topics and how you feel about them

Table 4.2 Ways to explore your research field

- General research trends as described in Chapter 3 in this book.
- Books on general research trends: see recommended reading in Chapter 3.
- Using reference lists: skim through reference lists in key publications.
- Read section on 'recommendations for further research': most articles and books give research recommendations in the final part.
- Professional bodies: discover trends via newsletters, conferences, workshops.
- Grant opportunities: funds often announce grant opportunities for specific and unspecified topics (see Online Table 4.2).
- Service providers: many health-care providers facilitate research projects to evaluate and improve their services, but these topics may be limited to audits of existing services.
- Societal trends: consider researching societal challenges, e.g., pandemics, to understand their impact on mental health, coping, and therapy. Find trends via GoogleTrends, TrendWatching, OfficeForNationalStatistics, Pew, PlumXMetrics. Vos, Roberts, and Davies (2019) review mental health and health services in societal contexts.
- Personal contacts: ask experts, placement providers, lecturers, supervisors.

Step 2: Use self-reflection and reflexivity

Definition

Epictetus claimed that the foundation of all research is self-knowledge: our interests, ignorance, and gullibility ought to be the first subject of our study. To prevent experiences and assumptions from disproportionally biasing their research project, many researchers reflect critically about themselves, their interests, and their research. Qualitative researchers usually engage in critical self-reflection and reflexivity from the start of their project, whereas quantitative researchers may engage in simpler self-reflections. If your research project and research/education institute are quantitatively oriented, you may only skim through this step and move to the practical applications in the next step.

Explanation

Whereas an insider may have the advantage of understanding a research topic from within, research is not a means to overcome personal traumas or obsessions. An insider researcher may unconsciously focus only on examples confirming the relevance and truth of their experiences while dismissing contradictory information (self-confirmation bias). For example, a researcher who had personally been discriminated against as an EU resident in the UK might interview other EU residents in the UK about their negative experiences of Brexit, without enquiring about positive and unchanged situations. Based on his biased interviews, he would conclude Brexit had had a negative impact. According to Karl Popper (2005), research needs to have questions that can be proven false (falsification). For example, the researcher could have formulated the generic question 'what are your experiences with Brexit', followed by asking for examples of positive, negative, and unchanged situations. Vos, Van Deurzen, and Tantam (2020) systematically reviewed 22 studies, and found that most, but not all, EU residents in the UK reported discrimination and negative emotions. Thus, we need to translate our personal interests into researchable questions that can be falsified and that are not disproportionally biased. We need to balance our connections and critical distance from our research. Critical self-reflection and reflexivity can help find this balance.

Components

Spectrum of self-reflection and reflexivity

Self-reflection and reflexivity seem to exist on a spectrum, ranging from simple self-reflection to critical self-reflection and radical reflexivity (Etherington, 2004). Research methodologies often differ in where they position themselves on this spectrum. Stereotypically speaking, most quantitative researchers (research based on a positivist epistemology) include simple self-reflection and sometimes critical self-reflection, but rarely radical reflexivity. Most quantitative methods do not require explicit self-reflection and reflexivity, except for discussion sections. Most qualitative researchers explicitly use critical self-reflection and reflexivity, sometimes radical reflexivity.

Simple self-reflection

Self-reflection means that researchers reflect on themselves, for example, how their experiences, perceptions, and life story may impact, transform, and limit their research. Researchers reflect on the knowledge they want to produce, their role and potential blind spots and biases in creating that knowledge (Braun & Clarke, 2012; Finlay & Gough, 2008). For example, a researcher may examine how their experience with depression has made them select depression as a research topic.

Self-reflection seems relevant for all types and stages of research, as everyone asks questions such as 'how can I interpret these findings?' and 'am I unbiased enough to make these conclusions?' Self-reflection seems particularly important when choosing the topic, searching for literature, relating with research participants and colleagues, analysing data, and selecting examples to include in a research report, thesis, or article. Many professional bodies, training programmes, and journals require researchers to acknowledge and manage their impact on the research process (Kasket, 2012).

Critical self-reflection and reflexivity

Stereotypically formulated, simple self-reflection may be described as superficial, non-intrusive introspection about our world without making logical connections with our out-side world. For example, a researcher may describe how they came up with the research topic, their initial thoughts, and later conclusions about the topic and participants (A/B/I in Figure 4.1). However, our relationships with the topic, participants, and our social context can be more complex than this (Figure 4.1). Therefore, simple self-reflection bears the risk of blind spots and self-confirmation bias, which critical self-reflection and reflexivity may help to overcome.

The word 'critical' is not meant in the daily life sense of a person inclined to find faults. It refers to critical theorists, such as the Frankfurt School using the word 'critique', like evaluating the merits of a piece of art. Similarly, critical self-reflection means judging the merits of one's own research. This self-judgment is also critical, i.e., an important and integral part of research. Although 'critical self-reflection' and 'reflexivity' have slightly different meanings, they are often used synonymously. The word 'reflexivity' has been derived from 're-flex', implying bending over (re-flexing) ourselves. Instead of passively observing and describing the world from our position, we acknowledge and judge our position and actively use this knowledge in our interactions with the world.

> Reflexivity generally refers to examining one's beliefs, judgments and practices during the research process and how these may have influenced the research. If positionality refers to what we know and believe, then reflexivity is about what we do with this knowledge. Reflexivity involves questioning one's taken-for-granted assumptions. Essentially, it involves drawing attention to the researcher instead of brushing her/him under the carpet and pretending they did not have an impact/ influence. It requires openness and an acceptance that the researcher is part of the research. (Finlay, 2006, p.15)

Critical self-reflection and reflexivity often consist of the following components:

1   **Awareness of assumptions and biases:** We are aware of our unconscious motivations and implicit assumptions about the topic and the participants more deeply than simple through self-reflection (A/B in Figure 4.1). For example, we recognise the true reasons we conduct this research, such as to improve our academic credentials or trying to prove our beliefs. To see our blind spots and become more critical in our self-reflections, we may need support from critical others, such as supervisors/therapists.

2   **Awareness of impact on others and interaction:** In our interaction with participants, we may bring a kind of academic armour, such as obscure academic language, professional clothing and physical demeanour, socio-economic privilege, and attempts to be neutral/objective (Lerum, 2001). Dropping this armour could help us collect richer and more authentic data. We acknowledge how we influence and interact with our participants and research topic (I' in Figure 4.1). In the first place, we

recognise how our position, perspective, and presence influence the participants and their relationship with the research topic. For example, a research participant may feel intimated by our open way of talking about depression, due to which they may find it difficult to speak freely about their experiences. In the second place, we understand our subsequent responses and interpersonal dynamics. For example, we understand that our expectations could make us feel frustrated about participants shutting down, and we also understand pressuring participants to open up does not work and that we need to ask interview questions sensitively.

3   **Awareness of societal context:** We take into account our societal context.

4   **Mutual shaping:** Whereas simple self-reflection reflects on ourselves, critical self-reflection and reflexivity actively reflects in relationship to our participants and research topic, and how we are shaped and shaping our social world. We understand how the participants, topic, and their experiences have been shaped by society, such as by dominant opinions in the society (II/III/6 in Figure 4.1). Researchers may ask themselves: 'how are the participants, and how am I influenced by the norms, values and opinions from society and the academic community?'

5   **Culture clash:** For example, we may find it easy to talk openly about mental health, due to the (sub-)cultural acceptance amongst people/researchers around us. However, participants may feel hesitant talking about such topics due to their age or culture.

6   **Powers:** Reflexive researchers critically consider the different powers in society of participants and researchers, e.g., 'How is it like to be in the socio-economic position of the participant, and how would they see me, a university-trained researcher? What impact does my socio-economic position have on my relationship with the participant and how they respond to the interview questions? Would individuals in other socio-economic situations experience the topic differently?' (C/4 in Figure 4.1).

7   **Public scrutiny:** Taking into account our societal context may imply opening our research up for public scrutiny (Finlay & Gough, 2008), e.g., by disseminating findings, public discussions, member-checking, and inviting stakeholders as co-researchers.

8   **Social justice:** Action researchers often ask, 'how can my research contribute to society and improve how society relates to this topic and these participants?' (C/4'/6' in Figure 4.1).

9   **Higher-level reflection:** The previous components showed how researchers may reflect on a higher level. Simple self-reflection means that a researcher has a one-dimensional understanding of the relationship between participants and the research topic. Simple-reflecting researchers may, for example, examine the research questions: 'what do participants say about this topic of depression' (participant → topic) and 'what impact does depression have on their life' (topic → participant). However, critical reflection means we recognise the bi-directional relationship between participant and topic (participant ↔ depression). We are aware of how the participant's background influences how they relate to the topic (1 in Figure 4.1). For example the participant's personality, life story, or socio-economic status may influence what and how they speak about depression. We also understand the topic may affect how participants relate to the topic (2 in Figure 4.1). For example, depressed individuals often talk in a depressed way about their depression due to the nature of depression. Thus, the research data may be influenced (social-constructivists would say 'co-constructed') by the dynamic interactions between the researcher, participant, and topic.

10 **Active reflection:** Whereas simple self-reflection means theoretically knowing our position regarding the participants and topic, critical self-reflection implies actively using this knowledge and moving away from our position. We translate our theoretical self-knowledge into practical action by adjusting how we speak sensitively with the interviewee about the topic and the research project, encouraging them to feel free to share their experiences and challenge our preconceptions.

11 **Continuous reflection:** We do not merely engage in critical self-reflection and reflexivity at one point in time, for example when writing a course assignment or thesis. Critical self-reflection and reflexivity require continuous active examination of moment-by-moment thoughts and feelings throughout the research process.

12 **Critical theories:** Some researchers use a critical-theoretical lens through which they look at the research topic, which may highlight underexposed topics and power dynamics in dominant research paradigms and society. Self-reflective researchers describe and justify their critical-theoretical lens at the start of their research project and any publications; in the discussion section of their publications, they reflect critically on the strengths and limitations of using this lens. Common critical-theoretical frameworks include critical theory, cultural studies, Marxist theory, critical-ethnography/discourse/grounded theory, critical race theory, and feminist, post-colonial, LGBTQI+/queer/quare, indigenous/ethnic, critical-pedagogy, critical-technology, and intersectional theories (Denzin & Lincoln, 2021).

These critical theories often share five assertions: (1) research fundamentally involves issues of power; (2) the research report is not transparent, but rather it is authored by a raced, gendered, classed, and politically oriented individual; (3) race, class, and gender [among other social identities] are crucial for understanding experience; (4) historically, traditional research has silenced members of oppressed and marginalized groups; and (5) systems of divisions and oppression were historically constructed and are continuously reinforced.

These [critical-theoretical] perspectives contain three injunctions: As researchers, we should (1) examine how we represent the participants – the Other or the subaltern – and search for their counternarratives and modes of domination in our work; (2) scrutinize the complex interplay of our own biography, power and status, interactions with participants, and the written word; (3) be vigilant about the dynamics of ethics and politics in our work. One implication is paying attention to the participants' reactions and the voice they use in their work as a representation of the relationship between themselves and their participants. Another is that the traditional criteria for judging the adequacy or trustworthiness of a work have become essentially contested. Those frustrated with traditional research may find greater flexibility of expression in [critical theories]. Each [critical theory] embraces changing existing social structures and processes as a primary purpose and, when framed by explicitly critical orientations, has openly political agendas and often emancipatory goals. (Marshall & Rossman, 2014, p.95)

In sum, whereas simple self-reflection means theoretically knowing our thoughts and feelings about the participants and research topic, critical self-reflection and reflexivity mean that researchers understand and actively use the dynamic multi-level interactions between their personal and professional experiences, participants, topic, and social context.

Radical reflexivity

Radical constitutive reflexivity is a more radical form of higher-level reflecting, based on the postmodern idea that there is not one objective reality. Individuals construct reality, and nobody's perspective has more value than any other. The research process constitutes a reality in itself, for example, through the subjective selection of the topic and interview questions. Therefore, we may invite our participants to become co-researchers (Chapter 9). Some authors criticise radical reflexivity for being non-pragmatic, anything-goes, narcissistic, and self-indulgent (Johnson & Duberley, 2003).

Procedures

Development

Critical self-reflection and reflexivity skills need to be trained. You may want to develop these skills from the start, particularly if considering doing qualitative research. Be patient and self-compassionate, as it may take time before you see any insights arising from self-reflection, as our intentions, emotions, and unconscious processes may initially be inaccessible to us (England, 1994). Reflective experiential self-development often includes moments of doubt, cycling through evaluation, analysis, and conclusions to then cycle back to reconsidering the subject from a different perspective/approach (Gibbs, 1988). These cycles should not be understood as vicious cycles but as positive spirals: the same topic is repeated at a more insightful level (Vos, 2017), slowly accumulating experiences and understandings to develop vital research competencies and knowledge about the research topic (Hullinger et al., 2019).

Reflective research journal

The most frequently used self-reflective tool is a reflective research journal or reflexive research diary. In this journal, researchers record each step in the research process, detailing what they did, how they did it and why. This creates a verifiable audit trail of the research process and the rationales behind each step, allowing retrospective quality checking and identification of errors. Reflective writing can also help researchers develop critical thinking and conceptualisation skills, as the researchers need to explicate and justify each step, which can make them aware of their blind spots and learn from them. Furthermore, by explicating each step, reflective journaling elucidates the legitimacy of the knowledge claims and increases the study's trustworthiness and ethical rigour. Diaries can be physical or on a computer file, written in the first person, often following an associative train of thought in the moment. Most researchers write in their journals each time they do research or at the end of a day; at minimum, they write after critical incidents or immediately after a research interview. Researchers regularly re-read diary entries, reflect on their development, and identify learning opportunities (see overview in Wright & Bolton, 2012).

Possible topics for reflection

- Day-to-day personal introspections, thoughts and feelings about the project
- Day-to-day research activities

- Methodological decisions
- Interaction with research participants
- Interaction with colleagues/peers/supervisors
- General self-reflections on the research topic, also beyond research activities

Self-reflective questions

The simplest self-reflective questions a researcher may ask include: what did I observe, experience, and do (observations); what could explain this (explanations); what do I want to do with this knowledge (implications)? Table 4.3 offers more comprehensive questions to REFLECT (report, experience, follow, label, explain, conclude, translate), which integrates self-reflective questions recommended by several authors (Denzin & Lincoln, 2021; Jasper, 2005; Wright & Bolton, 2012).

Numbers and letters refer to different relationships and levels of reflection (Vos, 2021a; Online Table 4.3 includes systematic self-reflective questions about each relationship).

Table 4.3 REFLECT questions

Report: Report factual observations:
- ○ What was the context (date, location)?
- ○ What happened?

Experience: Describe subjective experiences:
- ○ What did I think, feel, and do?

Follow: Describe what followed what:
- ○ What were the effects of my thoughts/feelings/actions on the situation/others?
- ○ What were the effects of the situation/others on my thoughts/feelings/actions?
- ○ How did the interactions between me and others evolve?

Label: Label the observations and experiences:
- ○ What was good/helpful/easy?
- ○ What was bad/unhelpful/challenging?
- ○ How open-minded/close-minded was I throughout the situation?
- ○ What are alternative ways of seeing the situation and experience?

Explain: Find possible explanations for the observations and experiences:
- ○ What could explain what happened in this situation?
- ○ What could explain what I thought, felt, and did?
- ○ How does this situation confirm/challenge my ideas and goals about the participant and research topic?
- ○ How does this situation fit the ideas and goals of my institute/supervisor/field/society?
- ○ How does my position in society explain what I observed and experienced?
- ○ If relevant, how did the personal and societal background of others influence how they responded in the situation and how we interacted?

Conclude: Conclude what you have learned from your observations and experiences:
- ○ What did I learn about the topic, participant, society, and myself?
- ○ What do I want to do differently?

Translate: Translate your lessons into a practical action plan:
- ○ How will I prepare myself for similar situations?
- ○ What will I practically do next time?

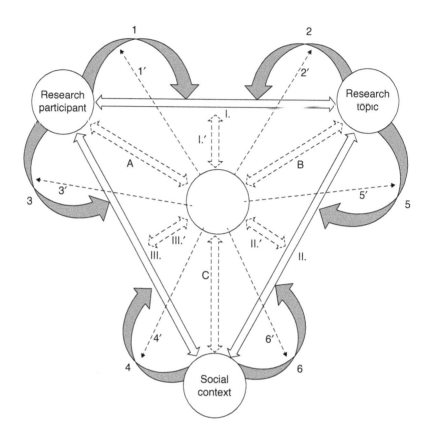

Figure 4.1 Model of systematic critical self-reflection and reflexivity

Step 3: Transform personal interests into a researchable topic

Definition

After identifying possible research interests in the first step, you may want to transform these personal interests into researchable topics. This section describes critical self-reflective questions to transform your interests into a personally feasible, unbiased, relevant, innovative, well-designed research project with a feasible plan for data collection and time planning.

Components

Transform into a personally feasible project

- Does this topic fit the requirements of your training programme, organisation, or funding body?
- Are you motivated enough to spend many months/years researching this topic?
- Will this topic be good for your CV?

- Can you get the right support from supervisors/others for this topic?
- Do you have the required knowledge and skills? What knowledge/skills do you need, and how can you develop this?

Transform into an unbiased research project

- Start a reflective research journal, and do exercises in critical self-reflection and reflexivity.
- When you have identified an initial research topic, analyse your relationships with the topic, participants, and society (Figure 4.1 shows all relationships; Online Table 4.3 offers self-reflective questions about each relationship). The following questions regard the most important relationships.
- How have your personal and professional experiences made you interested in this topic? How do these experiences bias/limit you? What would someone without your experiences be interested in? What does research say about your personal theories?
- What is your social position, and how has this influenced your interest in this topic? How does your socio-economic/political position bias/limit you? What would someone in a different position be interested in?
- What do different stakeholders say about this topic, e.g., mental health advocates, lobby groups, experts-by-experience?
- What have you learned about your biases, opinions, feelings, and intuitions over the years? What are your usual blind spots? How could you overcome your blind spots and biases?
- How will you identify, set aside, and/or constructively use your biases, opinions, feelings, and intuitions in this research project (e.g., start using a reflective research journal)?
- How will you prevent self-confirmation bias? Are your research questions falsifiable (i.e., can the research questions be disproven)? Are you searching for evidence pro and contra your intuition?
- How do researchers and therapists usually look at this topic? What are sensitivities, norms, and contexts in the research field? Which voices have been minimised? Critically reflect on the dominant research paradigms and your own preconceptions through critical-theoretical lenses.

Transform into a relevant and innovative research project

What makes this research (a) innovate and (b) relevant for:

- the practices of psychological therapies?
- the research field on psychological therapies?
- clients/individuals with mental health problems?
- society in general?

Transform into a well-defined project

The research project needs to be well defined:

- Is the initial research idea focused enough on one precise research area (instead of including multiple broad areas)?

- Are the key concepts clearly defined and described explicitly enough? Name the specific individuals, groups, or organisations you plan to study. For example, the research question 'why are students not achieving' is too general; a specific question is 'to what extent do IQ levels predict student marks?'

Transform into a project with a feasible data collection and timeline

Consider whether you can potentially collect sufficient data and participants (at a later stage, you can further specify the sample):

- How realistic is it to collect sufficient data or to recruit sufficient participants for your research project? For example, have other researchers collected similar data or recruited similar participants; what were their challenges (e.g., check decline rates and dropout in similar studies)?
- What is the time for this research project, what are formal deadlines (e.g., assignments/ proposals), and how much time do you need for each research stage? Develop a preliminary timeline or Gantt chart to regularly update, e.g., with the following components:

Months 1–2: Developing basic skills, getting an overview of the field, finding a topic and research supervisor (see Chapters 2–4)

Months 3–4: Conducting the literature review (Chapter 5)

Months 5–6: Writing the research proposal (Chapter 6)

Months 7–8: Waiting times for research committee, revising/rewriting research proposal

Month 9: Writing ethics proposal (Chapter 11)

Months 10–11: Waiting times for ethics committee, revising/rewriting ethics proposal

Months 12–13: Participant recruitment

Months 14–16: Data collection (e.g., interviews, survey)

Month 17: Data insertion/interview transcription

Month 18–19: Data analysis (Chapters 8–10)

Months 20–22: Draft thesis/report (Chapter 12)

Months 23–24: Final thesis/report

Months 25–...: Dissemination of findings (Chapter 12)

Step 4: Do a scoping review

Definition

Once you have identified an area of research via previous steps, you may want to read more about this specific topic. You do not need to read all articles in this research stage, as this scoping review aims to identify key trends and the most frequently cited authors and publications.

Example

You may want to search for the following publications on your topic: literature reviews, meta-analyses, meta-syntheses, and handbooks. Furthermore, you may want to identify the most cited publications and authors; to find these, you can order the search results according to the number of citations in many academic search engines. As you are merely scoping the literature, you may use generic search engines such as scholar.google.com (although generic search engines often show many irrelevant references and miss key publications; Chapter 5 introduces better search engines). You might, for example, limit yourself to the 20 most cited publications.

Step 5: Formulate a research interest statement

Definition

It can be helpful to write a research interest statement, for example to ask for feedback from peers/supervisors, or to guide your literature review (Chapter 5).

Example

An interest statement is not written in stone and will be refined during your literature review. As the tree-structure of your text, use Template A, 'Preliminary interest statement'.

━━━━ Reflective questions ━━━━

- Start a reflective journal (e.g., physical notebook, Word file), in which you can do the following exercises.
- Select three frequently cited articles in your field. Examine how they engage in critical self-reflection and reflexivity; how could they be more critically self-reflective and reflexive? What lessons can you learn?
- Practice reflection by answering the REFLECT questions (Step 2) about a meaningful situation, such as a meeting with clients/colleagues/supervisors.
- Ask self-reflective questions (Online Table 4.1).
- Identify at least ten intuitively appealing topics in Chapter 3, website/newsletters from relevant professional bodies, and societal trends.
- Select three interests from the previous exercises that intuitively feel meaningful and feasible. Reflect on how you can transform each interest Into a researchable topic with the questions in Step 3.
- Systematically analyse your relationships with each interest (Online Table 4.2).
- Based on previous exercises, select the most meaningful researchable topic. Find relevant publications on this: e.g., search scholar.google.com for literature reviews, meta-analyses, and handbooks. Identify the most cited articles and key authors.
- Use Template A to write an interest statement.

5

How to Conduct a Literature Review

Chapter aims

This chapter explains how to conduct a formal literature review. Before conducting a formal review, you need to know your general field and have scoped your general area of interest as the previous chapters described. A formal review can identify a gap in the literature that the research project aims to solve, as the next chapter will explain. A formal literature review is often included in its totality or in abridged form in research proposals, theses, and research articles. Popular introductions to conducting literature reviews include Gough, Oliver and Thomas (2012), Jesson, Matheson, and Lacey (2011), and Machi and McEvoy (2016).

Steps in chapter

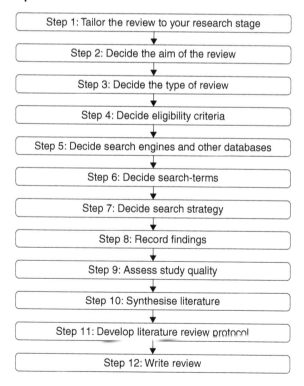

Step 1: Tailor the review to your research stage

Step 2: Decide the aim of the review

Step 3: Decide the type of review

Step 4: Decide eligibility criteria

Step 5: Decide search engines and other databases

Step 6: Decide search-terms

Step 7: Decide search strategy

Step 8: Record findings

Step 9: Assess study quality

Step 10: Synthesise literature

Step 11: Develop literature review protocol

Step 12: Write review

Templates

B: Literature review plan

C: Systematic literature review

Step 1: Tailor the review to your research stage

Definition

Literature reviews often serve different aims in different stages of the research process. For example, a scoping review suffices when formulating your initial research interest statement, but a comprehensive review may be required for a research proposal and thesis. This section gives an overview of the different aims of a literature review in various stages. After identifying the stage of your research in this step, you can formulate the tailored aims and methods for your literature review in the following steps.

Rationale

'It has been published; thus, it must be true!' Too often, social media and student theses use variations of this authority argument. If you want to find support for your idea, however crazy, you may find it via cherry-picking from the immense store of 50 million published scholarly articles (Jinha, 2010). However, some cherries are very sour. For example, many people in the late 2000s uncritically cited the studies from Stapel and Vonk, alleging that meat eaters have anti-social traits. The ball started rolling when critical reviewers asked questions because other studies had not found such strong correlations between personality and eating habits. The authors admitted they had faked the data. Thus, instead of focusing on single studies confirming our paradigmatic thinking, we should critically look at the entire body of literature. This is a basic rule of research: never base far-reaching conclusions on one study, but use critical systematic reviews of all relevant studies.

Mulrow (1994, p.16) wrote that a literature review 'separates the insignificant, unsound, or redundant deadwood in the literature from the salient and critical studies worthy of reflection'. The method to make this separation consists of systematic exploration, critical evaluation, and integrative synthesis. Systematic implies not only searching for studies confirming our ideas but also for studies rejecting or extending them. This is falsification: if we hypothesise that all swans are white, we should not only search for studies looking into white swans but also for studies looking for swans of other colours (Popper, 2005). 'Critical' means assessing the quality and risk-of-bias of the studies; Stapel and Vonk's studies, for example, were sponsored by animal rights groups, potentially biasing the study. The synthesis helps to summarise the field and draw conclusions about a topic. The synthesis can also show the gaps in the research about a topic, which may inspire researchers to develop their own project. A literature review can also indicate which research methodologies are trustworthy and helpful and which are not.

Thus, literature reviews can achieve multiple aims, but all use, at least to some extent, a systematic, critical, and integrative method. As will be described, reviews differ in how systematic, critical and integrative they are, often depending on their aims.

Examples

Finding a topic: Scoping mini-reviews

Chapter 4 described how a scoping review may identify the main trends within a topic, allowing the initial formulation of an interest statement. A scoping review is usually non-systematic, focusing on literature reviews, meta-analyses, handbooks, and most cited publications and authors (search engines such as Web of Knowledge and EMBASE allow the ordering of references according to number of citations). For example, if you want to examine CBT for cynophobia, search scholar.google.com with the terms 'cognitive behaviour therapy' and 'phobias'. However, this non-systematic method yields an overwhelming number of studies and misses crucial studies and nuances, including studies similar to yours. Therefore, while scoping reviews may be a good starting point for a preliminary interest statement or a student essay, they are insufficient for research proposals/theses/articles.

Introducing a theoretical/critical framework: Scoping mini-review and lenses

If you decide to use a theoretical framework or critical lens, as Chapter 4 introduced, explicitly describe this before you start any literature/background review, such as looking at treatments for cynophobia from an attachment theory lens (otherwise, skip this). You may describe this is in a section on your personal background with a critical-reflective and reflexive writing style. Name and justify your theoretical or critical-theoretical lens, mention key authors and most cited publications on the critical theory (found via scoping mini-reviews), describe how this lens will influence your selection and discussion of the topic and methods of your literature review, and critically reflect on its strengths and limitations. Using a theoretical or critical-theoretical lens does not mean that you can cherry-pick whatever studies you like, and blind yourself to the broader field beyond your position. You need to contextualise your position, and make the argument that the field so far has focused on topic X but you want to give voice to Y. The difference with a literature review without a theoretical/critical lens is that you will possibly run additional specific searches on topics that other researchers may not have thought of (e.g., LGBTQI+ and cynophobia, or therapy with LGBTQI+ clients in general). You will highlight these theoretical/critical topics, and be on the look out for implicit assumptions and omissions in the dominant research paradigms when describing and discussing the literature. Thus, like looking through coloured lenses, you may look at mostly the same studies but see these in slightly different colours.

Building the conceptual framework and writing the background sections: Scoping mini-reviews

Each research proposal, report, thesis, or article starts with a reflection on the conceptual and theoretical background before zooming into the specific topic of the study (Greetham, 2020). Chapter 3 described how researchers often start with a conceptual framework of their field. For instance, researchers may highlight the most important concepts, their relationships, and empirical evidence, regarding the clinical and aetiological phenomena, outcomes, therapeutic mechanisms, clients, therapists, therapeutic relationship, processes, and competencies. For most research purposes, it suffices to do non-systematic scoping mini-reviews for these conceptual models, e.g., via handbooks, key authors, literature reviews, and meta-analyses For instance, if your research project tests the outcomes of exposure therapy for cynophobia, you do not need to systematically review all studies published on the clinical or aetiologi-cal model of phobias because your primary interest is outcomes. However, you may want to introduce the broader field; for instance, give definitions of phobias, an overview of phobia types, diagnostic criteria, prevalence/incidence, and key ideas about the aetiology of animal phobias, the most frequently used treatment types and therapeutic mechanisms. This will help you create a logical conceptual framework, such as: individuals may develop cynopho-bia due to traumatic experiences and avoidance behaviour, and therefore exposure therapy may help to process the traumatic experiences and prevent avoidance. To contextualise your study, you may also briefly mention outcomes for CBT in general and for other phobias, and other therapies for cynophobia (in your major-review you will systematically review all stud-ies on exposure therapy for cynophobia). With these scoping mini-reviews, you have intro-duced the conceptual background of your study, and can justify your project's importance and innovation.

Becoming an expert and identifying the research aim: Major systematic literature review

After the non-systematic scoping mini-reviews of the background, you may want to do a major systematic literature review on the specific topic of your research project. A systematic literature review aims to comprehensively review all relevant and similar studies on your topic, critically assess their strength and weaknesses, and identify a potential gap in the field that your research project may fill. For instance, if your research project aims to test the out-comes of exposure therapy for cynophobia, you may want to conduct a systematic literature review of all clinical trials of exposure therapy for cynophobia. Sometimes, you may also want to broaden this scope when there are few or no studies on your topic, and you may conduct a systematic review of all outcome studies of CBT for all types of phobias. When the topic of your research project is complex, you may have to do two, three, or four major-reviews each with their own specific aim and method – as long as doing multiple reviews is feasible. It is important to be systematic, critical, and integrative in the method(s) of the major literature review(s) on the main topic of your research project. Amongst others, examiners and journal editors may question your academic authority if you have missed key publications. You do not want to hear your examiners or journal editors suggest you have wasted your energy because others have already conducted a similar or better study that you did not find because your review was not systematic enough.

Developing research/ethics proposals: Summarising highlights

Early in the research process, researchers conduct mini-reviews of the background and major-reviews on their main research topic. The more rigorous the literature reviews are at the start of the research process, the stronger are the justifications for this study, and the less work a student will have when writing the final thesis. However, often researchers cannot include their full literature review in their research or ethics proposals, or articles, due to word count limits. This does not imply that researchers can skip conducting rigorous reviews and cherry-pick: they still need to show they are an expert in their field, and that the study is conceptually embedded, relevant, and innovative. The limited word count forces researchers to focus on literature highlights, requiring them to be certain that they have picked the best references, which they can only know via rigorous reviews. Researchers may explicate that 'this text only discusses the most cited studies identified in a systematic literature review that I cannot present entirely due to the word limit'.

Selection of methodology: Scoping mini-reviews

To select your research method, you will need to have a general understanding of which methods exist, when they can be used, and their strengths and weaknesses. Chapters 7–9 give a generic overview of most methodologies in therapy research, which you may complement with overviews/handbooks on research methods. Do not only familiarise yourself with personally appealing methods but keep an open mind towards alternatives. In methodology sections, justify why you have selected this method and dismissed alternatives. In discussion sections, critically reflect on whether alternative methods would have led to different findings and conclusions.

Application of research methodology: Scoping mini-reviews

After selecting a method, you need to become an expert on this method, particularly on how to apply it. You may want to conduct four mini-reviews. First, search for the most recent handbooks on this method, which usually give an overview of the foundations and applications. Second, you may want to identify texts on this method's foundations, such as the first and most cited publications. Third, you may search for instruction manuals explaining how to apply the method (if this exists). Fourth, you may want to search for how other researchers have described and applied the method; for instance, read the most cited applications on similar topics like yours. Read these applications critically, and consider their strengths and weaknesses, and how you want to apply this method.

Writing the discussion: Focused mini-reviews

When analysing your data, you will most likely come across findings that surprise you, that you do not understand, or that raise new questions. You may also have stumbled upon methodological or organisational challenges that you may or may not have been able to solve, and that may influence the data interpretation. You may also wonder how your findings relate to other concepts and studies. Therefore, most researchers do new mini-reviews to answer these very specific questions, in addition to the literature reviews they conducted before data collection and have already mentioned earlier in their research thesis/report/article. In most methods, these mini-reviews are done after completion of the data analyses and are described in the discussion section (see Chapter 12), to differentiate between the participants' voices and the researchers' interpretative voices (some interpretive/hermeneutic methods include these extra mini-reviews in the findings section).

Writing a research article: Summaries and highlights

Most journals only accept articles between 3000 and 6000 words, leaving little space for discussing the literature. You will need to summarise the reviews, discuss the most representative and influential publications in the field and relevant to your study, to justify your research and explain your conceptual framework. You can only know which publications are worthy of mentioning after having systematically reviewed the literature, even if you cannot include the full review in your article.

Step 2: Decide the aim of the review

Definition

This and the following steps will focus on conducting major-reviews. This step outlines possible aims of systematic literature reviews and how to formulate aims.

Examples

Generic overview of the field

Many major-reviews aim to give a general overview of the field, such as: 'What is the nature and scope of research knowledge on this topic?'

Clinical aims

A major-review may help practitioners and service providers identify evidence-based concepts and bona fide interventions. A major-review may help policy-makers decide which therapies should be provided and/or funded. Frameworks of evidence-based competencies can be used as standards for training and practice. A review can also act as a political statement to make a particular point and prove that particular topics have been ignored. Example review questions include: 'What evidence exists for this therapeutic intervention?'; 'What types of interventions are effective for this psychological problem?'; 'How do clients experience this treatment?'

Methodological aims

A major-review may help identify the types of study design and methodologies used in a field and assess their strengths and weaknesses. For example, 'What kind of research has been conducted?'; 'How valid, reliable, or trustworthy are certain research methods?'

Conceptual aim

As described before, the mini-reviews and major-review can embed a research project in the broader research context. Each research project needs to be embedded in an evidence-based, coherent, logical conceptual framework (Chapter 3). For example, 'What is the prevalence/ incidence of this problem?'; 'What is known about the aetiology of this?'; 'What are the criteria of this disorder?'; 'What are the empirical foundations of this diagnosis?'

Identifying the gap in the literature

'Mind the gap!' Anyone using London's public transport is familiar with this phrase. Anyone reading research publications knows its academic equivalent: mind the gap in the literature! The last paragraph/section of a major-review, before the formulation of the aims of the research project, usually includes a sentence such as: 'In conclusion, this literature review has shown there is insufficient research on this topic. This review has also shown the importance of further investigating this topic. Due to this gap in the literature and the importance of the topic, I have decided to conduct this research project on this topic'. Subsequently, your research project's aims/objectives/questions/hypotheses logically follow from this gap in the literature (see Chapter 6). This review shows your project's relevance and innovative contribution to the field, which can justify you, your supervisors, and participants spending time and resources on it. For example, 'What are gaps in the literature?'

Implicit aims

Many literature reviews have implicit aims, such as becoming an expert on your topic, avoiding reinventing the wheel, and understanding common practices and standards in your field. Training institutions often ask students to conduct reviews to familiarise themselves with key trends, authors, theories, and concepts in a field. A review may demonstrate a student has reached a professional academic level, as shown by its academic rigour, critical synthesis, contribution to the debate, self-reflection, and reflexivity.

Procedures

1. Decide to conduct one/multiple major-reviews

A research proposal/thesis has usually only one major systematic literature review with one specific aim, as this often already involves much work. However, sometimes the literature review is divided into multiple major-reviews. A researcher may also decide to conduct multiple reviews if few studies exist on the specific topic or if multiple reviews are needed to explain the conceptual framework and justify the study. For example, few clinical trials have been published on CBT for cynophobia, so a researcher may want to conduct three major-reviews: clinical trials on CBT for any phobias; clinical trials on CBT for animal phobias; clinical trials on cynophobia (also non-CBT). If systematic literature reviews already exist, researchers do not need to repeat this but can discuss these and update with recent studies.

2. Formulate aim

A literature review can quickly become unwieldy without a focus. Therefore, before you search for literature, formulate a clear and specific aim for your review. Some researchers, particularly inexperienced individuals, criticise the idea that literature reviews need an aim and method (Online Table 5.1). Naturally, the aim and method should not become a straitjacket but should enable researchers to develop a rich and inspiring understanding of their field. However, all reviews should have an aim and method, albeit generic or narrative aims and snowballing methods – i.e., decide and transparently describe what you are doing and why you are doing this. A clear plan makes doing a review easier, and facilitates critical reflection on the review's strengths and limitations.

3. Formulate aim via conceptual frameworks

Many methods have been proposed to develop aims (Online Table 5.2). For example, the authoritative Cochrane network recommends using the acronym PICO to define an aim describing the types of population/problem, intervention, comparison group, and outcomes. A reviewer may also develop the aim by asking themselves the following reflective questions based on the conceptual steps and example from Chapter 3:

An alternative acronym for qualitative reviews is SPIDER: Sample, Phenomenon of Interest, Design, Evaluation, Research type.

- **Clinical concepts:** What clinical problem or psychological phenomenon? Cynophobia.
- **Aetiological concepts:** What aspects of the aetiology? N/A.
- **Outcomes-related concepts:** What types of outcomes/evaluations? Anxiety.
- **Therapeutic-mechanisms-related concepts:** What types of interventions, therapies, or therapeutic mechanisms? Exposure-therapies.
- **Client-related concepts:** What type of participants? Adults > 18 years.
- **Therapist-related concepts:** What type of therapists? N/A.
- **Relationship-related concepts:** What types of client–therapist relationship? N/A.
- **Process-related concepts:** Which processes? N/A.
- **Competencies-related concepts:** Which therapeutic competencies? N/A.

This example can be formulated as: 'This literature review aims to review the effects of clinical trials of exposure therapy for cynophobia on anxiety in adults'.

Step 3: Decide the type of review

Definition

Different types of literature reviews have different aims. This step describes the most common review types. If your review has multiple aims, you may use different review types for each aim.

Busting the being-unfocused-and-non-systematic-is-good myth

Often, researchers/lecturers have a semantic battle over whether a review should be systematic or not. From a pragmatic perspective, it does not matter what a review is called; what matters is that the review follows a precise, pre-determined, justified, replicable, and consistently applied method or strategy. For example, a narrative review uses a narrative method to search and select literature: this method should be consistently used. A scoping review uses a scoping method. Without a clear and consistently applied method, there is a large danger of cherry-picking, self-confirmation bias, and paradigmatic thinking. What demarcates academic literature reviews from well-intended layman's reviews is that the researcher not only tells what they have found but also explains how they arrived at these results and why they have used these methods, based on critical self-reflection and reflexivity. It may be hypothesised that the being-unfocused-and-non-systematic-is-good myth is caused by the researcher's misconceptions, unresolved personal issues, or academic incompetence (Online Table 5.1).

Examples

Review types frequently used in student research:

- **Scoping review (usually of study background):** Gives a quick-and-dirty initial overview of key trends, topics, authors, and publications. Introduces novice researchers to the field and helps identify a personal research interest or gap in the literature.
- **Review of the study background, structured according to the conceptual framework:** It may be argued that each review sketches the conceptual framework of the research topic. However, it is also possible to explicitly present the literature review according to the nine conceptual models in Chapter 3: clinical, aetiological, outcomes-related, therapeutic-mechanism-related, client-related, therapist-related, relationship-related, process-related, and competencies-related. The researcher searches for the most cited research and trends for each conceptual model in their field (i.e., nine scoping mini-reviews; note not all conceptual models may be relevant). The review could be finished with a synthesis, for example, possibly aided with a visual figure or mind-map.
- **Thematic review (usually of the study background):** Critically analyses all relevant research on a topic, organised in multiple organically emerging themes (each of which may be a review in itself). It aims to develop the conceptual framework and identify recommendations for the research project – the most common method in student theses.

- **Historical or narrative review (usually of the study background):** Describes how knowledge has evolved, such as changes in the dominant conceptual models of the research topic (e.g., evolution of different types of therapies for cynophobia). May discuss different schools, controversies, and socio-political influences. It aims to describe broad trends, not a comprehensive, in-depth understanding of a topic, which can help to justify and position a research project in the broader research field. Easily combined with a theoretical/critical framework/lens. Common as major-review in bachelor/master theses or as a background section in a doctorate thesis.
- **Systematic review of the specific research topic:** A systematic approach is used to find all relevant publications about one particular topic, such as all clinical trials on exposure therapy for cynophobia (see previous step). It does not need to be a systematic review *study* as described below (as this may be too time-intensive and unnecessary for the research project), but just a systematic review of studies closest to the study the researcher is doing. The systematic method ensures that the researcher does not miss similar studies, making a new study obsolete. If a similar study has been undertaken before, the researcher can learn from its strengths and limitations. A systematic review of the specific research topic often follows after a generic background review sketching the conceptual framework of the field. Sometimes a systematic-review of the specific research topic is impossible, for example because this is a new research field, and then only a background review may be conducted. The findings may be described via conceptual models, themes, narratives, or chronology.
- **Practice-friendly review:** This gives an overview of a body of research and can differ in comprehensiveness, aiming to identify implications for practice. For example, an evidence-based practice guideline is a comprehensive review by experts to inform policy-makers.

Formal systematic literature reviews

A formal review *study* strengthens the foundations of a research project, is more likely to be accepted by peer-reviewed journals, is transparent for peers/supervisors to give feedback on, and reduces uncertainty and bias via rigorous methodology. A formal review study can have strong authoritative power and help make firm conclusions, such as which therapy works best for whom, which can influence practitioners and policy-makers.

- **Systematic literature review study:** Systematically reviews all the available literature on a specific topic, according to the steps and assessment criteria discussed in formal frameworks, with the most frequently used being PRISMA (Moher et al., 2009) and Synthesis without Meta-Analysis (Campbell et al., 2020). Usually, the review protocol is pre-registered or published, e.g., via Cochrane (Higgins et al., 2019). A review study gives an authoritative review of the topic but can be time-intensive.
- **Meta-analysis:** Systematically synthesises findings of quantitative studies with a formal systematic method and statistical analysis (e.g., Borenstein et al., 2021; Erford, Savin-Murphy, & Butler, 2010). This helps to statistically combine the results of multiple studies. For example, a meta-analysis can calculate the mean prevalence or incidence of a clinical phenomenon, the mean pre–post effect size of treatments, or differences between two interventions; network meta-analyses can compare multiple interventions. Additional moderator analyses may examine which intervention works best for whom,

mediators and therapeutic mechanisms of change (Kazdin, 2007, 2009). Check APA-JARS publication guidelines for meta-analyses. Meta-analyses are often regarded as the most robust evidence on a topic, and could be a game-changer, such as the first ever published meta-analysis on psychotherapy (Smith & Glass, 1977). However, the generalisability of the findings of a meta-analysis depends on the homogeneity, quality, and ecological validity of the included studies, as well as on the quality of the sensitivity analysis in the meta-analysis (Baldwin & Imel, 2020; Cuijpers et al., 2017). Consequently, meta-analyses are not the panacea to all clinical and policy questions, and should be viewed as the beginning of a conversation rather than the end.

- **Meta-synthesis:** This systematically synthesises and interprets findings of qualitative studies with a formal systematic method (Paterson et al., 2001; Paterson, 2011; Timulak, 2009; Walsh & Downe, 2005).
- **Meta-narrative review:** Critically reviews and narratively summarises all available research on a topic, often carried out by experts (see Wong et al., 2013).
- **Mixed-review:** Combines review types and study types, usually by experts (Dixon-Woods et al., 2005).
- **Meta-ethnography:** Systematically reviews and interprets ethnographic data, developing theories and concepts (Noblit & Hare, 1988).
- **Grounded theory:** Develops theory, often combining literature and new research (see Chapter 9).
- **Systematic pragmatic phenomenological analysis:** Systematic phenomenological analyses of quantitative and qualitative studies, which may include new research (Vos, 2020, 2021a).
- **Data archive:** Instead of combining the summarised research findings, a reviewer may ask for the data or collaborate in a practice research network (Margison et al., 2000). Data archives may be a more powerful way to undertake detailed analysis.

Combination

A research proposal/thesis/article often consists of multiple literature reviews. Like a narrowing funnel, most research proposals/theses/reports/articles start with a very broad 'introduction' on the researcher's personal and professional motivation for the study, including their theoretical/critical framework (if applicable). For example, a researcher may explain and justify using an LGTBQI+ lens based on their experiences of treating cynophobia in gay men. This may be followed by a 'background' section, providing a thematic, historical, or narrative review of the conceptual framework of the research project, via multiple non-systematic mini-reviews on specific concepts or topics. For example, a background review on literature on clinical and aetiological concepts of cynophobia. Ideally, the subsequent 'literature review' section includes a systematic major-review of studies similar to this research project; sometimes, this literature review is divided into separate topics/reviews. For example, the major-review section includes all studies on exposure therapy for animal phobias, structured in different sub-sections for different phobias. (Sometimes, a 'literature review' section combines non-systematic mini-reviews of the study background/conceptual model and a systematic major-review of similar studies; this conflation is not recommended as these reviews have different aims and methods.) This usually ends with a summary of the main gap in the literature, highlighting the importance of the topic, such as reminding the reader of the incidence/prevalence. This logically leads to the formulation of the research aims (see Chapter 6).

Step 4: Decide eligibility criteria

Definition

The researcher explicitly decides the criteria about which publications to include and exclude. These criteria are less strict in practice-friendly, historical, and narrative reviews than in thematic reviews or meta-syntheses/meta-analyses. Do not only describe but also justify your decisions regarding each criterion. Not all criteria may apply to your project.

Components

General criteria

Specify which studies will help achieve the review aim, such as the population/problem (e.g., age, gender, type, psychopathology), therapeutic approach ('CBT'), specific intervention ('exposure therapy), group/individual interventions, short-term/long-term interventions, and control groups. Specify outcomes (e.g., 'depression' or 'perceived meaning in life') or instrument-names ('PHQ-9'). Specify study design (e.g., quantitative, qualitative, mixed methods, RCT, quasi-experimental).

Publication characteristics

Decide which types of publications you are interested in, such as language, publisher (journal/dissertation/book/chapter/report/self-publication), status (published/unpublished), peer-reviewed/non-peer-reviewed, year, study type (original article/systematic review/meta-analysis/meta-synthesis/comment/letter/case study).

Step 5: Decide search engines and other databases

Definition

Decide which search engines and other databases you will use for your search.

Examples

Use engines and databases sensitive and specific to your research topic (see Online Table 5.3. for search engines). Do not use search engines giving many irrelevant hits (e.g., scholar.google.com) or not specific to your field. Do not miss the most cited references.

- **Search engines:** e.g., scholar.google.com (all research fields; includes all types of academic publications including citations; many irrelevant hits; overwhelming; helpful for scoping reviews; rarely accepted for formal publications); Web of Science (social sciences, humanities, arts; extensive search tools; articles only; frequently used); PsycInfo/PsycArticles (psychology; extensive search tools; frequently used); PsycTest (psychological tests only); Medline/Embase/PubMed (medicine, psychiatry; extensive search tools; articles only); Frontiers in Psychology/PLOS-One/MicrosoftAcademic (psychology; free open-access publications only); Psychoanalytic Electronic Publishing (psychoanalysis); Psychology and Behavioural Sciences Collection (psychology, education, therapies); Sage Research Methods (articles, books, chapters on research methods); publishers' search engines.

- **Databases of literature reviews:** e.g., cochranelibrary.org, healthevidence.org, nice.org.uk, eppi.ioe.ac.uk, crd.york.ac.uk/crdweb, campbellcollaboration.org.
- **Governmental departments of statistics:** ons.gov.uk, usa.gov/statistics.
- **Researcher-profiles:** e.g., scholar.google.com, academia.edu, researchgate.net.
- **Gateways:** i.e., selections of web-based resources.
- **Theses and dissertations:** e.g., ProQuest US, dissonline.de Germany, www.theses.com UK.
- **Library catalogue:** may be used as a starting point. Library search engines are often limited to their onsite or subscribed resources. May include student dissertations, which have passed a module or degree, but may not be at the highest academic standard.
- **Snowballing:** e.g., check reference list in key publications, reviews, handbooks.
- **Personal contacts:** e.g., research supervisors, lecturers, experts.
- **Authors:** in formal systematic review *studies*, you may ask key authors for (un)published studies.

Step 6: Decide search terms

Definition

Decide which search terms to use in search engines.

Procedures

Trial and error

Find the best search terms by trying them. For example, add or delete words, formulate synonyms.

Suggestions

Use search terms that are not too broad (scope creep) and not too narrow (empty net). Use formal terms, such as 'depressed' instead of 'sad'. Use synonyms and different spellings (automatically included in advanced search engines). Save the search terms in a Word file to copy-paste/copy-adjust-and-paste again later (in a literature review process journal; see Chapter 2). Many search engines use asterisks at the beginning or end of a word to identify all options: psych* includes psychological, psychology, etc.

Search query

A search query usually includes multiple terms, such as only articles on clinical trials with CBT for cynophobia. Many search engines allow combining terms via Boolean search operators (AND; OR; NOT; NEAR). You may use parentheses to find an 'exact combination of words', and brackets to create sets of terms: ('clinical trial' OR 'controlled trial') AND ('behaviour therapy' OR 'cognitive therapy').

What is a good search-query result?

Whether a search query is good depends on the aims and feasibility of the review, i.e., how much time do you have to sift through all the results? If you aim for a comprehensive overview, you may accept a query result with many references, including many irrelevant references. A scoping/narrative/historical review usually only needs key publications, and thus does not require a comprehensive highly sensitive result. You may use a rule of thumb (depending on your review aims): a search-query result is relatively specific when more than 20% of all search results are relevant (10 of the first 50 references in search-query results); a search-query result is relatively sensitive when you find multiple relevant key publications in the first 50 search results.

How to limit

If you have too many hits or have little time, add search terms to limit the number of findings, for example by narrowing the field ('psychology', 'counselling', 'depression'), [Mesh]-terms in PubMed, publication year (e.g., >2000), reviews only ('review' OR 'meta-analyses' OR 'meta-synthesis' OR 'overview'), publication type (articles, books); English only. You may rank the search results in order of the number of citations and focus only on the most cited articles. If you feel overwhelmed, ask yourself what is needed to achieve your review aims.

How to broaden

If you have too few hits, add search terms (e.g., synonyms, associations), try other search engines, broaden the topic, and search in different disciplines. If few studies exist on a topic, this suggests a gap in the literature which can justify your research project.

Step 7: Decide search strategy

Definition

After a researcher has decided on search terms and the search engine, they decide a strategy for how they will search for articles. Most researchers do this informally.

Examples

Informal search strategy steps

1. **Trial-and-error development of search terms, engines, and eligibility criteria:** try out and improve search terms in different search engines until giving a sensitive, specific, and feasible result.
2. **Initial eligibility screening of search engine results:** include/exclude publications based on title, keywords, and abstract; print/save included publications.
3. **Snowball technique (also called 'root-and-branch search'):** search for new relevant references in reference lists of included articles.
4. **In-depth screening:** assess the eligibility for your study by reading full-text manuscripts.
5. **Identify initial pattern:** while reading, become aware of patterns of themes or a history line.
6. **Organise studies:** organise studies according to the identified pattern, check which studies do not fit, and how the pattern could be improved.
7. **Feedback:** describe the literature according to the pattern; ask for feedback from experts/supervisors and peers, about the coherence and logic of the review, and whether they recognise similar patterns in the literature.

Formal search strategy steps with multiple independent reviewers

1. Select a formal framework, e.g., Cochrane, PRISMA.
2. Pre-determine search terms, engines, eligibility criteria.
3. Initial eligibility assessment of search engine results, based on title/keywords/abstracts, done independently by two or more reviewers.
4. Reviewers share selection and discuss disagreements until agreement is reached.
5. Eligibility assessment of full-text manuscripts.
6. Reviewers share selection and discuss disagreements until agreement is reached.
7. Organise/structure discussion of studies.

Step 8: Record findings

Definition

Decide a strategy to record and organise the findings to save time and avoid getting lost.

Examples

- Literature review protocol describing decisions about Steps 1–9 (see below).
- Literature review process logbook describing the review process and saving search terms (see Chapter 2).
- Literature review content logbook summarising the content of publications, e.g., via tables/mind-maps (see Chapter 2).
- Referencing software (see Chapter 2).

Step 9: Assess study quality

Definition

A good research article makes clear points based on evidence acquired via sound research methodologies and a sound conceptual structure in a trustworthy context. Studies differ in quality. Decide how you will assess the quality of studies. In your literature review, do not only discuss the findings but also the quality of the studies, and base your strength-of-claim on the quality (see Chapter 2). Read Girden & Kabacoff (2010) on assessments.

Procedures

Informal quality assessment

Most informal research projects and student theses do not formally assess the quality of studies. When I asked my students and colleagues about how they informally evaluate the quality of publications, I noticed they often loosely appraise quality via the following steps (Online Table 5.4):

1. **Clear research aim and main findings:** e.g., has the study a clear focus; is the main message clear?

2. **Sound evidence:** e.g., strength, importance, relevance; do findings make sense?
3. **Sound methodology and rationale:** e.g., reliable, valid, trustworthy methods?
4. **Sound sample and rationale:** e.g., size, representative, relevant/coherent sample, unbiased exclusion/inclusion criteria, outliers and variation are discussed and are not too large?
5. **Logical and coherent structure of the text:** e.g., no logical fallacies; clear conceptual steps?
6. **Social/political/financial trustworthiness of publication and authors:** e.g., who funded the study?
7. **Critical self-reflection and reflexivity:** e.g., what is my bias; do I only read findings confirming my preconceptions?
8. **Relevance:** e.g., how relevant are the findings?

Formal quality assessment

A quality appraisal tool (QAT) is a checklist that readers can use to appraise the quality of a study. QATs can help inexperienced academics to develop their quality-assessment skills and ensure that they critically assess the publications in their literature review (e.g., train assessment skills by applying a QAT on studies and compare assessments with peers). CASP offers good QATs for inexperienced academics (casp-uk.net); formal systematic literature reviews require advanced QATs (Online Table 5.5 gives an overview of QATs). QATs for quantitative instruments, such as questionnaires, are discussed in Chapter 8 (and see, for example, cosmin.nl).

Step 10: Synthesise literature

Definition

Depending on the aims and type of the literature review, findings can be synthesised in different ways, informally and formally (e.g., Cochrane/PRISMA guidelines).

Procedure of informal synthesis

There is no perfect formula for informal synthesis: be creative and discover what works best for you. Usually, you will not immediately find the perfect structure/synthesis, and you will refine this over consecutive rounds. Gadamer (2013) called this process a hermeneutic circle in which we go back and forth between detail and overview, between the structure we initially identified and the literature. It can be helpful to use mind-maps and mind-mapping software (Chapter 2). Post-its are easy: write each relevant key message from a reference on a post-it (do not forget to report the reference number/author on the back to know the reference), put similar post-its together, and group the post-its until a coherent, logical structure of themes and sub-themes emerges (further instructions in Online Table 2.2). You may use the following informal synthesising steps inspired by Gadamer (2013 and Braun and Clarke (2012):

1. **Prepare yourself:** write the review process in a process logbook, summarise selected publications in a content logbook, save references in referencing software, save/print full texts.
2. **Read texts globally:** familiarise yourself with general content, e.g., title, abstracts, skim discussion and findings.

3. **Identify and write initial superordinate themes:** usually researchers skip this step, but sometimes an initial structure may intuitively arise, or you may use a pre-existing structure which may be refined later (e.g., write each initial superordinate theme on a separate post-it).
4. **Identify initial themes within each text:** each theme answers an aim/question of your literature review (e.g., write each theme on a post-it; write reference on the back).
5. **Create superordinate themes:** group initial themes/post-its and give each Superordinate theme a unique name (i.e., each group has one overarching name and multiple themes derived from various texts).
6. **Refine superordinate themes:** read each text again to find more examples and counter-examples of superordinate themes.
7. **Decide final superordinate themes.**
8. **Analyse strength of evidence for each superordinate theme:** e.g., number of studies, quality of studies, types of studies, sample sizes.
9. **Analyse relationships between superordinate themes:** How do topics relate? Can we logically explain their relationships? Is the structure coherent? Where are the literature gaps?
10. **Critically contextualise the superordinate themes:** How do superordinate themes fit the broader field (see Chapter 3)?
11. **Critical self-reflection and reflexivity:** How do themes reflect my biases, research paradigms, and social norms? Write in a reflective research journal (see Chapter 4).
12. **Summarise gap in literature/problem in field:** e.g., problems, incoherence, illogical relationships, lack of evidence; this gap may justify your research project.
13. **Visualise themes:** e.g., visual figures, mind-maps, tables (see Chapter 2).

Step 11: Develop literature review protocol

Definition

Develop a review proposal including your decisions for Steps 1–7. A review proposal increases the trustworthiness of your study by ensuring you remember and stick to your decisions. A review proposal can also be used for feedback by peers/supervisors. You may want to use Template B to develop the review proposal. If you conduct a review in multiple parts (e.g., a non-systematic background review and a systematic review on the topic/similar studies), you may want to give each part its own aim and method.

Step 12: Write review

Definition

The final step is writing the literature review.

Procedures

You may want to use Template C to write your review. Literature reviews usually include the following parts: introduction (e.g., personal and professional motivations for this review; key definitions), aims (Step 2), method (Steps 3–9), findings (Step 10), and a discussion (e.g., conclusions, explanations, strengths, limitations, implications). Often, the discussion leads to the formulation of a gap in the literature, which the new research project aims to solve (see Chapter 6). Depending on the aims and type of review, tell the review as a logical story with head/body/end, such as a historical overview from past to present day, or a funnel model from broad/theoretical to specific examples/applications. Paraphrase studies, describe both findings and the quality/trustworthiness of the findings, including a critical reflection on its methodology, give the text a logical structure and flow, show the connections between studies, and use the correct strength-of-claim reflecting the evidence (more tips in Online Table 5.6). End the review by highlighting possible recommendations for future research (Randolph, 2009). Whereas this chapter explained the components for a formal research project or publication, some authors may conduct a quick-and-dirty non-systematic scoping review, which they need to explain and justify (Table 5.1).

Table 5.1 Example justification of a non-systematic scoping review

This literature review aimed to develop an overview of the main research trends on topic A. This helped to develop a general understanding of the main findings and types of research and identify a gap in the literature that my overarching research project aims to fill. This review also helped contextualise the research project and build its conceptual framework. As this is a broad topic, the review was broken down into specific areas. The first area describes..., the second... Each area was examined with a new search query. As this review merely aims to develop a generic overview of the field, conducting a formal systematic literature review was deemed unnecessary. Therefore this review used a scoping review methodology to identify the most cited publications and main ideas by inserting keywords and synonyms in A, B, and C search engine Y and informally assessing their quality and relevance for this literature review. Additional references were identified by examining reference lists of key publications (i.e., snowball technique), and asking for recommended references from experts Y and Z. Due to the explorative scoping nature of this review, some details and publications were left out which appeared less important for this project. Consequently, this review is neither complete nor perfectly representative of the field. Therefore, the findings of this review need to be interpreted carefully; conclusions and implications need to be read tentatively as hypotheses. This limited aim and method seemed justified because this research stage merely requires a general understanding of the field. I will conduct a full systematic literature review in the next research stage.

▬▬ Reflective questions ▬▬

Learn from the masters

- Select three frequently cited literature reviews in your field (e.g., search terms 'literature review' AND topic in scholar.google.com). What are the strengths and weaknesses? What lessons can you learn?

Learn to assess study quality

- Download/print quality appraisal tools (QATs) for qualitative and quantitative studies (e.g., from casp-uk.net).
- Select one qualitative and one quantitative article.
- Assess the quality with CASP-QATs.
- Compare the quality assessments for these articles with peers

Practice conducting a literature review

- Formulate a simple aim for a literature review (e.g., CBT for cynophobia).
- Select maximum three search terms and a search engine (e.g., 'CBT' and 'cynophobia' in Web of Knowledge).
- Search and order search results according to number of citations.
- Select six frequently cited publications with different methodologies.
- For each publication: read and assess quality (e.g., use informal assessment or CASP-QATs); write one paragraph summarising this study's key findings and quality.
- Synthesise the findings from all the articles (e.g., via informal synthesis).

6

How to Develop Research Aims

Chapter aims

A research problem regards the broad issue that you aim to address with your research. This chapter describes how to formulate the aims, objectives, questions, hypotheses, and contributions of a research project to solve the research problem. This helps creating a well-formulated, focused, and feasible project. This aim logically follows the previous chapters, as it needs to fill a gap in the literature, solve a problem in the field, and conceptually fit and contribute to the broader research field. The aim will help to select the methodology as the next chapters will explain: the research methods will help to achieve the aim(s), answer question(s), reach objective(s), and test hypotheses. Recommended reading is mentioned within the relevant steps below.

Steps in chapter

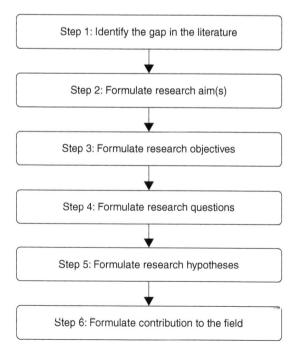

Step 1: Identify the gap in the literature

Step 2: Formulate research aim(s)

Step 3: Formulate research objectives

Step 4: Formulate research questions

Step 5: Formulate research hypotheses

Step 6: Formulate contribution to the field

Step 1: Identify the gap in the literature

Definition

This step regards the question: 'What is the problem in the field or the gap in the literature that this study aims to solve?'

Procedures

The research project aims to solve a problem in the field or fill a gap in the research literature. Therefore, you may want to end your literature review with a sentence such as: 'This review has found this gap in the literature, which has also been shown to be relevant and important for many people'. The literature review should logically lead to the formulation of your research aims. After reading the literature review, the reader should be able to formulate the aims, objectives, and questions of your research project. For example, all hypotheses logically follow from the review. All key concepts and terms have been defined. Nothing at this stage should come as a surprise. A paragraph/section on research aims often starts with a sentence summarising the gap and the importance of filling this gap; this could be followed with 'therefore, to answer this relevant and important problem, this study aims to examine...'

Step 2: Formulate research aim(s)

Definition

This step regards the question: 'What is the overall aim of this research project?'

Components

One aim

Many research projects, particularly student studies, only have one overall aim, as otherwise the project might be unfeasible. An aim describes the general direction of the research, which could be further specified with multiple specific research objectives/questions (note that there does not seem to be a consistent use of the terms 'research aim', 'research objective' and 'research question' amongst researchers; this chapter follows what seems to be the predominant usage of these terms, as identified in the analyses of the 200 most frequently cited studies in our field; Vos, 2014).

Formulation

The aim is formulated in general terms and often consists of an action-oriented verb (e.g., 'investigate', 'confirm', 'examine') combined with the problem identified in the literature review; the meaning of the research aim is to say 'this study aims to solve this problem'.

Relatively specific

Although formulated in relatively generic terms, the aim is not unfocused or undirected. This is why it is called an 'aim', like aiming a dart at a darts board.

Self-reflective questions in terms of conceptual steps

Similar to literature review aims, several frameworks may help formulate aims. For example, you may define your aims in PICOS terms: participants/problem, intervention, comparison group, outcomes, study type (Online Table 5.2). Qualitative researchers may use the SPIDER acronym: Sample, Phenomenon of Interest, Design, Evaluation, Research type. To formulate the aim, you may also ask yourself reflective questions in line with the conceptual framework (see reflective questions in Chapter 6, Step 2, derived from Chapter 3):

- Which clinical problems or psychological phenomena am I interested in?
- Which aetiological factors?
- Which outcomes?
- Which therapeutic mechanisms?
- Which population?
- Which therapists?
- Which therapeutic relationships?
- Which processes?
- Which competencies?

The aim should only include relevant components, such as 'this study aims to examine the effects of a five-week exposure therapy for cynophobia on the level of anxiety in adults'.

Generally feasible

Sometimes, researchers formulate ambitious aims, going beyond this specific research project, particularly in qualitative studies. For example, 'This study aims to contribute to a better understanding of topic X and develop better solutions'. However, it needs to be logical how this study could contribute. For example, 'this study aims to contribute to solving all mental health problems in the world' is too ambitious, but the following sounds more feasible: 'this study aims to create a better understanding of how clients with cynophobia can be treated more effectively'. Ask yourself whether the findings in your research projects can achieve this aim: what will happen after you have finished the research project, and how could this contribute to the field, users, and target community?

Step 3: Formulate research objectives

Definition

This step regards the question: 'What are the specific objectives this research project aims to achieve?'

Components

Multiple

Research objectives are not the same as project aims. Objectives are clear, focused, concise, complex, and arguable research statements with more concrete details than the generic aims, describing the specific actions you will take to complete your research. Objectives follow logically from the literature reviews and the research aim, and should therefore not surprise the reader. Do not introduce new concepts and terms which you have not explained before. Qualitative research projects often have between two and five objectives. Quantitative projects can have more because it may require less time to add another test in statistical software than analysing an additional objective in qualitative research (sometimes, one quantitative research objective is further specified into multiple research questions; for example, if a research project has many research questions, these may be grouped into a smaller number of research objectives). Be aware that the more research objectives/questions you formulate, the more complex the study becomes, not only for the researcher but also the reader; a single research article may only be able to address a small number of research objectives/questions due to the word count limit and the reader's attention span. Bear in mind Miller's Law, stating that the magical number of items that our working memory can keep at the same time is seven, plus or minus two (i.e., keep the number of clearly differentiated research objectives/questions in a short research publication preferably at five or lower, and maximum at nine in a larger research publication) (Saaty & Ozdemir, 2003).

Primary versus secondary research objectives/questions

Sometimes, researchers differentiate between primary and secondary research objectives/questions, particularly in grant applications, medical journals, and brief research reports. Primary research objectives/questions regard the main focus and the most important objectives/questions in their research, such as 'examining the effects of exposure-therapy for cynophobia on anxiety' (overall outcomes). This is often the main reason to conduct this research project. If you were to summarise the key findings of a study in one sentence, it would regard these primary research objectives/questions. Secondary research objectives/questions regard additional objectives/questions, that often zoom into more detailed topics that help to understand the primary objectives/questions better, such as exploring the influence of sociodemographic characteristics on the overall outcomes (moderation) and explaining the overall outcomes through the amount of exposure (mediation).

Specific and feasible

The research project needs to be able to answer the specific objectives. You may use the same reflective questions as for the research aim. However, objectives are more specific and closely connected with the methodology. For example, a quantitative objective of a non-controlled clinical trial could be: 'the first objective is to measure the amount of change in symptoms of cynophobia in adults, via self-report questionnaires before and after five sessions of exposure therapy'. Objectives in qualitative studies may be formulated closely to interview questions. Suppose you formulate the objective 'to examine the subjectively lived experiences of adults of what has been helpful in exposure therapy for cynophobia'; you may ask the interview question 'what did you find helpful in therapy?' Therefore, to formulate objectives, you may imagine the interview questions you want to ask. If you know the interview questions you want to ask your research participants, but you have not formulated the research objectives yet, ask yourself what objectives you hope to achieve by asking these interview questions.

Procedures

You may not find the right formulation at once. Use the following self-reflective questions to evaluate the formulations of your research objectives/questions:

- Clear/unclear?
- Focused/unfocused?
- Specific/non-specific?
- Simple/complex?
- Realistic/unrealistic?
- Original/unoriginal?
- Important/unimportant?
- Follows aims logically/illogically?
- More/similarly/less specifically formulated than aims?
- Clearly/unclearly explains the problems in the literature?
- Clearly/unclearly explained who will benefit from this study?
- All terms/concepts are clear/unclear and introduced/not introduced before?
- Have/do not have all resources and skills needed to achieve this?
- Personally really/not really interested in knowing this?
- Objectives are falsifiable/not falsifiable (i.e., could be disproven)?

Step 4: Formulate research questions

Definition

This step regards the question: 'What are the specific questions this research project aims to answer?' Despite differences, many researchers seem to treat research questions as objectives with question marks.

Components

Research questions regard the specific concerns in your field that you try to. answer (e.g., 'This study answers the question: how effective is exposure therapy for cynophobia?'). The difference with a research objective is subtle, as objectives are statements about what you will do to understand or solve these problems, that function like milestones that will help you to complete your research. Research questions ask how you can solve the research problem and achieve the research objectives in a feasible and specific way. Most researchers only report either questions or objectives but not both. Check the practice in your field. For example, many quantitative researchers formulate questions and not qualitative objectives; a research question seems to fit the specific focus of testing a quantitative variable (e.g. 'what is the impact of exposure therapy for cynophobia on a phobia questionnaire?') and the underlying positivist epistemological assumption that a clear-cut answer can be directly observed and answered for example by using a questionnaire (see chapter 8). Qualitative researchers usually formulate research objectives but not research questions, which seems consistent with the common assumption in qualitative research that reality may not be directly accessible, for example via questionnaires, and that answers may not always be as clearcut as in quantitative research (see chapter 9). You can use the same reflective questions to assess the quality of your research questions as for formulating objectives.

Special example: Service evaluations

The previous steps focused on studies aiming to contribute to the research field. In contrast, service evaluations or audits usually have practical aims. Professional bodies recommend that therapists and therapy services evaluate their services. However, many therapists and therapy services do not routinely evaluate/audit their services, as a result of which they may miss potentially valuable input for justifying and improving their practices. Without unbiased monitoring procedures, clients and authorities may find it difficult to know what happens inside the therapy room, how clients benefit, and trust that clients are not harmed. Providing therapy without evaluation may indicate the therapist's poor self-reflection and ethics. The overarching aim to 'routinely evaluate the service' may be separated into specific objectives/questions, such as 'what service is given', 'which population is the service reaching', 'how do clients experience the service', 'what impact do service users experience', 'how cost-effective is the service'? Different stakeholders may want to answer other questions; for example, therapists may want to get feedback about their clients' variation, satisfaction, and recommendations, whereas funders may wish to understand the extent to which the service covers the target population and how services are implemented. Service evaluation may include routine outcome monitoring, such as asking clients to fill in online questionnaires before each session (Chapter 7). (See Barkham and Mellor-Clark, 2003; Burgess and Moorhead, 2011; Mellor-Clark et al., 2016).

Step 5: Formulate research hypotheses

Definition

This step regards the question: 'What hypotheses are tested or explored in this study?'

Components

Quantitative research

Researchers usually formulate hypotheses when they conduct statistical tests, for example in experiments or clinical trials. Explorative quantitative studies, such as surveys describing a trend in a population without expectations, may not test specific hypotheses. If a researcher has an expectation about their findings, they usually formulate two hypotheses for each research objective/question: a null hypothesis and an alternative hypothesis. A hypothesis describes the expected outcomes. For example, the null hypothesis (H0) describes the expectation that no effect will be found: 'there will be no significant changes in anxiety symptoms measured with GAD-7'. Researchers often expect some change and formulate an alternative hypothesis (Ha; sometimes further hypotheses can be identified, e.g., H1, H2, H3), such as 'there will be significant changes in anxiety symptoms measured with GAD-7'. Each alternative hypothesis needs to be justified and follow logically from the literature review, and the hypotheses should not surprise the reader.

Qualitative research

Qualitative researchers usually do not test hypotheses. However, some qualitative researchers explicate their expectations and assumptions as part of their critical self-reflection and reflexivity. This is generally followed by explaining how they cope with possible biases that these initial expectations and assumptions may have been influenced by, such as phenomenological-bracketing (see Chapter 9).

Step 6: Formulate contribution to the field

Definition

The researcher needs to explain the possible contributions of their research project to for example the following (not all points may be relevant):

- individuals struggling with the central research problem/topic
- clients/individuals with mental health problems
- practitioners
- research field
- other stakeholders (e.g., advocacy groups)
- society in general
- the research participants (e.g., in action research; uncommon)
- the researcher (uncommon).

Each contribution needs to be:

- positive
- clear and specific
- innovative
- important
- solving a pre-identified problem/gap in the literature
- realistic, feasible, believable (e.g., dissemination plan; strategic steps for social change).

▬▬▬ Reflective questions ▬▬▬

- Select six frequently cited empirical studies in your field (not reviews; qualitative and quantitative).
- Examine how they formulate research aims, objectives, questions, and hypotheses. What are the strengths and weaknesses?
- For each article, formulate three alternative aims/objectives/questions/hypotheses.
- For each article, examine whether and how they describe their contributions. Do you agree with this description? Examine their impact (e.g., number of citations, cited in media, policies, PlumXMetrics).

7
How to Decide the Methodology

Chapter aims

This chapter guides researchers in deciding the overall methodology of their research project. The methodology helps them to achieve their research aims and solve a problem in the field, as previous chapters have explained. Specifically, this chapter explains how to select and justify a qualitative, quantitative, or mixed method. The methodological decisions logically lead to the study design, sample, recruitment, and practical organisation. After making these overall methodological decisions, researchers are ready to consider which specific analytical method will help them achieve their research aims, as Chapters 8–10 will specify. Recommended reading is included within the relevant steps below.

Steps in chapter

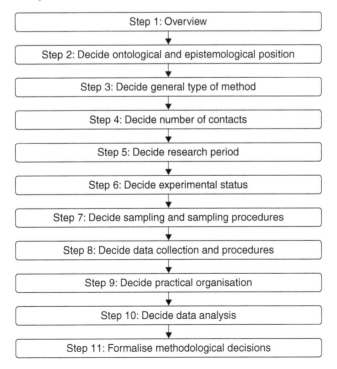

Step 1: Overview

Step 2: Decide ontological and epistemological position

Step 3: Decide general type of method

Step 4: Decide number of contacts

Step 5: Decide research period

Step 6: Decide experimental status

Step 7: Decide sampling and sampling procedures

Step 8: Decide data collection and procedures

Step 9: Decide practical organisation

Step 10: Decide data analysis

Step 11: Formalise methodological decisions

Templates

D. Essay on methodology

E. Essay on critical self-reflection and reflexivity

F. Research proposal

Research proposal checklist (online)

Research proposal presentation (online)

Step 1: Overview

Definition

The overall methodology describes how the researcher tries to achieve the research aims (Chapter 6), which serve the purpose of solving a gap in the literature or a problem in the field (Chapter 5). This section gives an overview of the main components of research methodologies. Chapters 8 -10 detail how to develop the specific types of methods: quantitative, qualitative, and mixed methods.

Components

Position in research project

Figure 7.1 visualises how the methodology follows logically from previous steps. For example, with the help of your basic academic skills and general understanding of the field, you have identified a researchable topic. You have reviewed the literature and identified an important problem or gap your research aims to solve. The methodology describes how you will try to achieve your research aims/objectives/questions. After deciding on the methodology, student researchers often write a research proposal and ethics proposal, which supervisors, examiners, or peers may assess. After approval, the researchers prepare the study, collect and analyse the data, and finish writing the report/thesis/article.

Methodological components

Before we decide on the specific methodology of our project, we often already have some implicit assumptions about the type of knowledge we expect to acquire. For example, many researchers seem to believe questionnaires are a good way to understand a topic. Others are not sure about this as they think that questionnaires are reductionist and cannot do justice to the totality and complexity of the subjective experiences of the research participants. Therefore, it can be helpful to start our methodology by critically reflecting on our assumptions (i.e., determine our ontological and epistemological position). Whereas most quantitative researchers do not systematically reflect and clarify their position regarding knowledge and reality, qualitative researchers usually do. Check with your research institution, journal, or key publications whether your text has to include an explicit reflection on your ontological and epistemological position (otherwise skip the second step).

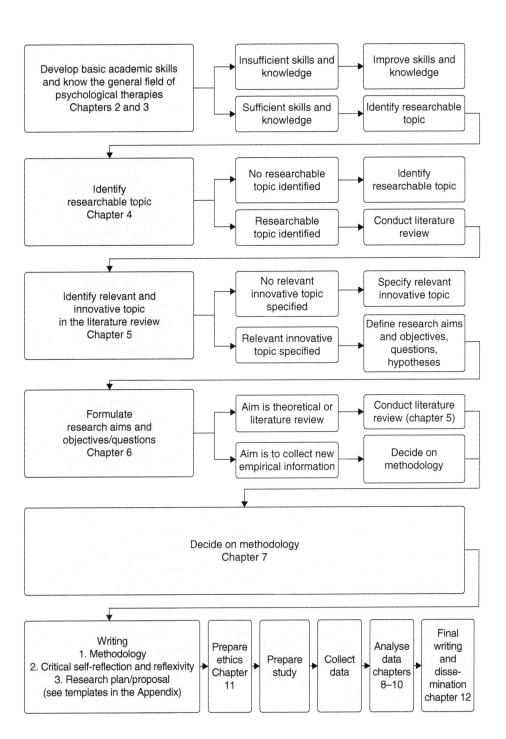

Figure 7.1 Flowchart of overall steps in a research project

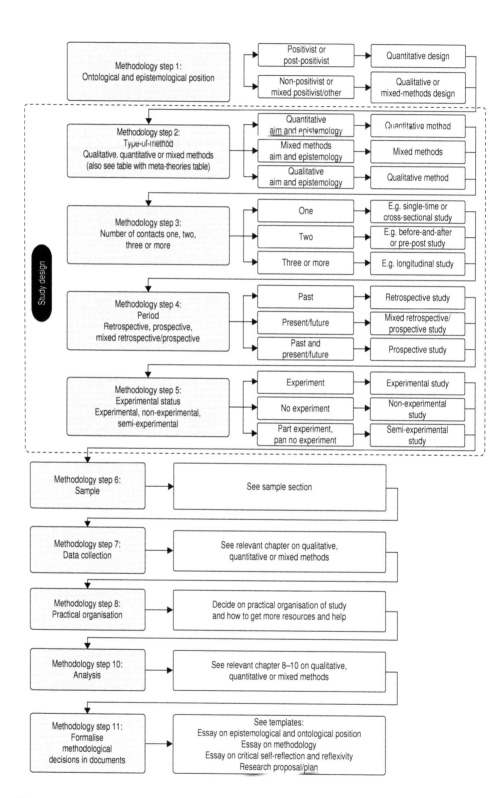

Figure 7.2 Flowchart of specific steps in deciding the methodology

Regardless of your ideas about knowledge and reality, you will need to explain and justify the study design. The study design describes the type of method (quantitative, qualitative, or mixed method), number of contacts with your research participants, duration, and experimental status of the study. Based on your study design, you will decide which individuals are eligible for your study, how you will recruit them, and how you will collect the research data (e.g., interview or questionnaire). Following the study design, sampling, and data-collection procedures, you will detail how you will analyse the findings. Chapter 8 gives a comprehensive overview of quantitative methods, Chapter 9 on qualitative methods, and Chapter 10 on mixed methods. This chapter explains each methodological step.

Step 2: Decide ontological and epistemological position

Definition

It is common practice that qualitative researchers, and sometimes quantitative researchers, start by explicating their position towards 'reality' (ontology) and how we can get knowledge about reality (epistemology). While ontology and epistemology are branches of philosophy, this section will give an overview of popular positions in therapy research. Researchers usually use critical self-reflection and reflexivity to develop their ontological/epistemological position (see Chapter 4). Do not use stereotypes and straw man arguments when describing your position.

Relevance

All researchers may benefit from reflecting on how their research is positioned, as different ontological and epistemological positions may lead to different methodological decisions (Goertz & Mahoney, 2012). In recent years, increasing numbers of training institutions, journals, and professional bodies, particularly in humanistic therapies and counselling psychology, require researchers to reflect on their position. However, many therapy researchers do not explicate their position, particularly quantitative researchers. Therefore, consider whether you need to read this step. This chapter excludes the countless philosophical theories (Moser, Mulder, & Trout, 1998) and focuses on applications in therapy research (see introductions: Pernecky, 2016; Ponterotto, 2005; Willig, 2012, 2019). Online Table 7.1 gives further explanation; Online Table 7.2 offers reflective questions for individuals or classroom discussion.

Components

Ontological position

The word 'ontology' combines the words 'logos', which means study, knowledge, or understanding, and 'ontos' referring to 'being'. Thus, our ontological position describes how we understand the nature of being: how do we understand reality?

1 **Realism–relativism spectrum:** In a very simplified explanation, we could place ontological theories on an (incomplete) spectrum ranging from realism to relativism.
    1A **Realist ontological position:** There is a reality independent from our beliefs and knowledge. There are multiple variations of realism. Naïve realism assumes that our senses give direct objective knowledge of reality. Scientific realism assumes that the rigorous use of scientific tools gives direct objective knowledge of reality. Critical realism assumes a reality exists, although our knowledge of this is filtered through our subjective senses; we may get a slightly better understanding of reality via critical self-reflection and reflexivity (thus, critical realism seems near the middle of the realism–relativism

spectrum). A realist ontology often goes hand-in-hand with an objectivist epistemology, such as the belief we find knowledge via systematically observing facts and universal laws with replicable, reliable, and valid methods in a sample representing the entire population. Many quantitative researchers seem to have a realist position.

1B **Relativist ontological position:** Reality depends on our minds. We can only know the world via subjective experiences and socially constructed meanings. We could systematically examine our perceptions and biases and understand better how individuals make sense of their subjective experiences, but may never be able to explain objective reality. Relativism could lead to a subjectivist epistemology, as individual differences in perceptions and experiences can lead to different types of knowledge. Many qualitative researchers have a relatively relativist.

2 **Essentialism/existentialism spectrum:** We may also place ontological theories on an (incomplete) spectrum from essentialism to existentialism (Vos, 2021a).

2A **Essentialist ontological position:** As long as we use trustworthy methods, we can identify true essences. For example, after interviewing many individuals, we can boil down all different stories to one or a few key points/universal laws.

2B **Existential ontological position:** We cannot find an essence because our human senses and subjective perceptions limit us. No theories or models can do perfect justice to the totality and dynamic complexity of individuals' lived experiences of their daily life existence: 'existence precedes essence' (Sartre, 2021). For example, researchers are limited by their biased perceptions, and research participants are limited in what they share during the research process by their biased perceptions: researchers need to make sense of how clients make sense of the world (called the 'double hermeneutic'). The only thing we can say for certain is that we cannot be certain that essences exist. We can only report how individuals try to make sense of their experiences and how we make sense of their sense-making, and thus we can use our critical self-reflection and reflexivity to try to do justice to the idiosyncrasies of individual research participants. Whereas many quantitative researchers seem to have an essentialist position, many qualitative researchers seem to have an existentialist position. The existentialist position has been popularised by critical psychiatrists, feminists, and critical queer/quare theorists who question the idea of fixed, rigid labels and identities (e.g., Butler, 2011). Authors on intersectionality have argued how identities are fluid and may interact (Collins & Bilge, 2020). (See Vos, Roberts, & Davies, 2019, for an overview of critical psychology/psychiatry.)

2C **Pragmatic/pluralistic position:** Many researchers seem to have a pragmatic or pluralistic position. This means that they seem to assume that, although we may never know for certain whether true essences and universal laws exist, we may find in our research project that some people report essences whereas others do not (Goss & Mearns, 1997; Vos, 2021a).

Epistemological position

A research method – such as a questionnaire or interview – may help achieve our research aims. However, how can we be certain that this method gives us the type of knowledge we aim for? We need to have a sense of the nature of knowledge and the scope, validity, reliability, and trustworthiness of our claims to knowledge. Epistemology answers the two questions 'what can we know?' and 'how can we know?' For example, a simple definition says that knowledge is justified true beliefs: we believe that we have evidence that we have gathered justifiably. The stress lies on 'justified': how do you justify what you believe to be true? Researchers can have different beliefs about what type of knowledge is justified; in other words, they differ in their epistemological position. It can be helpful to reflect on our episte-mological position because our position about knowledge influences which types of methods we may consider for our research project. For example, I may decide to use a questionnaire in my project if I believe psychometric instruments can give reliable and valid knowledge about reality. However, I may prefer interviews if I believe questionnaires cannot do justice to my research participants' subjective experiences and social constructions.

Philosophical epistemologies: Some realist philosophers argue that a belief is true if it matches reality (correspondence theory). In contrast, some relativist philosophers say that we cannot check our beliefs because we do not have direct access to 'reality'; instead of comparing our beliefs with a presumed reality, a belief is justified if it is internally consistent or logically non-contradictory (coherence theory). Other philosophers argue a third position: a belief is true if it is practical (pragmatist-utilitarian theory) or reflects a consensus (consensus theory). You can imagine the vast implications for research methods: correspondence researchers may want to test whether their hypotheses are true – correspondence researchers describe the consistency/coherence of experiences and beliefs, and others the utility and consensus of our beliefs. How do therapy researchers position themselves? To simplify, we may place their epistemological posi-tions on an (undoubtedly incomplete) scale ranging from objectivism to subjectivism.

Objectivist epistemological position: There is a reality we can objectively know. For example, researchers with a positivist or empiricist epistemology believe we can directly access reality, as long as we use good research instruments. For example, we can use a ther-mometer to directly know the objectively true temperature. Similarly, a reliable and valid questionnaire may give objectively true information about our research participants.

Subjectivist epistemological position: There is no objective reality due to the subjec-tivity of our individual experiences. Theories on the subjectivist side of the spectrum include post-structuralism, post-positivism, hermeneutics, symbolic interactionism, phenomenology, and constructivism. Constructivism means that individuals construct their sense of reality (see overview in Raskin, 2002). Constructivism gained prominence through Kelly's Personal Construct Theory and Mahoney's Constructivist Therapy, based on the idea that humans construct the realities in which they live. Social constructivism means that individuals may share some experiences they may label 'intersubjective reality' but never an 'absolute objec-tive reality'. Constructivists vary in how radically they apply their constructivist position; radical constructivists are sceptical about the possibility that people can go beyond the limits of their subjective and intersubjective constructions. Critical constructivists combine a sub-jective epistemology with a social-political critique, such as critical theories, which focus on how social powers, oppression, and paradigmatic forces influence the research participants and the research process (Stanley & Wise, 2002).

Overview of common research paradigms

An individual's ontological position and epistemological position should be logically connected. For example, an objectivist ontology may not fit a radical-constructivist epistemology. This combined ontological-epistemological position is also logically tied with the methodology. For instance, a relativist/constructivist would not choose experiments, randomised samples, questionnaires, and statistical analyses. Thus, our ontological position informs our epistemo-logical position, which subsequently informs our methodology (Figure 7.2).

Meta-theories: Although this is an enormous oversimplification, we may boil down all possible connections between ontology, epistemology, and subsequent methodological deci-sions to a small number of popular meta-theories in psychological therapies, like the most popular package deals in therapy research (see Table 7.1, inspired by Sousa, 2010; Guba in Denzin & Lincoln, 2021). For example, stereotypically speaking, many quantitative studies seem based on an objectivist ontology and positivist epistemology. Qualitative studies are often based on a constructivist/subjectivist ontological position and various epistemological positions; e.g., the interpretative phenomenological analysis method is often based on constructivist or critical-realist epistemologies (Shinebourne, 2011).

Historical change of dominant meta-theories: The history of science can be described as periods in which different meta-theories dominate. For example, many early researchers on psychological therapies seemed to have a positivist position like their colleagues in medicine. Later research was positioned more in post-positivist and constructivist paradigms, influenced by an increased psychological understanding of human biases, cognitions, and group dynamics. Critical meta-theories evolved in response to critical theory, humanistic and empowerment movements, such as critical ethnography, discourse analysis, grounded theory, Marxist theory, critical race theory, and feminist, post-colonial, LGBTQI+/queer/quare, indigenous/ethnic, critical-pedagogy, critical-technology, and intersectional theories (Denzin & Lincoln, 2021; Stanley & Wise, 2002). Since the turn of the millennium, postmodern ideas such as radical relativism and constructivism seem to have become less popular in society, which also seems reflected in the increasing popularity of critical realism in humanistic therapies and counselling psychology (Archer et al., 2013; Pilgrim, 2019). Critical realism sits between radical positivism and radical constructivism (cf. post-positivism/post-post-positivism). Critical realists believe in an objective reality, which we cannot directly know because all our knowledge about reality is filtered through our limited and fallible perceptions and experiences. It may be helpful to describe people's experiences and perceptions of reality, for example, to differentiate more-meaningful from less-meaningful descriptions of reality. Our experiences are constructed on three levels: the empirical (what we perceive through our senses), the actual (events happening in a time and place), and the real (foundational mechanisms that underpin events).

Practical use of meta-theories as shortcut: It is recommended to reflect on your ontological and epistemological position via systematic critical self-reflection and reflexivity (Figure 7.2; e.g., do the warming-up exercises in Online Table 7.2). However, many researchers seem to use the shortcut of following the dominant meta-theories in their field. Examine the meta-theories in Table 7.1 and identify which one fits your research best. Consider the following crude steps to identify your meta-theoretical position:

- **Identify methodological expectations/requirements:** Your institution/field may have methodological expectations limiting your options. For example, if you are expected to conduct quantitative research, this may limit you to a relatively positivist/post-positivist/critical realist position.
- **Read frequently cited researchers in your field:** Which meta-theories and epistemological/ontological positions do they explicitly mention or implicitly assume?
- **Read meta-theories in Table 7.1:** Examine which 'package deal' sufficiently fits your position, field, and project.
- **Search for explanatory texts:** You may want to deepen your understanding of your meta-theory or ontological/epistemological position, particularly in qualitative research.
- **Explicate your position in your research texts (may not be required):** When describing your position, refer to key thinkers, and reflect on limitations and alternatives. Show how your position logically leads to methodological decisions, like in Figure 7.3. Describe how your position fits within the dominant meta-theories in your field (use Template D).

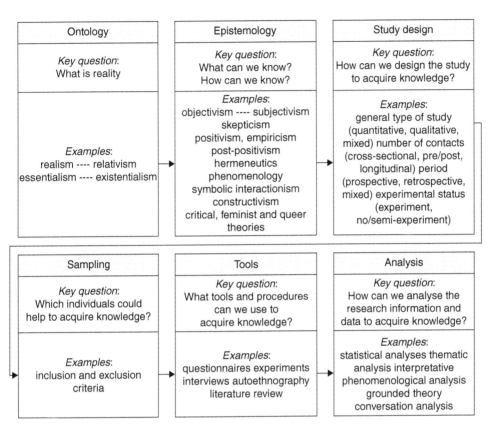

Ontology	Epistemology	Study design
Key question: What is reality	*Key question:* What can we know? How can we know?	*Key question:* How can we design the study to acquire knowledge?
Examples: realism ---- relativism essentialism ---- existentialism	*Examples:* objectivism ---- subjectivism skepticism positivism, empiricism post-positivism hermeneutics phenomenology symbolic interactionism constructivism critical, feminist and queer theories	*Examples:* general type of study (quantitative, qualitative, mixed) number of contacts (cross-sectional, pre/post, longitudinal) period (prospective, retrospective, mixed) experimental status (experiment, no/semi-experiment)

Sampling	Tools	Analysis
Key question: Which individuals could help to acquire knowledge?	*Key question:* What tools and procedures can we use to acquire knowledge?	*Key question:* How can we analyse the research information and data to acquire knowledge?
Examples: inclusion and exclusion criteria	*Examples:* questionnaires experiments interviews autoethnography literature review	*Examples:* statistical analyses thematic analysis interpretative phenomenological analysis grounded theory conversation analysis

Figure 7.3 Connections between ontology, epistemology, and methodology

Step 3: Decide general type of method

Definition

There are three general types of methods: quantitative, qualitative, and mixed methods. Do not only describe which type you are using but also justify this: argue this is the best way to achieve your research aims and solve the problem in the field identified in your literature review.

Components

Coherence

Table 7.2 describes stereotypical differences between quantitative, qualitative, and mixed methods. The type of method you select should be coherent with the ontological/epistemological position (Step 1), and the following methodological decisions (Steps 2–10). Your research project's aims, objectives, questions, and hypotheses (Chapter 5) should be formulated in terms of the chosen methodology. A quantitative study may aim to 'test the effects of exposure therapy for cynophobia on anxiety measured with GAD-7', whereas a qualitative study may aim to 'describe the subjectively lived experiences of clients after exposure therapy for cynophobia'.

Table 7.1 Simplified overview of popular meta-theories in psychological therapies (inspired by Sousa, 2010)

Meta-theory or research paradigm	Ontology (what is reality: realism – relativism)	Epistemology (what is knowledge and how can we acquire it: objectivism - subjectivism)	Example study designs (what design helps to acquire knowledge)	Example sample (which individuals could help acquire knowledge)	Example research tools (which tools and procedures could help acquire knowledge)	Example analytic methods (how can we analyse the research information or data to acquire knowledge)	Quality criterion of good research	Example of popular applications
Positivism	Radical realism: There is an objective reality and single truth which can be directly studied and understood. Based on empiricism, e.g. reality can be accessed by human senses and research tools	Radical objectivism: There is a difference between knower (subject) and known (object). Research methods can directly access reality and discover facts, natural laws and cause-effect relationships. Research leads to progress in knowledge Minimise researcher's bias Researchers do not engage in post-research policy-making/ action	Experiments Verification of hypotheses Observation Survey with standardised questionnaires	Random sample representative of the target population	Replicable methods Inductive methods (e.g. observation) Hypothetico-deductive methods (e.g. test hypotheses) Standardised questionnaires Experiment Observation Structured interviews	Statistical tests Positivist analysis of qualitative data (e.g. positivist grounded theory or content analysis) Meta-analysis	Reliability and validity of tools Validity of study design	Traditional quantitative 'hard' research, for example, in physics, medicine and psychiatry

Table 7.1 Simplified overview of popular meta-theories in psychological therapies (inspired by Sousa, 2010) *(Continued)*

Post-positivism	Nuanced realism:	Nuanced objectivism:	Modified experiments	Homogeneous sample	Questionnaires with exploratory and open questions	Modern statistical theories	Trustworthiness	Contemporary
	There is a reality, but this may never be completely understood	We can only approximate reality and truth Research may help making decisions with incomplete data The researcher is the method to acquire knowledge; try to minimise researcher's biasing influence, and improve their skills. We can reason and describe patterns, generalise and ground theory General belief in (fallible) scientific methods and some progress in human knowledge	Falsification of hypotheses Most quantitative methods Some rigorous qualitative methods	Preferably representative of target population although all sampling is limited	(Semi-) structured interview schedules Focus groups Transcripts and video recordings of conversations Observation Public narratives, conversations and dialogues	theories (e.g. Bayesian, Item Response Theory, bootstrapping, models based on complex systems) Post-positivist narrative analysis, discourse analysis, conversation analysis, thematic analysis, or grounded theory Narrative literature reviews, meta-synthesis	(e.g. credibility, transferability, dependability, confirmability) Sometimes reliability and validity of tools and study design	quantitative researchers in medicine and social sciences Many contemporary qualitative researchers

(Continued)

Tab e 7.1 Simplified overview of popular meta-theories in psychological therapies (inspired by Sousa, 2010) (*Continued*)

| **Constructivism** (sometimes considered example of post-positivism; sometimes not seen as a meta-theory) | **Radical relativism:** Relativist and sceptic rejection of absolute notions of truth ('multiplicity of truths') Different individuals have different experiences and constructions of reality. They may share some intersubjective experiences but not an absolute objective reality (note similarities with post-structuralism) | **Radical subjectivism:** Knowledge is a human fallible, transactional and contextualised construction The researcher and research participant co-construct how they understand reality. We may examine cases, narratives, interpretations and reconstructions Does not aim to progress knowledge, but for example describe current local experiences and positions and delegitimise prevailing knowledge claims | Hermeneutic and dialectical Naturalistic qualitative methods such as case studies, narrative and discourse analyses | Homogeneous sample | Semi-structured and unstructured interviews Focus groups Transcripts and video recordings of conversations Observation Public narratives, conversations and dialogues | Interpretive, participatory and dialogical analysis Narrative analysis Discourse analysis Conversation analysis Constructivist thematic analysis Constructivist Grounded Theory Constructivist ethnography Some phenomenological methods Meta-synthesis, meta-ethnography Usually includes critical self-reflection and reflexivity | Intersubjective agreement Trustworthiness Authenticity | Many qualitative studies in social sciences and humanities |

Table 7.1 Simplified overview of popular meta-theories in psychological therapies (inspired by Sousa, 2010) *(Continued)*

	Realist and relativist aspects:	Subjectivist and objectivist aspects:				Trustworthiness	
Critical realism (sometimes considered example of post-positivism)	There is a reality but this is like a stratified open system that may never be perfectly known. Some realist and some relativist assumptions	Researchers may develop theories about reality which are fallible and contextualised, but experiences and knowledge can be more than mere social constructions. Some theories may appear more congruent with reality, with more explanatory power Knowledge may be applied and some progress may be possible	Many quantitative, qualitative and mixed methods study designs are possible	Depends on study-design, bearing in mind that all research is contextualised	Many quantitative, qualitative and mixed methods are possible, bearing in mind their limitations	Many quantitative, qualitative and mixed analytical methods are possible Often includes critical self-reflection and reflexivity	Critical-realist applications of the concepts of validity and reliability	Many contemporary researchers across disciplines, including psychological therapies

(Continued)

Table 7.1 Simplified overview of popular meta-theories in psychological therapies (inspired by Sousa, 2010) (*Continued*)

Post-structuralism	Radical relativism: / Radical subjectivism:		Study design			Trustworthiness
Post-structuralism	**Radical relativism:** There is no outside reality of independently knowable facts, as we construct reality **Radical subjectivism:** No truth to be known; all knowledge is contextual Questions and problematses ideas and assumptions in research and society, e.g. via human action, discourses, narratives and conversations	Deconstruction and genealogies of discourses, narratives, and conversations Multi-voiced studies e.g. with co-researchers Transformative research designs Action research Foucauldian Discourse Analysis	Study design depends on the context	Public narratives, conversations and dialogues Unstructured or semi-structured interviews Focus groups Transcripts and video recordings of conversations Observation	Narrative analysis Discourse analysis Conversation analysis Ethnography Some post-structuralist applications of other methods Often includes critical self-reflection and reflexivity	Frequently found in literary analysis, gender studies

Table 7.1 Simplified overview of popular meta-theories in psychological therapies (inspired by Sousa, 2010) (Continued)

Critical theories	Relativism:	Subjectivism:						
(e.g. Frankfurt School of Critical Theory, Cultural studies, Marxist, Critical Ethnography. Critical Discourse Critical Grounded-Theory, Critical Race-Theory, Feminist, Post-colonial, LGBTQI+, queer, quare, indigenous/ethnic, critical-pedagogy, critical-technology and intersectional theories) (may overlap with post-structuralism and post-positivism)	How we understand our world is influenced and influences the social structures, political powers and oppression (e.g. differences in class, race/ethnicity, gender, sexual orientation, age, soioeconomic status, religion).	Knowledge is always subjective, historical and political All research is value-driven. Researchers should critically reflect on the lenses through which they look at the topic, participants, society and themselves. Researchers should critique power structures, give voice to muted voices, follow emancipatory and liberating social-justice values, and suggest resistance towards oppressing powers. Researchers have an educational and empowering role	Participatory, dialogical and dialectical, which empowers the oppressed and fosters social change. Transformative inquiry Action research Foucauldian Discourse Analysis	Homogeneous sample of individuals with a usually-silenced or critical voice	Semi-structured and unstructured interviews Focus groups Transcripts and video recordings of conversations Observation Public narratives, conversations and dialogues	Critiquing, dialogical, participatory, empowering and revolutionary analyses Critical narrative analysis, discourse analysis, conversation analysis thematic analysis, or grounded theory Some phenomenological methods Includes critical self-reflection and reflexivity	Trustworthiness Authenticity Catalyst for action	Critical studies on diversity, political powers and oppression, often in sociology and political sciences

Table 7.2 Stereotypic differences between quantitative, qualitative, and mixed methods

	Quantitative method	Qualitative method	Mixed method
Dominant ontology	Realism Essentialism/reductionism	Relativism Existentialism/holistic Pragmatic/pluralistic	Critical realism Pragmatism Pragmatic/pluralistic
Dominant epistemology	Positivism Post positivism (Critical realism)	Constructivism Critical theories Post-structuralism Post-positivism	Constructivism Critical theories Post-structuralism Post-positivism
Example research aims	• Hypothetico-deductive • Observing attitudes and opinions in population • Testing hypotheses • Examining correlations • Testing effects and statistical significance • Describing frequencies and means • Testing influences (predictors/moderators) • Testing mechanisms (mediators) • Testing models • Developing and testing the validity and reliability of psychometric instruments • Often in standardised controlled setting to limit bias and external influences	• Explorative-inductive and critical-deductive • Exploration • Subjective experiences • Trends/patterns • Narratives • Ethnographies • Case studies • Coherence • Theory building • In-depth understanding of a concept • Generate new ideas • Identify unknown phenomena • Active involvement and co-creation by research participants • Often in natural settings with attention to daily life experiences and external influences	• Knowledge that is broad/ generalisable as well as in-depth • Building and testing theory • Simultaneously achieving quantitative and qualitative aims
Example sample	Random, representative sample of population	Purposive sample in the natural world	Sample depends on research aims
Example data-collection tools	Questionnaire Experiment Clinical trial Closed/multiple-choice questions Simple self-reflection	Methods respecting the humanity of participants Emergent/non-fixed methods Interpretative analyses Interview Focus group Open questions Text/image/video analysis Theory development Critical self-reflection and reflexivity	Concurrent, sequential, transformative or systematic combination of quantitative and qualitative tools

Stage-of-field

Therapies are often developed in multiple stages with different methodological accents (see Chapter 9). Therefore, ask yourself which type of method fits the stage of your research field. For example, qualitative methods may help explore a new topic to generate ideas for future research or give more in-depth information about a topic that has previously only been broadly or superficially studied with quantitative research instruments. Quantitative research may help examine the incidence/prevalence of a phenomenon in the population, and test specific hypotheses or effects.

Step 4: Decide number of contacts

Definition

How many times will you contact your participants? The answer depends on your study aim, objectives/questions.

Examples

Quantitative research

Quantitative researchers may contact participants one or multiple times (Kumar, 2018):

- **Cross-sectional/one-shot/status studies:** Examine the prevalence/incidence of a phenomenon, situation, problem, or diagnosis at one point in time. This design may suffer from retrospective recall bias, and may not be conclusive regarding timelines (what happens after what?) and causality (what causes what?).
- **Trend studies:** Explore a trend in opinions/attitudes in the population over time.
- **Cohort studies:** Examine a group with specific characteristics, e.g., birth year or diagnosis at one or more measurement-moments.
- **Before-and-after or pre-test/post-test studies:** Examine changes between two measurement-moments, e.g., impact/effects of an event/intervention/treatment.
- **Longitudinal studies:** Measurements at three or more measurement-moments to examine change over time. For example, session-per-session measurement in clinical trials may reveal that the effects of individual therapy sessions represent partial 'takeaways' that may together build longer-lasting therapeutic change (Greenberg, 1986; Orlinsky & Howard, 1986).
- **Panel studies:** Longitudinal prospective cross-sectional or cohort studies in which the same participants are asked questions at multiple measurement-moments.

Qualitative research

In qualitative studies, data can be collected at one or more moments, such as in one or more interviews, focus groups/participant observations:

- **One interview**: Most researchers conduct only one interview, as this is easy to organise.
- **Multiple interviews**: Some researchers, such as in grounded theory, invite participants for a second interview. This allows researchers to ask new questions which

have arisen after the interview, for example during data analysis or conversations with colleagues. Participants may also have reflected on what they said in the first interview, share new insights, or give additional information. Conducting multiple interviews increases the risk of self-confirmation bias as the second interview may be less spontaneous, more deliberate, and more reflected. It may be uncertain whether the information from the first and second interviews can be treated equally and synthesised; therefore, the interviewer needs to interpret the hypothetical impact of time and self-reflection. An alternative format is to do member-checking which can improve the study's trustworthiness: after the first interview, the researcher analyses the data, and in the second interview, the results of these analyses, interpretations, and conceptualisations are shared with the participant for feedback.

- **Longitudinal qualitative data:** Some qualitative studies include information collected over a longer period, such as cases, online forums, public narratives, or discourses.

Step 5: Decide research period

Definition

Research can be retrospective, prospective, or mixed retrospective/prospective.

Examples

In retrospective research, participants reflect on previous experiences. In prospective research, a participant is followed over time; they may be invited to describe their experiences immediately after they experienced predictable events – an intervention/treatment. In mixed retrospective/prospective research, participants are both followed over time and asked to reflect on past experiences.

Step 6: Decide experimental status

Definition

A study could have an experimental, semi-experimental, or non-experimental design.

Examples

Non-experimental design

In naturalistic or passive-observational studies, no experiment or clinical trial is conducted. For example, a descriptive study design can help to understand a concept in more detail, and a correlational design may examine the relationships between concepts. An epidemiological population survey may describe how many people are depressed (descriptive research). A survey may also show how depression correlates with income (correlational research). A consumer-satisfaction study may show clients' satisfaction with a mental health service. Descriptive and correlational studies can be conducted with questionnaires and interviews and analysed with qualitative analysis/descriptive statistics such as frequencies, means, and correlations. However, descriptive and correlational studies cannot prove causality (e.g., low income causes depression or therapy causes symptom reduction): correlation does not equal causation. The non-experimental study design should logically follow the conceptual framework and literature review (see Chapters 3–5).

Experimental design

Causality may be studied with a study design such as experiments or clinical trials. Imagine the hypothesis that a strong therapeutic relationship (variable A) improves the client's well-being (variable B). To use a loose guideline: to conclude that A causes B, researchers must have evidence for the following conditions (Bradford-Hill, 1965; Höfler, 2005; Kazdin, 2021; Ward, 2009):

1. **Strong association (covariation):** The two variables have a strong association. For example, the researcher finds significant, large correlations between an intervention (A) and outcomes (B). Correlational studies may give some evidence for this condition.

2. **Consistency:** The same findings are found across studies, samples, and conditions. Inconsistencies between studies may be caused by a moderator, such as different sample characteristics.

3. **Specificity:** The findings are specific. For example, the intervention has a specific effect on a specific outcome instrument or a specific mediator instrument; for example, relationship-oriented therapy has a specific effect on improving the therapeutic relationship. These specific effects are in line with the conceptual framework, and are not explained by other plausible concepts.

4. **Logical timeline:** There must be a logical timeline. Outcome (A) must reliably precede outcome (B). For example, improvements in the therapeutic relationship happen before improvements in client well-being. Note that we would expect that the quality of the therapeutic relationship correlates with well-being; however, this correlation does not prove that A precedes B (A → B), as clients who improve (B) may also be functioning better in relationships (A) (B → A).

5. **Gradient:** A stronger dose leads to larger effects (cf. dose-response research). For example, the stronger the therapeutic relationship (A) is, the larger the outcomes (B). Dose-response effects can be linear or non-linear.

6. **Plausibility or coherence:** There is a plausible, coherent, and reasonable process explaining the conceptual steps (see Chapter 3 for the conceptual framework). For example, during relationship-oriented therapy, the therapeutic relationship improves over time, which predicts the client's ability to share and deepen their experiences in therapy, which subsequently improves their emotional well-being.

7. **Experiment:** There is a clear experimental study design: a well-defined intervention or treatment is delivered and this leads to changes in the outcomes (or key components in the intervention are changed to increase its effects).

8. **Analogy:** Are there similar causal relationships in other areas? For example, improvements in relationships with friends have been shown to improve one's well-being.

9. **No alternative explanations:** This condition is already assumed in the other conditions. It may for example look as if there is a relationship between A and B, but this may be a spurious relationship because both may be explained by a third variable C, such as psychological mindedness, as clients who are more psychologically minded may both have better outcomes and have better relationships. Correlational studies may show the relationships between A, B, and C, but this may not be conclusive evidence as the researcher may have forgotten also to include other variables. Furthermore, it is possible that A does not predict B directly but indirectly via a

'mediator' D. For example, a better therapeutic relationship (A) may help the client to explore their experiences at a deeper level (D) which may improve their well-being (C). The values of A and B may also both depend on a moderator variable E. The gender of the client (E) may moderate the relationship between A and B, as the therapeutic relationship may only predict the client's well-being in women and not in men. Statistical tests (e.g., regression analysis, structural equation modelling) in longitudinal/experimental studies may help to reject some alternative explanations.

To test several conditions of causality at once, researchers may conduct an experiment. In an experiment, the researcher may test the effects of the experiment, possible confounders, mediators, and moderators (Kazdin, 2007, 2009). An experiment is usually called a clinical trial if this involves a clinical intervention such as therapeutic treatment. Researchers need to consider several decisions when designing an experiment, such as adding control groups. For example, a researcher may train one group of therapists in therapeutic relational skills (called 'independent variable', 'experimental condition', or 'experimental manipulation'). They may compare these therapists with a group of therapists without this training ('control group') in their effects on the client's well-being (called 'dependent variable' or 'outcome'). The experimental design should logically follow the research aims and may also depend on the organisational feasibility and sample size. Chapter 9 will detail how to develop experimental designs.

The experimental design should logically fit with the study's conceptual framework. A researcher may only test the outcomes of an intervention (outcomes-related hypothesis), but they will need to justify how its therapeutic mechanisms may address the underlying aetiological causes of the clinical problem (see Chapter 3). For example, to justify that exposure therapy causes significant decreases in cynophobia via the therapeutic mechanism of reducing behavioural avoidance, a researcher needs to prove the following: behavioural avoidance correlates with and precedes cynophobia; exposure therapy precedes a reduction in behavioural avoidance; the reduction in avoidance correlates with and precedes a decrease in cynophobia; there are no alternative explanations.

Special example: Service evaluation

Service evaluations or audits are usually 'quasi-experimental' as mental health services often lack the rigour of full experiments, such as randomised allocation to treatments (see Chapter 8). Although these studies may strongly indicate that these services are associated with client improvements, they cannot conclusively prove causality because the study design does not control for alternative explanations. Service evaluations may risk experimenter bias if conducted by in-house auditors. Despite these design flaws, service evaluations may give rich ecologically valid information about client experiences and recommendations, particularly if mixing quantitative and qualitative methods (see service evaluation study designs: Rossi, Lipsey, & Freeman, 2004; Shadish, Cook, & Leviton, 1991).

Step 7: Decide sampling and sampling procedures

Definition

Based on their study aims, researchers need to explain and justify which participants to include and exclude, and how participants will be recruited.

Explanation

Researchers use different terms for four groups:

- **Country population:** e.g., UK.
- **Research population:** e.g., all individuals diagnosed with cynophobia in the UK.
- **A *priori* sample:** e.g., intended number and inclusion/exclusion criteria for participants in your research project (mentioned in research proposal and methodology section in report/thesis/article); define your a priori sample in relation to the research population (e.g., is the potential research population large enough for you to recruit the number of participants that you want for your sample?).
- **A *posteriori* sample:** e.g., actual number of participants in your research (usually mentioned in findings section).

Procedures

Decide inclusion/exclusion criteria

Each research project has specific inclusion criteria for participants, following logically from the research aims, e.g., 'eligible participants fulfil the DSM-V criteria of animal phobia'. Each project has exclusion criteria; for example, eligible participants should not suffer from neurocognitive and linguistic problems which make participation difficult (e.g., not speaking the language, dementia, delirium, psychosis). Participants may be excluded for ethical reasons, such as minors and individuals legally unable to make decisions; parents or legal guardians may be asked for informed consent. Inclusion/exclusion criteria need to be formulated to be as specific as possible. Each criterion needs to be justified, particularly sensitive socio-demographic criteria such as gender, age, sexual orientation, religion, and ethnicity, as selecting participants based on these characteristics could be considered discrimination..

Decide sample in quantitative studies

Quantitative researchers often aim to generalise the findings and conclusions from the research project. For example, a researcher surveying the aetiology of cynophobia hopes that the results in this sample can be extrapolated to the entire population. To generalise, the study participants need to be a random sample representing the total research population. Random selection means that each individual in the population has a similar probability of being selected for the research project, and thus there is no bias in who was selected and the study findings may be generalised to the general population (external validity). For example, if you aim to understand a phenomenon in the full country, you do not only want to invite individuals from one village. You need to define your population to be able to define your random sample. In your study, you will need to describe the socio-demographic characteristics of your *a posteriori* sample and compare this with the socio-demographic characteristics of the population: is there a difference, and if so, does this limit the interpretation and generalisability of your findings? Furthermore, researchers may not want a too-heterogeneous sample as participants may differ too much from each other to make general conclusions; thus, researchers often balance heterogeneity and homogeneity. The research proposal will need to explain and justify the recruitment strategy. (See randomisation in Chapter 9.)

As samples are usually an imperfect representation of the total population, your findings and conclusions will be imperfect. You may observe an effect in your sample that does not actually exist in the population. Before starting an experiment/clinical trial, you want to know that the effects you will find in your study are actually there and not mere chance. Therefore, you may want to statistically calculate how many participants your study needs (*a priori* sample size) to detect the actual effects you expect. After conducting a study, you may also want to calculate the likelihood that the findings are actually true based on the *a posteriori* sample size (which may differ from your anticipated *a priori* sample size). Chapter 9 explains the steps to calculate *a priori* sample size and *a posteriori* power statistically.

Decide sample in qualitative research

Qualitative researchers usually do not aim to generalise their findings but may aim to develop an in-depth understanding of the research topic: quality over quantity. Consequently, many qualitative studies aim for a purposive and homogeneous sample, a sample of individuals with relatively homogeneous characteristics. Researchers may, for example, focus on critical, confirming, disconfirming, extreme/deviant/intense, typical, or politically important cases. Individuals may be selected for their elite status in an organisation or community, such as being considered influential, prominent, and well-informed in their field (Delaney, 2007).

There seems little consensus about the required sample size for qualitative studies, and the sample size often depends on the researcher's subjective opinion (Marshall et al., 2013). On average, qualitative doctorate projects have 31 participants (Mason, 2010). (See tips in Emmel, 2013.) It has been recommended to justify the sample size on the basis of the data required to achieve the research objectives (Boddy, 2016). Some researchers have developed the term 'information power' for qualitative methods, similar to 'statistical power', an extension of the concept of 'saturation' in grounded theory. The size of a sample with sufficient information power depends on the narrow/broad aim of the study, sample specificity/non-specificity, applied/no established theory, weak/strong quality of dialogue, and case/cross-case analysis strategy (Malterud, Siersma, & Guassora, 2016). The sample size also depends on the feasibility of recruitment and in-depth analysis of each case; for example, part-time professional doctorate research students using a time-intensive in-depth analytical method may want to limit themselves to a maximum of eight to ten participants (Smith & Fieldsend, 2021). Whatever sample size you choose, give a clear justification, and check the recommendations and requirements from other authors in your field.

Justify convenience sample

In an ideal world, quantitative researchers would have a perfectly random and representative sample and qualitative researchers a perfectly purposive homogeneous sample. Reality often differs. For example, the research population may be so small that the researcher cannot have many rigid exclusion criteria: beggars cannot be choosers. Alternatively, a researcher may only have limited recruitment resources or depend on one specific recruitment location (e.g., service evaluation). Consequently, many studies use a convenience sample. For example, many studies are conducted in WEIRD students: Western, educated, industrialised, rich, from democratic cultures, which may not be generalisable to non-WEIRD people (Henrich, Heine, & Norenzayan, 2010).

Researchers need to explain how their convenience sample relates to the population and justify that the findings can be interpreted. Convenience samples risk self-selection bias and under-representing minority populations. To interpret the results, researchers often use socio-demographic information, such as age and gender (e.g., see socio-demographic questions in Online Table 7.2).

Decide recruitment procedures

Table 7.3 provides an incomplete overview of recruitment opportunities. Asking people to participate requires proactive reaching out. When considering recruitment, consider why individuals would be motivated to become participants. For example, an engaging marketing poster, social media post, or website makes participation look interesting. An individual may want to participate because they feel the study is important, they want to contribute to social change, they feel bored and are killing some time, or they feel an obligation towards an institute/researcher/peer. Participants must feel that their participation will influence something they care about and that their opinions will be listened to and acted upon. Some participants may do research for a reward, such as study credits, money or a shot at a prize, which may be unethical and bias the findings.

Be aware of the ethical considerations of recruitment, such as no disproportionate pressure or misusing leverage. For example, asking your friends or clients to participate may be unethical as they may feel pressured to say 'yes', and what they share may influence your relationship. Recruiting clients from colleagues or in your department may be biased and unethical, as clients may reveal (or feel hindered from disclosing) information about your colleagues that could put you in an awkward position. Often, recruitment involves gatekeepers, such as a head of department; the relationships with these gatekeepers and their clients/participants may be symbiotic. Recruitment via health service providers may be effective but formal approval procedures may be time-consuming. Imagine how it would be like to walk in the shoes of your potential participants: consider the potential impact of research.

Furthermore, regarding recruitment materials: proofread them, find a balance between an accessible/friendly and professional tone, be brief and to the point, practical about next steps, sensitive, and convincing but not pushy. In verbal communication, be friendly, personalise your explanations, and be enthusiastic. Respond quickly to emails/calls/messages. Build empathic-supportive, and collaborative relationships. Recruitment often fails due to researchers not being proactive enough, not using relevant marketing resources, being shy, and not having a realistic and detailed recruitment plan. Reflect on underlying causes of failure, ask for supervision, and broaden your recruitment plan. Search for articles and blogs on recruiting in your field.

Step 8: Decide data collection and procedures

Definition

Data can be collected in many ways, such as via interviews, questionnaires, observations, and secondary and creative resources. Mixed methods use multiple data-collection methods and analyses (see Chapter 11). Use a valid and reliable or trustworthy method, and justify this as the best way to answer your research questions/objectives.

Examples

Questionnaires

- **Popularity:** Most frequently used quantitative data-collection method in therapy research.
- **Examples:** Paper/online, send by post, complete in a public space, mental health service.
- **Pros:** Standardisation, reduction of bias, anonymity, lower costs in large samples.

Table 7.3 Recruitment opportunities

Recruitment by researcher
- **Poster/leaflets:** mental health service, universities, GP surgeries, pharmacies, libraries, charities, charity shops, supermarkets
- **Snowballing:** send email, give poster/leaflets to colleagues/friends/influencers to share
- **Research institute/university:** advert in newsletter, website, social media, noticeboards
- **Social media:** Facebook (professional profiles, groups), Twitter (add e.g., @BPSOfficial, @BACP, #counselling), Instagram, YouTube
- **Dedicated website:** make sure search engines find this (SEO)
- **Professional network:** LinkedIn, ResearchGate, Academia.edu
- **Professional bodies:** advert on website, newsletter, conference
- **Forums:** Reddit (topic-specific subreddits), discussion forums, topical websites
- **Service-user groups, networks, charities:** see overview of the UK on www.nhs.uk/nhs-services/mental-health-services/
- **Research websites:** psychology research websites, findparticipants.com
- **Blogs**
- **Conference attendees**

Recruitment of paid participants by paid services
(NB: note costs, ethics, risk of bias, quantitative focus)
- **Recruitment services:** respondent.io, testingtime.com, surveymonkey.com, positly.com, prolific.io, cloudresearch.com
- **Paid crowdsourcing websites:** mysurvey123, Amazon/MTurk, Prolific, Sona, MindSwarms, SurveyCircle, Craigslist, Fiverr, Clickworker, Gumtree

---

- **Cons:** Literate participants only, lower participation rates and more dropouts with long questionnaires, self-selection bias, difficult to control context of filling in questionnaire online or at home, limited freedom/space for open answers
- **Procedure:** Select existing questionnaires with proven reliability and validity, develop your own survey/questionnaire (see Chapter 9).
- **Norm group:** Compare outcomes with cut-off points of a norm group; e.g., PHQ-9 scores larger than 13 may be interpreted as 'depression'.
- **Benchmarking:** Compare outcomes with benchmarks from other studies or health services (e.g., digital.nhs.uk). This can help to evaluate how much better/worse the outcomes are compared to other services. Minami et al. (2012) explain how to compare your study with other studies or benchmarks; Minami et al. (2007) give benchmarks for common instruments.
- **Details:** See Chapter 8.

Interview

- **Popularity:** Most frequently used qualitative data-collection method in therapy research.
- **Pros:** Explore new/complex topics, provide in-depth information, offer freedom to participants, explain questions.

- **Cons:** Time-consuming, travel costs for in-person interviews. Interview transcription requires 1–2 days per hour of interview. Interview quality depends on the quality of the interaction between participant and researcher and the interviewer's quality and biases.
- **Procedure:** Develop your interview schedule or use or adjust pre-existing interview schedule.
- **Interview-types:** Interviews can be fully-structured, semi-structured or unstructured. A fully-structured interview follows a pre-determined interview schedule with questions in a specific order. An unstructured interview offers participants the space to share their experiences in response to a general introduction of the topic, and often with the help of a list of possible topics. Other types include focus group interviews, narrative interviews focusing on life stories, and oral history interviews.
- **Details:** See Chapter 9.

Observation

- **Popularity:** Infrequently used in therapy research, e.g., analysis of video recording of non-verbal behaviour in a session or public observation.
- **Pros:** Verifiable, quantifiable, little need of interpretation.
- **Cons:** Behaviour may not reflect subjective experiences, risk of bias such as the error of central tendency (an assessor systematically giving average scores), elevation effects (systematically scoring everyone higher), halo effect (scores on one aspect influence other scores).
- **Procedures:** Develop or use standardised observation schemes.

Secondary sources

- **Explanation:** Secondary sources are existing sources not created by researchers, e.g., governmental documents, client records, online forums.
- **Popularity:** Common in narrative/discourse/conversation analysis, less common in psychotherapy research.
- **Pros:** Relatively easy to find, particularly online.
- **Cons:** Available data may be biased (e.g., governmental lack of transparency), challenging to verify the validity/reliability/trustworthiness of sources.

Creative tools

- **Explanation:** Research data can be non-linguistic, unconscious, embodied, experiential, aesthetic, intuitive, or sympathetic, e.g., drawing, pictures, art, music, videos, psychodynamic projective tests (Morrow, 2005).
- **Popularity:** Uncommon, sometimes used in psychodynamic, art, and drama therapies.
- **Pros:** Rich data, examine implicit/unconscious phenomena and attitudes, evidence-based coding schemes for some projective tests.
- **Cons:** May be difficult to interpret, risk of bias, rich data.

Step 9: Decide practical organisation

Definition

The success of a research project depends on its practical organisation. A researcher can be brilliant in developing study designs and analysis, but horrendous in data collection. Consider what is required for this study, what you can do yourself, and which resources/people you may involve.

Examples

- **Timeline:** Realistic timeline, preferably visualised with a Gantt chart, as proposed in Chapter 4.
- **Safety net:** Plans for worst-case scenario, e.g., alternative recruitment-methods.
- **Details about data collection:** Such as participant's home, research lab. Since the COVID-19 pandemic, many interviews have been taking place online, e.g., via Skype/Zoom, which has pros and cons (pro/con arguments in Online Table 7.5).
- **Coding/scoring schemes:** Some questionnaires/interview schedules/data use coding and scoring schemes, norm groups, or anchors, which need to be explained and justified. A researcher may need professional training.
- **Software:** Decide on writing, editing, and research software (overview: Online Table 7.4).
- **Interview-transcription procedures:** Before interviews can be analysed, they need to be transcribed. As Chapter 10 will explain, interviews can be transcribed with coding schemes including details such as pauses, ums, etc. Some researchers use external transcribers; however, many experts advise against this, as transcribing an interview helps researchers to get an in-depth understanding of the interview, which facilitates analytical and interpretative processes.
- **Codebook:** In questionnaire studies, researchers may want to create a standardised procedure and template for how to code all questions and answers, and how they transform the raw data (i.e., direct answers of the participants) into data that can be used in statistical analyses. It is recommended to give each variable a logical name and record in a codebook the names and items they refer to.
- **Preparatory statistical analyses:** Quantitative data sometimes need preparatory analyses, such as checking for statistical assumptions and testing reliability and validity of questionnaires (see Chapter 8).

Step 10: Decide data analysis

Definition

Chapters 8–10 will help you decide which specific method to use to analyse the research data, such as a t-test to compare outcome measures (T1) with a baseline (T0) in a clinical trial, or reflexive thematic analysis of interviews. You will need to explain the chosen analytical technique and justify how this answers the research questions/objectives. Often, the research questions/objectives are formulated in terms of how you will do the analysis; for example, if 'a study aims to test the difference between groups A and B', it makes sense to use a student's t-test. The analytical method needs to be coherent with the ontological/epistemological position, study design, sample, and data-collection tools.

Step 11: Formalise methodological decisions

Definition

Before you build a house, you create a blueprint to identify potential flaws before building starts and justify your investment of time and resources. It is good practice to write all your methodological decisions in a research journal to create a verifiable audit trail of the research process and the rationales behind each step, allowing retrospective quality checking and identification of errors. For each document, researchers should not only explain in detail *what* they have decided (content) but also *why* they have made these decisions (rationale/justification) and *how* they will apply these decisions practically throughout the research process (implications/applications).

Examples

- **Brief research reports/articles:** Always include a part/section on methodology, explaining and justifying the main methodological steps.
- **Formal reports/theses:** Formal research reports/student theses usually require explication, justification, and specification of each methodological step.
- **Education assignments:** Often, university programmes use exercises or assignments to help students develop their methodology, e.g., essays on methodology, critical self-reflection, and reflexivity. Use Templates D–E as the tree-structure of essays.
- **Research proposal:** A research proposal 'is an argument for your study. It needs to explain the logic behind the proposed research, rather than merely describing or summarising the study, in a way that non-specialists will understand' (Maxwell, 2012, p.119). Template F may be used as the basis for writing a research proposal (downloadable Word files can be found online). You may check whether you have included all the relevant aspects in the proposal with the online proposal checklist. This proposal template closely follows Chapters 1–7, thus ensure to consult these chapters when writing your proposal (see also Coley, Scheinberg, & Strekalova, 2021; Locke, Spirduso, & Silverman, 2013).
- **Research proposal presentation:** It is good practice to present your research proposal to your colleagues and supervisors/examiners to get their feedback and suggestions, which may help you improve the research proposal. You may use the online PowerPoint template.
- **Reflective research journal:** Record and reflect on each methodological step (see Chapter 4).
- **Grant application:** Funds often require applicants to prepare a grant application, which resembles the research proposal and steps in Chapters 1–7. A grant application can include a longer-term plan with multiple sub-projects and co-researchers; it is essential to explain and justify who will do what. Funders need to be convinced of this

project's success, which can be argued by a good proposal as well as a convincing track record of success by the researchers. Carefully consider who should be included in the research team and how the team will be managed (Baer et al., 2011; Wyatt in Denzin & Lincoln, 2021). A feasible budget needs be prepared, often with the help of financial experts. (Read more in Pequegnat, Stover, & Boyce, 2011; Reif-Lehrer, 2005.)

━━━ Reflective questions ━━━

- Select three frequently cited articles in your field (qualitative and quantitative). Examine how they describe and justify each methodological step. What are the strengths and weaknesses? What lessons can you learn?
- Do the exercise in Online Table 7.2 to identify your ontological/epistemological position in daily life (also useful for a class discussion).

PART III
SPECIFIC SKILLS

8

How to Conduct Quantitative Research

Chapter aims

This chapter explains how to read, develop, and conduct quantitative research. A quantitative method helps to answer a quantitative research question, for example to calculate the correlation between two phenomena or to test the effects of a treatment. Whereas Chapter 7 gave an overview of all methodological steps, this chapter zooms into developing a quantitative mindset, building quantitative study designs, applying quantitative analytical methods, and developing and using psychometric instruments such as questionnaires. Some researchers may want to combine quantitative with qualitative methods, as Chapter 10 will explain. Like all research projects, quantitative studies need to be designed and conducted ethically and discussed critically (see Chapters 11–12). Helpful books on quantitative methods include Field, 2013; Kazdin, 2021; Kumar, 2018; Langdridge & Hagger-Johnson, 2009; Little, 2013; Stevens, 2012.

Steps in chapter

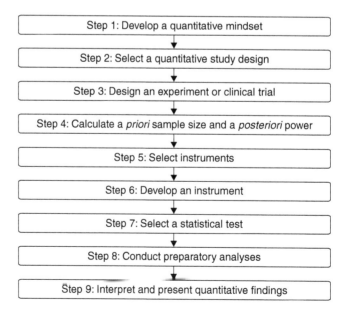

Step 1: Develop a quantitative mindset

Step 2: Select a quantitative study design

Step 3: Design an experiment or clinical trial

Step 4: Calculate a *priori* sample size and a *posteriori* power

Step 5: Select instruments

Step 6: Develop an instrument

Step 7: Select a statistical test

Step 8: Conduct preparatory analyses

Step 9: Interpret and present quantitative findings

Step 1: Develop a quantitative mindset

Definition

Doing quantitative research starts with developing a quantitative mindset, such as a quantitative ontological-epistemological position, and a mindset focusing on testing, probabilities, errors, reliability, validity, generalizability, and replication. This quantitative mindset will guide researchers in their subsequent methodological decisions, analyses, and writing.

Components

Ontological-epistemological position

Many quantitative researchers seem to assume that universal laws, such as cause-and-effect, can be relatively directly measured with the help of instruments and expressed in numbers. For example, a quantitative researcher gives participants a therapeutic intervention, tests outcomes with questionnaires, and statistically analyses the data with a statistical correlation test or a t-test. As long as the selection, collection, and analysis of data are done accurately, the researcher is assumed to have a relatively small influence on the research process. Chapter 7 described this position as a positivist meta-theory, realist ontology, and objectivist epistemology, although quantitative researchers may have other positions (e.g., post-positivist, or critical-realist).

Testing mindset

Thinking as a quantitative researcher means thinking about hypotheses, such as:

* **Testing correlations/covariations**: We could hypothesise that two or more events are related or cluster in a pattern, but we do not know which event causes which. This is the basis of research into correlations and analyses of covariation. For example, we could discover that male clients experience therapy as less satisfying than female clients, as indicated by significantly smaller scores on a satisfaction scale. This finding only says we observe two things simultaneously – gender and satisfaction scores – but this does not say that gender causes the difference in satisfaction. Correlation is not causation.
* **Testing predictions**: We could hypothesise that one factor, such as gender, predicts another factor, such as therapy effects. To test this hypothesis, we will need a study design that allows us to test causality. For example, we could give the same therapy to male and female clients, and at the end, the effects in both groups are compared. If we were to conduct such an experiment, we might have some initial indications that therapy may have different effects in both groups.

Probabilistic mindset

We can be confident that the sun rises in the east or that water boils at about 100 degrees Celsius. However, we cannot be as sure about human behaviours, feelings, and thoughts. Humans seem less predictable, interacting in complex social and physical contexts and prone to individual variation – possibly thanks to what philosophers call 'human will'. Concepts such as depression and anxiety may not be as precisely defined as boiling water. Therefore, researchers talk about the *likelihood* that humans respond in particular ways. Whereas a physicist could state, 'heat will make water boil at 100 degrees' (abstractly formulated: 'x causes y under condition z'), a psychologist could say, 'there is a large likelihood that CBT reduces anxiety in clients with cynophobia'. Thus, researchers talk about *probabilities*: 'there is a low/medium/large probability that x causes y under condition z'. This probability can be found in statistical reports as a p-value, where the consensus is that a finding is credible if it happens by chance in less than 5 of 100 times ($p < .05$): the significance level is 5%.

Variation-oriented mindset

Individuals differ. Therefore, individuals answer questions differently, have different sum-scores in questionnaires, and have different outcomes in experiments or clinical trials. Often, quantitative researchers seem less interested in individual differences than in the average experiences across individuals. Ultimately, they hope to generalise their findings to the general population, with the mean score in their sample reflecting the true mean in the population. Therefore, quantitative researchers report both means and variations.

How to report means: Quantitative researchers often assume that there is a mean effect across all individuals. An individual's score on a question in a questionnaire (called 'variable' or 'item') is the combination of the mean score and their individual difference from this mean. Therefore, researchers report average scores in their study, such as a statistical mean, and sometimes the modus (the most frequently reported number) or median (middle value in a range).

How to report variation: Researchers report how much individuals differ from the mean, for example by describing the full range of scores, e.g., 'scores ranged between 7.2 to 23.6'. However, what does this range mean: is this large or small? Therefore, researchers often standardise the variation by calculating the standard deviation (SD). A large SD means that individuals differ greatly from the mean within one dataset, whereas a small SD means small variation (NB: as will be explained later, if you have multiple datasets for different samples drawn from the same population, for example in a meta-analyses of multiple studies, the variability between these samples is called Standard Error, SE)

How to calculate confidence intervals: In many situations, when we examine the scores in a sample, we see many participants with scores around the mean, some with larger and smaller scores than the mean, and a few with much larger and much smaller scores. This distribution of frequencies is called a 'normal distribution', often visualised as a bell curve. You can describe how many people have scores around the mean. For example, more complex statistical tests, as discussed in Step 7, automatically report the 95% confidence interval, which refers to the lowest score and the largest score of 95% of all individuals who fall within two standard deviations from the mean (e.g., '95% CI = 9.2–21.6'). However, not all variables are normally distributed, for example many participants might have reported extremely large scores. Some statistical tests (see Table 8.3) assume that variables are normally distributed. Step 7 explains this in more detail.

Error-oriented mindset

Thinking in terms of probabilities also implies thinking systematically about the likelihood of error. Imagine a doctor investigating a patient with high-fever symptoms, such as hot skin and cold sweats. The doctor tests their body temperature with a thermometer, indicating 37.1 degrees Celsius. The doctor is puzzled and gets a second thermometer which shows 39.2 degrees. The doctor examines the first thermometer and finds a crack in the housing, which may explain the measurement error. Does this mean that 39.2 degrees is the patient's true body temperature? Not necessarily, because the second thermometer may also be faulty, the doctor may have used the thermometer incorrectly or have misread the temperature. Thus, our observations may differ from the true values in reality (note the positivist language).

Some measurement instruments and measurement procedures seem to have structurally larger errors, e.g., forehead thermometers are less reliable than anal thermometers. The risk of error may even be larger when we measure individual subjective experiences. For example, two therapists are likely to have at least small differences in their assessment of the precise symptoms and severity of anxiety in a client, even though training, step-by-step instructions, and diagnostic manuals may reduce potential error. Therefore, research project will have some measurement errors, observation error, or experimental errors, although the researchers will try to minimise these. There are two general groups of errors, random and systematic:

- **Random error:** Our observations differ from the true values at random. The error is mere chance, unpredictable and could lead to an overestimation or underestimation of participants' scores. Examples:
  o **Natural variations:** e.g., participants' memory is better early in the day than later
  o **Individual differences:** e.g., individuals respond differently to an electric shock due to different pain levels
  o **Reliability/precision of instruments:** e.g., unreliable and imprecise questionnaires are answered differently by the same participant at different points in time
  o **Poorly controlled experimental conditions:** e.g., there is no standardised treatment manual, training, and adherence by therapists in a clinical trial
  o **Solutions:** e.g., precise and reliable instruments, larger sample size, controlled measurements/experiments so extraneous factors do not randomly influence results
- **Systematic error (also 'bias', 'skew'):** There is a consistent difference between the observed and true values on a scale. The results are systematically biased and skewed in a particular direction. Each time we measure the same phenomenon, the measurements will differ from true scores in the same direction, sometimes even by the same amount.
  o **Response bias:** e.g., a questionnaire has biased/leading questions (e.g., due to social desirability and conformism) due to which all participants have high scores
  o **Offset errors and scale-factor errors:** e.g., a researcher has systematically given all specific answers from all participants too high scores
  o **Experimenter bias:** e.g., the researcher treats the experimental group differently from the control group (besides the different content of both groups)
  o **Halo effect**: e.g., interviewers/assessors may rate participants disproportionally high due to a generally positive impression of that participant
  o **Lake-Wobegon effect:** if individuals are asked to compare themselves with others, almost every individual is inclined to claim they are better
  o **Repeated-testing effect:** e.g., when the same questionnaire is given, scores tend to be closer (see also response shift, explained in step 9)
  o **Regression towards the mean:** e.g., participants with initially extreme low/high scores regress to the mean
  o **Mortality/attrition bias:** e.g., researchers base their conclusions only on participants participating from the first until last measurements

- ○ **Rivalry/demoralisation effect:** individuals in the experimental condition may do better when they know they are in the experimental group (rivalry), and those in the control group may have worse scores (demoralisation)
- ○ **Solutions:** e.g., select reliable, valid questionnaires; in experiments, use randomised, controlled, blinded control groups, train therapists to give therapy with a (semi-)standardised treatment manual, test adherence, and triangulate (i.e., use multiple instruments and assessors)

Testing-error mindset

Next to paying attention to variation and error, the quantitative mindset includes using statistical techniques to calculate the probability that observations are actually true. Remember that quantitative researchers formulate both a null hypothesis and an alternative hypothesis (see Chapter 6):

- **A null hypothesis (H0)** says that there is no effect, e.g., 'exposure therapy for cynophobia does not have statistically significant effects on anxiety'.
- **An alternative hypothesis (Ha/H1)** says that there is an effect, e.g., 'exposure therapy for cynophobia has significant effects on anxiety'.

Of course, a researcher hopes to reject the H0 hypothesis that there is no significant effect. Simply said, they want to conclude that exposure therapy changes anxiety. However, a researcher may find by error that exposure therapy changes anxiety, or they may find by error that it does not change anxiety, for two reasons (see Table 8.4):

- **Type I error:** Rejecting the null hypothesis of no-effect when it is actually true. The researcher concludes exposure therapy changes anxiety when it actually does not.
- **Type II error:** Not rejecting the null hypothesis of no-effect when it is actually false. The researcher concludes exposure therapy does not change anxiety when it actually does.

The level of statistical significance or significance level (α) regards the probability of a type I error, which means the probability of inaccurately rejecting the null hypothesis when it is actually true. Often, researchers decide before they do a statistical test how much likelihood of a type I error they will accept, and usually this is set at 5% (as we will see later, you may reduce this if you have many assumptions/estimations in your study). This means accepting that in less than 5% of the cases, we may find an effect that is actually not there. As Step 4 will explain, statistical power is the likelihood of avoiding a type II error: the higher the statistical power, the lower the risk of making a type II error.

Reliability and validity mindset

Quantitative researchers use the terms 'reliable' and 'valid' to describe how sound the methodology in their study is. A method is reliable if it gives consistent findings, e.g., each time a person fills in a questionnaire, they provide the same answers. A methodology is valid if it correctly measures the concept that the researcher wants to measure – e.g., an anxiety questionnaire truly measures how depressed clients are. Researchers select the most reliable and valid psychometric instruments, study designs, and statistical methods, as step 5 explains.

Generalisability and replication mindset

Quantitative researchers often aim to generalise the findings from their sample to the general population. Even though a study may include 500 participants, the researchers still need to justify that these findings in this sample for example represent all the millions in the population. Therefore, their sample must be a good representation of the entire population; to achieve this, researchers need to recruit a random sample with characteristics matching the general population. Researchers often conduct replication studies to confirm findings in other samples;a replication study can be a precise copy of the original study, or an extension in a different sample/context. Replication can increase the credibility of the generalisability or universality of the results and reduce the probability that the initial findings are caused by chance, fraud, specific context, or the researcher.

Know the quantitative lingo

When reading and writing quantitative research, note the quantitative terminology. For example, quantitative researchers often avoid the words 'we' and 'I', although this tendency has become less rigid in recent years. Questions in a questionnaire are called 'items', but when used in statistical analyses 'variables'. Questionnaires are often called 'scales' like in physics or medicine; they are 'psychometric instruments' as they measure psychological phenomena. 'Research participants' or 'respondents' are standard terminology. 'N' stands for number of participants or sample size.

Step 2: Select a quantitative study design

Definition

Chapter 7 described the general steps in developing qualitative, quantitative or mixed methods study designs. This step gives an overview of possible quantitative study designs. You may want to use the flowchart in Figure 8.1 when selecting a quantitative design.

Examples

Decide whether your study aims are mainly clinical, research, or both

You will need to decide what the primary aims of your project are: do you want to do academic research or do you have clinical aims? (although often both overlap). An example of a clinical aim regards a psychological assessment of the mental health or personality of individual clients. The next sections will describe study designs with clear research aims.

A specific examples of clinical research are service evaluations or audits, which regard the evaluation of existing services, usually without the addition of a new intervention/treatment. Service evaluations or audits often measure the following (Rossi, Lipsey, & Freeman, 2004; Shadish, Cook, & Leviton, 1991; https://nhsevaluationtoolkit.net/):

- **Population coverage:** The extent to which the target population is served, e.g., service users' socio-demographic characteristics, dropout analysis.
- **Service implementation:** For example, number of clients treated or on waiting lists, online/face-to-face sessions, session cancellations, onward referral, therapy dropout, waiting-list period.

- **Client experiences:** For example, client-satisfaction surveys (e.g., Client Satisfaction Questionnaire) or qualitative client helpfulness interviews (see Chapter 9). As self-evaluation forms and client interviews are often positively biased, researchers may ask about both positive and negative changes, both helpful and unhelpful aspects, attribution, importance, and size of changes. Ideally, researchers also invite third parties to confirm the changes that clients report themselves, such as partners and relatives.

- **Outcomes:** Quantitative case-tracking or client-focused research, e.g., via pre–post-therapy questionnaires or session-per-session Routine Outcome Monitoring (ROM) with standardised instruments relevant to the service population. To implement clinical measures feasibly, questionnaires need to be brief with quick, automated scoring and interpretation. For example, the British NHS-IAPT services often administer PHQ-9, GAD-7, CORE-10, IES (frequently used alternative scales are for example SCL-90, HADS, POMS, BDI, BAI). Specific services may use their own specialised instruments, for example therapists helping clients on the autistic spectrum may use questionnaires specifically designed for their population. Ideally, individual scores and changes over time are fed back to therapists via an outcomes-management system (feedback-informed treatment), to flag-up individuals with significant decline, suicidal risk, and satisfaction (e.g., Session-Rating Scale, Outcome-Rating Scale). Benchmarking may compare findings with other studies or mental health services. Sometimes, clients are asked to formulate their therapy goals in their first session, and later in therapy they rate to which extent they have achieved each goal (Goal Attainment Form). Some services ask questions about general quality in life and the impact of mental health problems on their daily life (e.g. WSAS, WHOQOL, SF-6D). Some therapists use questionnaires about the therapeutic relationship to check their working alliance with the client and identify possible areas of improvement (e.g. WAI, ARM-5).

- **Psychological assesment:** Some services conduct systematic psychological assessment with (semi-)standardised questionnaires and interviews, to develop a psychological profile of clients (Butcher, 2002; Groth-Marnat, 2003; Kaplan & Saccuzzo, 2017). The primary purpose of assessing an individual client may be clinical, although the service may combine the data from all their clients to develop an in—depth review of their population. Clients are not necessarily expected to change on these scales, but it may explain some of their daily life struggles, and give a focus for therapy. Examples include questionnaires about personality (NEO-PI, MMPI), intelligence (WAIS), neuropsychological tests (e.g. about brain impairment, motor ability, or executive functions), coping (COPE), clinical interview (SCID, Attachment Interview), cognitive schemas (Young's Schema Questionnaire), projective tests (Rorschach, TAT), object-relations (IPO), questionnaires about relationships, marital satisfaction, family systems and group dynamics, and a biographical interview. To develop a comprehensive profile of the client, it is important to also assess client's strengths and positive well-being (RLOT, RSES, SPWB, MLQ, PANAS, SWLS) (Lopez & Snyder, 2003). Practitioners do not merely describe the individual findings of each (sub)scale but try to understand how the different findings dynamically interact and offset each other's weaknesses and strengths (e.g. Eurelings-Bontekoe & Snellen, 2010). Overall, research indicates that if a well-trained practitioner uses a multi-method test battery, that this may yield equally valid and reliable findings as medical tests and possibly improve treatment effects (Bornstein, 2017; Meyer et al., 2001).

- **Cost-effectiveness:** The trade-off between financial costs and benefits of therapy. Policy-makers are often interested in whether treatment is not merely effective but also cost-effective. Direct costs may include salary and rent of therapy rooms. Direct benefits include the client's increase in quality of life, indirect benefits include less sickness leave, health services expenditure, etc. Research indicates that psychological therapies reduce medical costs and may annually save 9,000GBP per client; for each 1GBP investment in mental health care, society may get approximately 2–3GBP back (Vos, Roberts, & Davies, 2019). Researchers may calculate dose-response relationships to determine the number of sessions specific client populations require to improve significantly. For example, more than 50% of all clients experience significant change between 13 and 18 sessions (Hansen, Lambert, & Forman, 2002); routinely delivered therapies may require between 4 and 26 sessions, varying according to setting, population, and outcome measures (Robinson, Delgadillo, & Kellett, 2020). Clients seem to experience the largest improvement within their approximately first 12 sessions; although 12 sessions may not solve all problems, this may be a 'good enough level of improvement' (Barkham et al., 2006). Recent 'aptitude-treatment interaction studies' examined the suitability of specific therapy types for clients, as different treatments may work better for different clients with different problems (Snow, 1991). However, cost-effectiveness, dose-response, and aptitude-treatment-interaction studies have been criticised for being too narrowly focused on financial savings, using irrelevant outcome measures, and neglecting subjective experiences and political powers (Vos, Roberts, & Davies, 2019).

Decide experimental or non-experimental research

A key decision is whether or not researchers want to test the effects of an intervention, such as a laboratory experiment or treatment. This will be further explained in the next steps.

Decisions in non-experimental research

Non-intervention research usually does not focus on measuring causality but on trends, frequencies, and correlations. These could include surveys (e.g., panel, cohort. or trend), instrument development (e.g., development or replication studies) or case studies. In Q-sort tests, participants put cards with specific words or descriptions into piles ranging from 'most' to least' important characteristics.

Decisions in experiments/clinical trials in a research laboratory

In an experiment, the effects of an intervention can be tested, such as the effects of sublimi-nally showing emotive words or pictures on a computer screen or the effects of one specific therapeutic intervention. An experiment could investigate the efficacy of a complex treatment on clients, called a clinical trial. Clinical trials could test the change between pre-treatment and post-treatment scores, e.g., the effects of CBT for cynophobia on anxiety question-naires before/after treatment. By adding control groups, researchers can test whether these changes are smaller, equivalent or larger than other interventions or natural improvements.

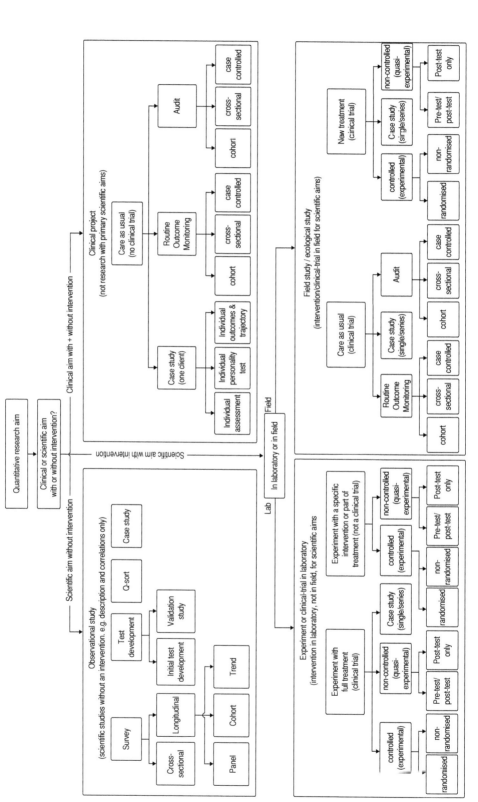

Figure 8.1 Decision-tree for frequently used quantitative study designs

The random allocation of participants to either experimental or control conditions may reduce bias. Step 3 in this chapter explains how to design clinical trials. Research in research laboratories, universities, or research institutes can give information about the efficacy of treatments under controlled circumstances where daily life influences and variations are controlled as much as possible, but may be limited due to the lack of ecological validity and generalisability.

Decisions in ecologically valid field studies in daily-life settings

This study design may give information about the effectiveness of treatments in clinical practice. This design resembles clinical research and service evaluations, as this also happens, for example, in a mental health service and not a laboratory or university; the difference is that these studies test research hypotheses and do not merely evaluate how well existing services are doing. For example, researchers may use Routine Outcome Monitoring (ROM) to test specific hypotheses about the general sample/service, care-as-usual, or a new treatment with/without control groups and randomisation. This can be in a particular cohort, cross-sectional, or case controlled. Research can be one-time-only or longitudinal. As these studies are conducted in daily-life contexts, they are more prone to influences from extraneous factors and comorbidities than laboratory research.

Step 3: Design an experiment or clinical trial

Definition

The previous step gave an overview of quantitative study designs. This step zooms into designing an experiment or clinical trial. However, trials on psychological therapies may have several limitations, such as the impossibility of blinding, influence from client preferences, and therapist Organising complex clinical trials is often challenging and expensive, and recruited samples may not reflect ecologically valid client populations. Therefore, in recent years, some researchers have argued that clinical trials may have been overvalued in therapy research, and instead they recommend collecting or combining large natural datasets in therapy services.

Procedures

1. Identify the stage of the research field

Psychological therapies are usually developed and validated in multiple stages, comparable to medical trials (Carroll & Nuro, 2002; Rounsaville, Carroll, & Onken, 2001; Vos, 2023; Vos & Van Rijn, 2023). When designing your trial, examine which study designs fits the current phase of the field.

- **Phase-0/proof-of-concept study:** This study describes whether the treatment may work in theory. For example, before they conduct a phase-1 study, researchers develop an evidence-based, coherent, logical conceptual framework, for example highlighting clinical needs, aetiology, therapeutic mechanisms, and therapeutic competencies (see Chapter 3). Population surveys may confirm the incidence/prevalence/relevance of the clinical problem in the population, which may justify the subsequent research phases. This phase may include literature reviews, qualitative interviews, focus groups, theoretical proof-of-concept studies, systematic treatment manual development based on empirical research, and case studies. A proof-of-concept study can for example focus on developing and exploring the face/construct validity of key clinical concepts and therapeutic mechanisms. This is an essential research phase, as this forms the basis of all next phases.

- **Phase-1/feasibility study:** This screens for safety, acceptance by clients, therapists, and researchers, treatment adherence, suggestions for improvement, the feasibility of research procedures – e.g., recruitment, questionnaires – checking for negative side effects, and identifying preliminary effectiveness. This may combine qualitative methods (interviews) and some preliminary quantitative measurements (although the sample size is often too small to generalise findings). The preliminary effects may be used in *a priori* sample-size calculations to determine the sample size in efficacy/effectiveness studies. A feasibility is limited due to its small sample size, but it may be helpful to explore the feasibility and validity of the treatment and data collection and evaluation procedures, and consider negative side-effects and ethical issues. This phase is essential to identify potential design flows that may impact subsequent large-size phase 2/3-trials.
- **Phase 2/pilot study/pilot RCT efficacy study:** This is a controlled study in a research laboratory or university clinic into the efficacy of the treatment, usually compared with a placebo control group such as those on a waiting list (e.g., RCT). Often uses mixed methods. The RCT design helps to conclude whether the effects may be caused by the experimental intervention/treatment, as other potentially influencing variables are controlled for. (See Leon, Davis, & Kraemer, 2011.)
- **Phase 3/RCT effectiveness study:** This is a confirmation of safety and effectiveness, usually at multiple sites, preferably in ecologically valid contexts such as mental health services. This often focuses on quantitative methods, although qualitative methods may explore subjective experiences of change and helpfulness. The larger sample size may help understand which intervention works best for which individuals with which characteristics ('moderators') and for what reason ('mediators'). The sample size is determined *a priori* and statistical power calculated *a posteriori*.
- **Phase 4/replication studies:** The treatment is validated in other populations, including quantitative, qualitative, and mixed methods, and cost-effectiveness analyses.

2. Build a conceptual framework

Before deciding on the experimental study design, researchers build a conceptual framework (Kazdin, 2007, 2009; Vos, 2014). This includes at least concepts related to aetiology, the clinical problem, therapeutic mechanisms, outcomes, and their relationships (see Chapter 3). Causality may, for example be implied when the concepts associate/correlate/covariate and precede each other logically, without alternative explanations (explained in Chapter 6, Step 5). One research project may not test all relationships and concepts, but the researcher may justify the other conceptual assumptions via a literature review. For example, a researcher may only study the outcomes of exposure therapy on cynophobia, and they may justify using exposure by citing other studies showing how behavioural avoidance causes cynophobia and how exposure reduces behavioural avoidance.

3. Decide experimental intervention/treatment

Researchers want to know whether the effects can be attributed to the experimental intervention/treatment and not to other variables, such as different therapists giving different interventions to different clients. Therefore, researchers standardise the treatment and treatment procedures. Standardisation increases construct validity and reduces risk of bias.

- **Fully/semi/unstructured treatment manual:** A treatment manual can be fully structured or semi-structured instead of unstructured. Structured means that the therapists give the same interventions in the same order. Due to the subjective nature of psychological therapies, it is often difficult to create fully structured treatment manuals. Most trials are semi-structured, allowing therapists to tailor interventions to clients (i.e., therapist's appropriate responsiveness).
- **Adherence:** To ensure therapists give the treatment manual as expected, they often get training and clinical supervision. Some studies use an adherence protocol to check the extent to which therapists adhere to the treatment manual (e.g., assessment of session recordings by independent assessors), or adherence questionnaires.

4. Decide the number of participants

- **Multiple participants:** The required sample size is calculated with power calculations (see Step 4).
- **Single-case experimental design:** An experimental intervention is tested on one individual, preferably with repeated-measures and rich mixed data (Barlow, Nock, & Hersen, 2008; Kazdin, 2021; see case studies in Chapter 9). This study design assumes a systematic case formulation based on a systematic analysis of the causal mechanisms and context (see Chapter 3). The client is measured at a baseline or a phase without any treatment (A) and receives one or more interventions/treatments (B, C, D). The AB design examines changes after one intervention, whereas the reversal design assumes that the client receives the intervention twice with a non-treatment phase in-between (ABAB). In the reversal design, the client functions like their control group (A1–B1 change versus A2–B2 change). Changing-criterion designs measure, for example, a gradual reduction in the number of cigarettes/alcohol units/drugs. In a time-series design, multiple instruments are measured for longer to examine their correlational and hypothetical-causal relationships. Single-case experiments are limited by their idiographic nature, which may be countered with replication studies, or cross-sectional case-control design (i.e., cases and control-cases are selected, evaluated, and compared).

5. Decide number of contacts

Decide the number of contacts in your study, as briefly introduced in chapter 7, step 3.

- **After-only design:** One-shot retrospective measurement after an intervention/event. Insufficient to conclude causality, as this would involve the logical fallacy known as *post hoc ergo propter hoc*: 'because B happens after A, B must be the result of A'. However, after-only designs may be the only feasible study design and may give some clues about causality if there is sufficient contextual information.
- **Before-and-after design:** One prospective measurement is taken before the beginning, one immediately after the end. This does not test potential long-term decreases in effectiveness and relapse.

- **Repeated measures/longitudinal:** Three or more measurements. Most clinical trials compare the scores of clients on questionnaires administered before the first therapy session (baseline measurement, T0) with more measurement-moments after the last session (outcome and follow-up measurements T1, T2, T3).

6. Decide experimental or semi-experimental/quasi-experimental design

A semi-experimental with or quasi-experimental study may have a control group, but participants are not randomly allocated to experimental with or control groups, and there is no blinding and matching. The control group is usually a naturally occurring group, like a waiting list or a treatment chosen by the client. This study design is often used in audits with and evaluations of mental health services, as it may be unethical to use an experimental design and deny clients their preferred treatment when they are randomly allocated to study conditions. A non-randomly assigned or non-equivalent control group can help to control for variables such as testing and maturation. It may be difficult to derive conclusions about the treatment effectiveness, as the effects may also be caused or mediated by extraneous variables such as experimenter bias and the client's therapy preferences. To sketch the study's validity and generalisability, the sample characteristics and study findings may be compared statistically with other studies or benchmarks in comparable samples in the same period (Minami et al., 2007, 2012; e.g., compare with NHS data https://digital.nhs.uk/).

7. Decide the control group design

- **No control groups, 'uncontrolled-trial' (also called 'open-clinical trial'):** An experiment/clinical trial without control groups tests the hypothesis that participants have changed during an experimental treatment. The independent variable is 'client change'. However, it cannot be concluded that the treatment caused these changes, as it cannot be ruled out that clients would not have had these effects without treatment, such as spontaneous remission or natural maturation. The effects may be caused by the artificiality of the research context (e.g., Hawthorne effect), extraneous factors (events in the client's life or society), long-term social trends (secular drift), the inclination of clients with extreme scores on the baseline to shift towards the mean (regression to the mean) or changed perception of the measures (response shift). This study design may also have low construct validity due to possible confounders, expectancy or placebo effects and experimenter effects. However, uncontrolled trials may be the only feasible study design and give some initial indications of outcomes. Additional qualitative research may provide rich information about participants' subjective experiences of concepts related to therapeutic outcomes, processes, relationships, clients, and therapists.

- **One non-intervention or waiting-list control group, 'non-equivalent-groups':** Clients receiving the intervention/treatment are compared with those not receiving any intervention or those on a waiting list. This study design tests the hypothesis that clients receiving the experimental treatment experience significant positive effects and that these effects are larger than/equivalent to the effects in clients not receiving the treatment. Thus, the independent variable is whether or not participants receive an intervention. This design has also been described as an experimental study design with two levels (the experimental group and the control group). Any effects in the non-intervention group may be attributed to spontaneous remission, natural maturation, secular drift, regression to the mean, and extraneous variables; this study design may indicate that the effects in the intervention/treatment group are larger than such variables. However, this does not rule out the possibility that the participants improved due to expectancy effects, Hawthorne effects, and response shift, as clients may, for example, change because they expect to change. Clients may deteriorate because they know that they are not receiving treatment (nocebo effect). An alternative is a no-contact control group, in which participants are unaware they are participating in a study and have no contact with the researchers. Participants on a waiting list may be less inclined to fill in questionnaires than those receiving an intervention/treatment.

- **More than two control groups, multifactorial design:** Some studies include more than one control group. This is called 'multifactorial' as it measures more than the between-groups factor that examines differences between one experimental group and one control group. For example, a four-level clinical trial could test the effects of behavioural activation, cognitive-restructuring, anti-depressants, and placebo.

8. Decide parallel, crossed, and stratified study designs

- **Parallel-groups design**: Each participant is randomly assigned to one group, and all participants in this group receive/do not receive one intervention (most common).
- **Crossover design:** Participants receive with and do not receive multiple interventions in a random sequence.
- **Cross-over comparative-experimental design**: Two or more groups are compared with each other where they receive two interventions in a different order (intervention sequence 1-2 compared with intervention sequence 2-1).
- **Replicated cross-sectional design**: Individuals in a mental health service are followed from beginning to end with the same measurement instruments.
- **Cluster design:** Pre-existing groups of participants (e.g., villages, schools) are randomly selected to receive/not receive an intervention.
- **Stratification:** Participants are sorted into different groups before allocation, e.g., 'low-level depression with or high-level depression'. This may test for moderators or balance the groups on crucial variables.

9. Decide superiority trial or non-inferiority trial design

Decisions about control groups depend on whether you aim to conduct a superiority trial (assuming one treatment is best) or a non-inferiority trial (assuming your treatment is not worse than leading treatment options). The treatment control group needs to be bona fide (Wampold & Imel, 20015, active (e.g., more than reading a leaflet), and therapists need to believe in the treatment (Cuijpers et al., 2010).

- **Gold-standard control group:** This tests the hypothesis that the experimental treatment creates significant positive effects and that these effects are larger than the gold standard in the field. This design may indicate equal or larger effectiveness than existing treatments, which can be a powerful conclusion for policy-makers.
- **Care-as-usual control group:** Similar to the gold standard, but the control group may not necessarily be gold standard, such as receiving usual care in a health service.

- **Placebo control group**: A placebo is a non-specific intervention which does not contain any active ingredients expected to be effective, such as a psychopharmaceutical drug with no active ingredients. This tests the hypothesis that the experimental treatment creates significant positive effects and that these effects are larger than placebo effects. In psychological therapies, examples of placebo effects may include common therapy factors such as empathic listening, emotional support, and emotional expression (e.g., supportive-expressive therapy).

10. Decide randomisation of control groups

Participants can be randomly allocated to either the experimental group or the control group. Randomisation minimises selection bias as the researchers cannot consciously with or unconsciously preferentially enrol clients between treatment arms. Randomisation aims to maximise statistical power, particularly in sub-group analyses. However, RCTs may be biased due to the researcher preferring one condition (researcher-allegiance effects) or due to the experimental groups not staying equivalent. For example, in in-patient settings, clients in different study conditions may talk with each other, or therapists influence each other, and thus the effects from one condition may leak to other conditions. RCTs may also not take account of client preferences and clients dropping out due to not being allocated to their preferred treatment group. When designing clinical trials, consider the possible risks of bias, as described by authoritative guidelines (e.g., www.consort-statement.org).

- **Simple randomisation**: e.g., literal/digital coin-tossing
- **Restricted randomisation:** e.g., block-randomisation (an entire group is randomly allocated, e.g., one location in a multicentre trial)
- **Other:** e.g., adaptive biased-coin, covariate-adaptive, response-adaptive and outcome-adaptive randomisation

11. Decide blinding or no blinding

The allocation to either experimental or control condition can be concealed to prevent the participant, therapist, or researcher from knowing which treatment they receive. This prevents selection bias and confounders, and can be done via sequential numbers, sealed envelopes, or randomisation by an independent researcher. In medical research, blinding can be simple, as clients/doctors/researchers cannot see whether the active ingredients are in an unmarked pill or not; in psychotherapy research, blinding can be difficult because participants see/experience the therapeutic interventions.

- **Blind studies**: Participants do not know their condition.
- **Double-blind studies:** Experimenters and participants do not know the condition.
- **Triple-blind studies:** Experimenters, participants, and third-party outcome-assessors/statisticians do not know the condition.

12. Decide matching or no-matching

To improve comparability between participants, matched control groups match participants on particular characteristics. Matching may allow analysing the matched-variable, change, and attrition, with increased statistical power

13. Single-centre or multi-centre trials

To improve the ecological validity and generalisability and recruit more therapists with and clients, RCTs often include multiple sites or centres. Statistical tests (e.g., multi-level analysis, structural equation modelling) can test differences between sites. Researchers may also develop practice research networks involving many clinicians agreeing to collaborate in collecting and reporting data (Margison et al., 2000). The comparability of sites needs to be justified to prevent effects from being merely attributed to between-site differences.

14. Consider alternatives

Consider important, less-frequently used alternative experimental study designs. For example, improve ecological validity by embedding the trial in routine practice. Instead of focusing on comparing group means, examine variability, individual clients, time, personalised therapy, therapeutic responsiveness, treatment availability, ROM, assimilation studies, and number of sessions (Barkham, Hardy, & Mellor-Clark, 2010).

15. Record all effects

Do not merely include the primary measures you are interested in, but also other secondary measures.

Positive effects: Most likely, you are primarily interested in the positive effects of a treatment (e.g., 'how much improvement do clients experience in anxiety scores?'). Frequently used instruments to measure general distress include CORE-10, Outcome Questionnaire-45, and SCL-90; specific instruments measure depression (PHQ-9, BDI), anxiety (GAD-7, IES), or combined depression/anxiety (HADS, DASS-21, POMS). See Online Table 8.1 with frequently used questionnaires.

Validating instruments: As described in step 5, include multiple instruments to measure the same constructs to cross-validate your findings, particularly for your primary outcomes.

Negative effects: Always record and report adverse effects and critical incidents (Ioannidis et al., 2004), such as frequency, severity, reasons for withdrawal, and safety procedures. Consider questionnaires such as the Negative Effects Questionnaire.

Well-being with and quality-of-life instruments: A reduction in negative symptoms, such as anxiety, does not imply an increase in positive experiences, such as meaning in life or happiness. Consider questionnaires measuring positive affects (e.g., Meaning in Life Questionnaire; Positive Affect Negative Affect Scale; Life Optimism Scale; Scales of Well-Being; Satisfaction with Life Scale), self-esteem (Rosenberg's Self-Esteem Scale), and quality of life (WHO-QOL, SF-6D).

Social and behavioural instruments: Clients may improve in social and behavioural functioning (e.g., Inventory of Interpersonal Problems; Work and Social Adjustment Scale) or coping (e.g., COPE, Coping Flexibility Scale), although it has been argued that such scales may be less sensitive to detecting therapy change.

Therapy satisfaction: Consider examining how satisfied clients are with therapy, e.g., whether therapy has improved their life, their problems were solved, their perception of the therapist, and recommendations to others (e.g., Client Satisfaction Questionnaire).

Approach-specific instruments: Consider measuring changes in outcomes specific to your intervention, such as Young Schema Questionnaire in schema therapy or Meaning in Life Scale in meaning-centred therapy.

Client-tailored instruments: Standardised questionnaires may not reflect the client's goals. Therefore, clients may be asked to identify their therapy goals in the first session and rate the extent to which these have been achieved after the final session (e.g., Goal Attainment Form). Battle's Target Complaints and Shapiro's Personal Questionnaire instrument have also been used to examine clients about their most troublesome problems. Note that setting and measuring goal attainment positively impacts therapy outcomes (Harkin et al., 2016).

Expert-rated outcomes: Instead of asking clients to fill in questionnaires, experts could use a structured clinical interview (e.g., SCID), or rate clients, or ask therapists to evaluate their client's progress.

Significant others' ratings: Significant others may give valuable insight into client changes, particularly when clients may find self-evaluations difficult, such as with children (e.g., Child Behaviour Checklist; Youth Outcome Questionnaire), substance abuse, partner relationships (Dyadic Adjustment Scale), and group therapy (Group Session Rating Scale).

Cost-effectiveness instruments: Consider using cost-effectiveness instruments, for example, to measure health-care usage and loss of productivity (e.g., PRODISQ) in addition to general and health-specific quality-of-life instruments (e.g., SF-6D, WHOQOL, CORE-10, SCL-90, PHQ-9, GAD-7, IES, BDI).

Neurocognitive/biophysical-instruments: Consider adding neurocognitive or biophysical measures, such as body mass index (BMI), heart rate, skin conductance, fMRI with, CT/PET/SPECT/EEG/MEG scans, and hormone levels (e.g., stress-related) in saliva or blood, which may cross-validate other subjective measures (Mohlman, Deckersbach, & Weissman, 2015; Naji & Ekhtiari, 2016). However, some neurocognitive/biophysical tests may not be sufficiently sensitive to detect subtle changes, or they may not strongly correlate with subjective-psychological instruments. Do not go on an unfocused broad fishing-net expedition, as this may reduce your study's validity and statistical power. Instead, have specific hypotheses based on a clear conceptual framework explaining how the intervention/treatment may have the hypothesised neurocognitive/biophysical effects.

Cheating: You can design your study in such a way that you are guaranteed to detect large effects, even if such effects do not exist in reality: cheating by study design. Unfortunately, many therapy researchers seem to artifically increase the likelihood of false positive study results by having flawed study designs. The consequence can be big, as artificially inflated study results may be used by ignorant therapists and policy-makers. If we were to remove the artificial inflation of study findings, the conclusions about the effectiveness of certain therapy outcomes may be radically different (Cuijpers et al., 2012; Cuijpers & Cristea, 2016; Vos, Roberts & Davies, 2019). For example, if you want to positively bias your findings, use external raters who know whether an individual participates in therapy or not, use gross rating scales (e.g., change/no-change) instead of a nuanced score on a larger range of answer options, include only the worst clients who can only improve (ceiling effects), focus only on specific symptoms expected to change in therapy, do not include measures about negative side-effects and daily life changes, present correlations between questionnaires that (partially) measure the same underlying construct ('tautology') as important and unexpected findings, use a control group that you know will be ineffective (e.g. no-intervention or waiting-list group) or that is delivered by therapists who do not believe in the control intervention or have only been briefly trained in, therapists and researchers are the same person, directly or indirectly suggest to clients in the experimental condition that they are doing better than other groups, suggests to clients in the control condition that they are receiving an inferior intervention, selectively allocate clients to the experimental or control group, have a small selective sample, collect findings only immediately post-therapy, do not ask participants for their subjective experiences with open questions or interviews, avoid neurocognitive/biophysical measures, present only statistical signifance and not stastical effect size, do no not calculater eliable and clinically significant improvements after an intervention, or do not publish negative findings (cf. Cuijpers & Cristea, 2016; Lambert & Hill, 1994). Obviously, any form of cheating violates the scientific integrity and ethics, and is possibly even illegal. See the Likelihood of False Positive Results by Design Index, or Cheating Index, in Online Table 8.3.

16. Record mediators, moderators, and confounders

Researchers need to give convincing evidence for the causality in their clinical trial and reject alternative explanations. Therefore, consider measuring a range of possible mediators, moderators, and confounders (Garber & Hollon, 1991; Kazdin, 2007, 2009, 2021; Kraemer et al., 2001). Ideally, all variables are tested via complex statistical models, such as Structural Equation Modelling (SEM), although this could also be done via regression analysis (Baron & Kenny, 1986). However, using too many questionnaires may demotivate participants to fill in all the questionnaires and may decrease the statistical power of the study (consider adjusting statistical significance levels, e.g., via Bonferonni correction, and using powerful analytical methods such as SEM, Bayesian analysis, bootstrapping). This may include the following variables (Chapter 3 gives more examples):

Moderators: Client factors, e.g., socio-demographics, psychological-mindedness, self-insight, mentalisation, personality, and therapy preferences. Therapist factors, e.g., expertise, type of therapy. Moderators may include different sites/centres/research groups; ideally, such 'nests' are tested via multi-level analysis.

Mediators: Mediators explain the effects as hypothesised by the conceptual framework, such as measures of the therapy process (e.g., Helpful Aspects of Therapy, Session-Impact Scale, Session-Reactions Scale) and the therapeutic relationship (Working-Alliance Inventory, Session-Rating Scale, Relational-Depth-Frequency Scale). Test underlying therapeutic mechanisms and assumed aetiological models, such as the client's emotion regulation and ability to tolerate/accept difficult experiences (e.g., Acceptance-and-Action Questionnaire, Coping-Flexibility Scale, Cognitive-Emotion-Regulation Questionnaire). Therapists may fill in a therapist-competencies questionnaire for each session to examine the extent to which changes can be explained by the hypothesised therapist competencies (e.g., CBT-Competencies Scale). You may include measures for the extent of adherence to the treatment manual (e.g., Adherence-and-Competence Scale). For example, meaning-centred therapy seems to improve psychopathology and quality of life, and the client's improvements in meaning in life mediate these improvements (e.g., measured with meaning questionnaires); these mediated effects seem to confirm the assumed aetiology that a lack of meaning leads to psychopathology and that greater meaningfulness leads to better-well-being (Vos & Vitali, 2018).

Confounders: Test for possible confounders, for example, by measuring changes in socio-demographic questionnaires (Online Table 7.2) and the Stressful-Life-Events Questionnaires before and after therapy.

Open questions: Consider adding open and multiple-choice questions about the size, importance, and attribution of therapeutic change, for example in line with Elliott's Clients-Change Interview. This may further validate, extend and deepen the findings, and include the subjective perspectives of participants, that you may not completely grasp via pre-selected questionnaires with limited answer-options.

17. Pre-register

Many research journals expect researchers to pre-register or publish their research proposal before starting the clinical trial. Pre-registration stimulates transparency and validity, and prevents researchers from retrospectively changing their methods according to their findings. Example: OpenScienceFramework, ClinicalTrials.gov, EU Clinical Trials Register, WHO-ICTRP.

Step 4: Calculate *a priori* sample size and *a posteriori* power

Definition

Researchers want to conclude that the study findings are actually there and not caused by random or systematic error. One factor influencing the likelihood of error is sample size: we are more likely to find an effect caused by chance in a small sample. Therefore, before they conduct an experiment/clinical trial, quantitative researchers usually calculate the *a priori* sample size to identify findings that are actually there and not caused by error. After they have conducted the trial, they also calculate whether the actual sample size was large enough to interpret the research findings as highly likely true scores. This step is relevant when conducting statistical tests or clinical trials.

Explanation

Statistical power says how likely it is that a study has distinguished an actual effect from one by chance, i.e., the likelihood of avoiding a type II error. The higher the statistical power, the larger the chance of detecting a true effect, and thus the lower the risk of making a type II error and the more likely your findings are valid. For example, a power of 80% means that if there are true effects in 100 studies with 80% power, only 80 out of 100 statistical tests will actually detect them (i.e., 80% chance of finding significant results). If your study has low power, you have a small chance of detecting a true effect, and the results are questionable and possibly distorted by error. Many clinical trials are underpowered, so it may be difficult to derive reliable, and conclusions (Cuijpers, 2016). However, if your study has too much power, your tests are over-sensitive to true effects, including very small ones, such as statistically significant but non-clinically relevant effects. Therefore, researchers aim for a balanced power of 80%.

The following steps may increase the power. Increase the sample size. Use repeated measurement instruments, reducing effect size errors. Reduce sources of possible variability in the study design and sample. Use more precise psychometric instruments; a reliable and valid questionnaire is powerful because it detects any effects, even small ones. Change the significance level (α), which is the probability of a type I error, which means the probability of inaccurately rejecting the null hypothesis when it is actually true; e.g., describe 'statistical trends' between p = .10 and p = .05. Use directional tests (e.g., one-tailed significance instead of two-tailed).

Procedures

First, researchers need to make some hypotheses:

- **Anticipated effect size:** Expected standardised effect sizes derived from a previous study or feasibility study. Ideally, anticipated effects are adjusted for confounders; e.g., when considering therapist effects, you may need larger samples and specific measures tailored to the research setting (Schiefele et al., 2017).

- **One-tailed or two-tailed effects:** Change is expected in any direction (you do not know yet whether this will be positive or negative; 'two-tailed') or effect is expected in a specific direction (you expect a positive effect but not a negative effect, or vice versa; 'one-tailed').
- **Desired power**: 80% by consensus.
- **Significance level:** The significance level, usually 5%. As explained in step 9, reduce if you have many estimations in your study (e.g., Bonferroni correction).
- **Other information:** In multiple regression: number of predictors; in hierarchical regression: number of predictors in both sets; in SEM: number of latent and observed variables.

Second, researchers insert this information into statistical software or an online *a priori* sample calculator (e.g., G*power, danielsoper.com). This tells the required number of participants to detect the anticipated effect size with sufficient statistical power.

Step 5: Select instruments

Definition

Instead of reinventing the wheel, researchers often use pre-developed measurement instruments (Online Table 8.1 shows the most frequently used questionnaires in therapy research). This step starts with an explanation of the five types of quality criteria defining a good measurement instrument: validity, reliability, sensitivity, specificity, interpretability/understandability, and item response theory (Figure 8.1) (see cosmin.nl). Move to the next section for practical applications (see Online Table 8.4. for an example how to describe an instrument)

Explanation

Imagine a researcher wants to understand a sample's mean intelligence level. We call a psychological concept such as intelligence a 'construct' (Chapter 3 used the more generic term 'concept'). Most constructs are not known directly ('latent'). For example, we cannot directly see someone's intelligence. First, the researcher needs to formulate the construct in terms that can easily be measured, e.g., deciding the type of intelligence they are interested in and the type of performance they would expect for different intelligence levels. This definition needs to be operationalised precisely to ensure this is what the researcher wants to know. Second, they use this definition of the construct to select or develop a measure such as an IQ test, which may give indications about a latent construct like intelligence. Questionnaires could measure many constructs, such as:

- **Cognitions:** e.g., thoughts, attitudes, expectations, opinions, memories
- **Affects:** e.g., emotions, feelings, moods, bodily experiences
- **Complex constructs less accessible for direct self-reflection:** e.g., personality, IQ, projective tests
- **Intensity:** e.g., pain level
- **Behaviour**: e.g., actions, social interactions, skills, performance, behavioural observation
- **Neurocognitive/biophysical:** e.g., heart rate, skin conductance, brain activity, hormonal levels, immune functioning

Components

The selection or development of a measure should be made carefully to ensure that you measure the construct you are interested in and can rely on the findings.

Reliability

A reliable instrument consistently measures what it has to measure: it does not suffer from measurement errors. Imagine we are wearing magic glasses and see the true temperature we are measuring; a completely reliable thermometer reports the true temperature every time we use it. 'Reliable' means that the scores are similar for repeated measurements under different conditions. An instrument can be unreliable due to systematic bias (e.g., skewed/leading questions in the questionnaire) or random bias (e.g., researcher misreading data); in both cases, the instrument will not show the true scores. The following are common types of reliability:

- **Internal consistency:** The degree of inter-relatedness between items/parts in the questionnaire. Example: Cronbach's alpha for overall scale, scale if item deleted; split half reliability (i.e., consistency between two halves of an instrument); Kuder-Richardson for dichotomous items.
- **Test-retest reliability:** Consistent findings over time, e.g., correlations between two measurements.
- **Intra-rater reliability:** Consistent findings for the same assessor on different measurement-moments (e.g., correlations).
- **Inter-rater reliability:** The agreement between two or more assessors (e.g., Kappa).

Validity

An instrument is valid if it measures the construct(s) it aims to measure, so inferences made from it are appropriate, meaningful, and useful: a valid instrument measures what it claims to measure. There are many different types of validity, with some overlapping. Validity includes aspects requiring conceptual reasoning that may not be proven by testing.

- **Content validity:** The degree to which the questions, tasks or items in the questionnaire are representative of all possible content:
  - **Face validity:** The instrument looks valid to relevant stakeholders, e.g., researchers, therapists, clients, focus groups, and interviewees. A rule of thumb is that if a test is frequently cited in the literature, people will likely believe in its face value.
  - **Content validity of instrument development:** This is not a formal type of validity but may be helpful to consider. Use your general knowledge of your field: e.g., a questionnaire on depression should not leave out any diagnostic symptoms/criteria stated by authorities (e.g., DSM/ICD), and have been developed by experts, based on systematic literature reviews.
- **Construct validity:** The degree to which the scores of an instrument are consistent with hypotheses: when you apply the instrument, you find the expected results. For example, you find that items are homogeneous, individuals experience an expected change in scores over time, and individual pre-/post-differences in experiments are as expected.

- o **Structural validity:** Some instruments have multiple scales/sub-scales, explaining the structure/dimensions of the underlying construct. Exploratory factor analysis identifies factors in your dataset that you may not have considered before (e.g., via principal-components analysis; the number of factors is usually decided by Eigenvalues > 1, factor number before elbow in scree plot, total variance explained, meaningfulness/interpretability; factors are interpreted with Varimax rotation). Confirmatory factor analysis tests whether a hypothetical factor structure, such as sub-scales in a pre-published questionnaire, can be found in the data (e.g., via SEM).
- o **Ecological validity:** The instrument has been developed and can be used in real-life settings, e.g., developed with clinical experts, therapists, and clients, and tested in clinical settings.
- o **Cross-cultural validity:** The instrument has been tested in multicultural groups in multiple countries.
- o **Hypotheses testing (sometimes called external validity):** The ability to generalise findings, for example to other situations and individuals, e.g., replication studies.
- **Criterion validity:** An instrument significantly correlates with someone's performance on other tests and time (= 'criterion'):
  - o **Concurrent validity**: For example, different questionnaires in one survey correlate with each other (e.g., GAD-7 and PHQ-9). Different instruments can measure similar constructs (convergent validity, expecting large significant correlations) or dissimilar constructs (divergent validity, expecting not-significant or small correlations). This may be shown in a multi-trait multi-method matrix.
  - o **Predictive validity:** For example, baseline scores significantly predict outcome scores (e.g., regression analyses/repeated measures, longitudinal study).

Sensitivity, responsiveness, and precision

Researchers want to select an instrument sensitive enough to detect a phenomenon or clinically relevant changes. Formally said, a sensitive instrument reports true-positive findings (e.g., the instrument shows a participant is depressed who is actually depressed) and does not show false-negatives (e.g., the instrument shows a participant is not-depressed who is actually depressed; Figure 8.2). A sensitive instrument does not only detect large changes, for example between baseline measurement before the first therapy session and a follow-up measurement at the end of all sessions, but can also detect small changes, such as changes in scores between each therapy session. Researchers can check that an instrument has detected subtle effects in similar studies.

Although sensitivity to change and responsiveness are often used hand-in-hand, responsiveness does not merely regard the detected effect sizes in clinical trials but also its association with standards in the field. For example, an anxiety questionnaire may detect an improvement in anxiety symptoms, which therapists may confirm via clinical interviews, client change interviews or client-based transition scales. Even though responsiveness may be clinically relevant, responsiveness is rarely systematically examined (see Chapter 3).

The precision of an instrument describes the accuracy of its scores in different samples, free from measurement error. A researcher wants the instrument only to detect the phenomenon they are interested in and nothing else, like a precise body thermometer only picks up body temperature, not room temperature. In therapy research, this is usually described with reliability or item response theory. In medical research, this can be discussed separately, alongside the terminology 'false-positives' and 'false-negatives' (Table 8.1). Receiver operating characteristic (ROC) curves show false-positive rates on the x-axis and true-positive rates on the y-axis, which can be helpful to predict rare binary events (SPSS:analyze>ROC).

Item response theory

Most novice researchers may not use item response theory (IRT), but IRT is nowadays often regarded a gold standard for instrument development (Van der Linden, 2017). IRT is a modern test theory assessing how well a questionnaire works as well as individual items while taking into account differences between participants filling in the questionnaire. For example, classical tests insufficiently consider the problem that answer items on a Likert scale often have unequal intervals; participants may, for instance, interpret the difference between 'a bit' (score '1') and 'moderate' ('2') as larger or smaller than the difference between 'very much' ('3') and 'moderate' ('2'). IRT takes into account the different levels or characteristics of the items and how participants perform, e.g., individuals with varying levels of intelligence or attitudes answer items differently. IRT is also more flexible than classical test theory, as it allows item banking (i.e., participants can be given different sets of items, for example, to prevent cheating) and adaptive testing (i.e., tailoring the difficulty of items to each individual).

IRT uses mathematical functions to model how participants respond to items. The item response function (IRF) gives the probability that a person with a given ability-level will answer correctly (IRF is lower in participants with lower abilities and higher in participants with larger abilities). The simplest IRT model, Rasch analysis, use the parameter 'difficulty of an item' to predict at which difficulty level a participant will select this item (e.g., '3' on a 1-to-5 scale). Rasch analysis helps to develop unidimensional instruments in which items range from easy to difficult. This can help researchers to select the best rating scale categories, differentiate clinical groups ('strata'), order, delete, or add items, and examine whether different populations have different interpretations of the items and rating scale categories. As the Rasch model is created from the data, look for the statistical significance (p < .05).

Whereas Rasch analysis only includes the parameter 'item-difficulty' (1-parameter-logistic-model; 1PL), other IRT-models also include item discrimination (the extent to which the item is measuring the underlying construct (2-parameter-logistic-model; 2PL), and the extent to which candidates can guess the correct answer (3-parameter-logistic-model; 3PL). Before they collect data, researchers develop the ideal 2PL/3PL model and subsequently test how well this ideal model fits the data; therefore, in a 2PL/3PL study, look for the author's description of goodness-of-fit (e.g., Chi-Square p > .05).

Procedures

Socio-demographic variables: Do not forget to ask socio-demographic questions to be able to describe the sample, interpret data, and justify generalisability.

Informal shortcut: Researchers often select instruments popular in their field, to enable comparison (e.g., Online Table 8.1). Search for the most cited publications on topics similar to yours, examine their instruments, check their methodology sections, and assess how the instruments work in their study (e.g., check sensitivity, face validity, interpretability, concurrent/predictive validity).

Formal instrument selection: Figure 8.3 describes a possible formal procedure to select an instrument. After defining the construct, decide whether you want a measure that is nomothetic (i.e., with clinical/non-clinical norm groups to compare scores), includes criteria references, or is idiographic (without norms/criteria, e.g., Q sorts, repertory grids). When scrolling through titles and abstracts in search engines, informally assess the instruments' face validity and interpretability. Search for literature reviews on the instrument and/or validation studies, and read the full text to assess reliability and validity (e.g., assess with the help of checklists such as cosmin.nl). Also search for studies applying this instrument in similar samples as yours, to examine its sensitivity. Try out the instrument in an informal or formal feasibility study to explore its preliminary acceptability, reliability, concurrent and structural validity, and sensitivity (although the sample size may be too small to detect significant effects).

Table 8.1 Overview of sensitivity and specificity

		The truth		
		Positive (e.g., has disorder)	Negative (e.g., does not have disorder)	
Finding with instrument	Positive (e.g., has the disorder)	True positive (TP)	False positive (FP)	Positive predictive values (PPV) = TP/TP+FP
	Negative (e.g., does not have the disorder)	False negative (FN)	True negative (TN)	Negative predictive values (NPV) = TN/TN+FN
		Sensitivity = TP/TP+FN	Specificity =TN/ TN+FP	

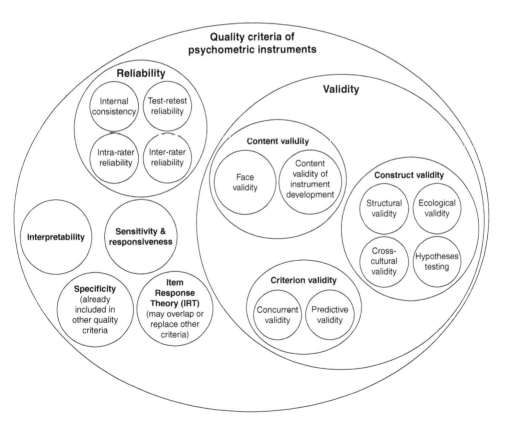

Figure 8.2 Quality criteria of psychometric instruments

Step 1: Operational definition of construct
- Formal term & synonyms
- Specific: what is it
- Sensitive: what is it not
- Defining criteria/dimensions (if relevant)
- Indication what different levels mean (e.g. few versus many symptoms)

Step 2: Decide selection of nomothetic, norm-referenced or idiographic measures
- Nomothetic: norm-group available
- Criterion-reference: criteria/cut-off-scores available
- Idiographic: no norm-groups or criteria

Step 3: Search literature for relevant instruments
- **Check lists of popular instruments** (e.g. online table 8.1.)
- **Search-engines dedicated to instrument studies** (e.g. PsycTest)
- **General scientific search-engines** (chapter 5)
- **Google:** websites giving an overview of instruments on a topic *
*Search terms = topic + (questionnaire OR instrument OR scale OR inventory)

Step 4: Informally assess content-validity & interpretability in any article
To get an initial impression and informally assess the instrument, any article in which the instrument was reviewed, developed, tested or used can be used in this step
- **Face-validity:** e.g., Does it make sense? Is the questionnaire used frequently?
- **Interpretability:** e.g., Can I understand and interpret findings?

Step 5: Formally assess reliability & validity in an instrument-development/validation/review study
Prioritise any formal psychometric review of the instrument which will summarise the quality-criteria; alternatives are a recent validation-study or application-study which will most likely start with a literature review of the quality of this instrument
- **Instrument development:** e.g., Developed by experts? Follows evidence & guidelines?
- **Internal reliability:** e.g. split-half reliabiliy, Cronbach's alpha, Kudar-Richardson
- **Test-retest reliability:** e.g. correlations between time-measurements
- **Intra-rater & inter-rater reliability:** relevant for instruments with multiple raters
- **Structural validity:** dimensions/sub-scales, e.g. factor-analysis/SEM, reliability sub-scales
- **Concurrent-validity:** e.g., correlations with other instruments as expected
- **Item Response Theory** (IRT studies not always available): e.g. significant Rasch-model; 3PL-model fits the data well (e.g. Chi-Squared p>-05)

Step 6: Formally assess reliability & validity in application-studies or validation-studies in which instrument is used
Select a study that validated or applied the instrument, preferably recently published in a sample similar to your research-project
- **Extra info:** these studies may confirm or give additional evidence for step 5 (e.g. confirmatory factor analysis whereas previous studies only did exploratory factor-analysis)
- **Ecological validity:** does this instrument work well in situations and samples outside the lab, like the context and sample of my study?
- **Cross-cultural validity:** is the study replicated in other cultures & culture of my study?
- **Predictive-validity:** can questionnaire predict outcomes, e.g. longitudinal or clinical trial?
- **Sensitivity and responsiveness:** studies that used the questionnaire found small, medium and large effects, particularly in a sample and intervention similar to my study?

Step 7: Evaluate previous steps & search for specific studies for unclear specific quality-criteria
The previous steps may not have given sufficient or convincing information for each of the quality-criteria. You may want to search in academic search-engines for specific studies that report this quality-criterion of this instrument.

Step 8: Synthesise information
Examine all the information you have found about the instrument.
- **Informal assessment and synthesis:** use your common sense and academic skills to conclude whether the evidence is sufficient for the quality of this instrument (there are no strict guidelines about when an instrument is good enough to use in your study)
- **Formal assessment and synthesis:** Use a quality assessment tool for psychometric instruments, e.g. COSMIN (c)osmin.nl

Step 9: Decide which instrument to use in your study

Step 10: Feasibility study
Try-out the questionnaire in a small sample (feasibility study), e.g. before you conduct a large survey or clinical-trial based on these findings, decide to use this instrument in a larger study, or continue looking for a better instrument.
- **Qualitative experience:** Ask participants how it was for them to fill in this questionnaire (e.g. use Three-Step-Test Interview from Hak et al.)
- **Preliminary face validity:** e.g. can you understand the findings
- **Preliminary reliability:** e.g. test-retest, split half, scale-if-item-deleted, intra/inter-rater
- **Preliminary concurrent validity:** e.g. correlations with other questionnaires
- **Preliminary structural validity:** e.g. factor-analysis, reliability of sub-scales
- **Preliminary sensitivity and responsiveness:** e.g. variation in scores between participants, any effects (NB: due to the small sample-size, you may not pick up small effects)

Short-cut

Check recently published studies on topics and samples similar to your research-project:

- **Instrument selection:** which instrument have they selected

- **Face validity:** does this instrument make sense

- **Interpretability:** can you interpret the findings with this instrument?

- **Quality description** how do they describe the quality of the instrument (they may have already done steps 4-10 for you)?

- **Concurrent-validity** do they report correlations of this instrument with other instruments as you would expect?

- **Predictive-validity:** does this instrument predict outcomes or effects in this study?

- **Ecological and cross-cultural validity:** is this instrument used in a similar sample and culture as your study?

Figure 8.3 Procedures for selecting instruments (see explanation in text)

Limitation: Researchers may be overenthusiastic and add many questionnaires. However, each extra question/item adds approximately 7.5 seconds to the total time that it takes a participant to fill in the questionnaire. The longer a questionnaire is, the less likely research participants are to participate and to fill in all questions. It may also not be needed to use multiple questionnaires due to the high correlations between instruments (e.g. high correlations between scores on anxiety, depression and general distress questionnaires). For example, different mental health questionnaires may measure one common factor 'general mental health' and not all questionnaires may be needed to measure this (Bohnke, Lutz & Delgadillo, 2014; De Beurs, Boehnke & Fried, 2021). To detect change, it may also not be needed to for example use all questionnaires at each measurement-moment, for example only after each fourth therapy session instead of after each session.

Step 6: Develop an instrument

Definition

Researchers may want to develop an instrument to conduct a one-time-only survey or create an instrument that can be used in future studies (Figure 8.1). This section explains how to develop a psychometric instrument (Figure 8.4). Good books on scale development include Carpenter, 2018; DeVellis & Thorpe, 2021; Gregory, 2014; and on surveys Blair, Czaja, & Blair, 2013.

Procedures

1. Define constructs

Clearly define the constructs and sub-constructs you aim to measure (Chapter 3): 'This questionnaire aims to measure [construct X], including sub-scales for [sub-constructs X1, X2, ...]'. A construct refers to a latent concept you are interested in. The construct can be defined based on a systematic literature review (Chapters 3, 5), focus groups or interviews with stakeholders (clients, researchers, therapists). Delphi-groups may help develop agreement about a definition in multiple iterations (Haynes & Shelton, 2018; Keeney, McKenna, & Hasson, 2011).

2. Decide open/closed questions

Consider whether you want to use questions with pre-determined answer options or have open answer options. For closed questions, consider whether you want to give the answer option 'prefer not to answer' and an option 'other: ...' followed by their own answer.

3. Decide scale of measurement

- **Nominal scale:** Answers can be named but not ordered. Can be used for statistical description, e.g., means and frequencies. For example, the question 'what is your gender' could have the options 'male', 'female', 'other', but these options cannot be ordered as no gender is larger/smaller.
- **Ordinal scale:** Answers can be named and ordered, but the distance between answers is unequal/unknown. Can be used for statistical description, e.g., means and frequencies. For example, the question 'what is your highest education' could have the answer options 'primary school', 'secondary school', and 'higher education'.

- **Interval scale:** Answers can be named and ordered with equal distances. A ratio scale is the same as an interval scale and has a value of '0', such as 'number of years in education'. Interval/ratio scales can be used for most statistical tests. Many questions on nominal/ordinal scales are treated as if they are interval/ratio. However, we do not know whether the differences between answer categories are equal distances (e.g., five-point scale: 1, completely disagree; 2, somewhat disagree; 3, neither agree nor disagree; 4, somewhat agree; 5, completely agree); it is uncertain that each participant perceives the difference between 'completely disagree' and 'somewhat disagree' as equally as large as the difference between 'somewhat agree' and 'completely agree'.
- **Binary/dichotomous scale:** Two answer options (0, 1). For example, a researcher creates a dichotomous dummy variable to code 'included in analysis' (1) and 'excluded from analyses' (0). Often requires specific statistical analysis, e.g., Loglinear regression. Sometimes treated as an interval variable.

4. Decide question format

- **Bullet points, tick boxes:** For questions on nominal/ordinal scales.
- **Rating scales, visual scales:** For questions on interval or ratio scales.
- **Rating scales:** For questions on ratio scales, can be used in most statistical tests. Includes a summated rating score, known as a Likert scale (e.g., the participant is asked to give a score on a range between 1 and 5), semantic differentials (two poles with numbers in between), a scale with equal-appearing intervals, also known as a Thurstone scale (e.g., the participant is asked to select an answer from agree/disagree), or a cumulative scale, also known as a Guttman scale (e.g., the answers from participants are ordered in cumulative order). Rating scales either assume a categorical order (ordinal) or equal distances between categories (interval), even though it may not be proven that this is the participant's actual perception (Online Table 8.5 shows frequently used Likert scales).
- **Visual scales:** For questions on ratio scale, useable with most statistical tests. Includes visual numerical scales, visual categorical scales with or without pictograms, and visual analogue scales.

5. Generate initial pool of items

It is not easy to develop good questions. A good question meets the following quality criteria as Step 3 in Chapter 9 explains: falsifiable, non-leading, non-assumptive, clear, non-ambiguous, specific but open, as simple as possible, not double barred, requires little self-insight/self-awareness, ethical, non-intrusive, not triggering of defence mechanisms or socially desirable answers, non-comparing, with correct word use, and preferably with the option of not answering. Poorly formulated questions could lead to unreliable and invalid findings, and supervisors/reviewers/examiners may reject all the questionnaire data and may require the researcher to develop or select new questionnaires and collect new data.

- **Derive questions from personal expertise** (not recommended)
- **Derive questions from systematic literature review** (recommended)
- **Invite experts/stakeholders to generate items** (recommended; e.g., invite researchers, therapists, clients in a Delphi study; Carpenter, 2018)

6. Assess the quality of items and select the best items

The researchers assess the aforementioned quality criteria for each item.

- **Researcher's informal assessment and selection (not recommended)**
- **Researcher's formal assessment and selection:** e.g., see self-reflective questions in Online Table 8.2
- **Invite experts/stakeholders to rate items:** (recommended) e.g., assess each item with evaluation questions (on a five-point Likert scale: 1, not at all, to 5, completely): 'to what extent does this item measure the concept?', 'to what extent is this a good formulation (e.g., non-ambiguous, clear, no double-barred question)?', 'to what extent would you recommend including this item in the questionnaire?' (Develis, 2016). Alternative questions regard clarity, representativeness, and comprehensiveness.
- **Delphi method:** Two or more iterations of questionnaires are administered to an expert panel (Keeney, McKenna, & Hasson, 2011). In the first iteration, experts are asked their opinion about a topic in an open manner (e.g., to develop a definition), which may subsequently lead to the generation of questions; in the next iteration, questions are rated until consensus is achieved. Modified Delphi methods may use structured questionnaires with Likert scales based on literature reviews (Hsu & Sandford, 2007). Although no strict guidelines exist, researchers often use between 10 and 50 experts (Linstone, Turoff, & Helmer, 2002), although smaller samples may be more practical. Consensus may be assumed when between 51% and 80% of experts agree or when stable over multiple iterations (Keeney, McKenna, & Hasson, 2011). Experts may be given the findings from previous iterations for feedback. Findings can be calculated via descriptive statistics (e.g., means, SD, Kappa).
- **Content validity index:** This describes the number of experts rating an item favourably divided by the number of experts (Lynn, 1986).

7. Conduct feasibility study

The researcher tries out the instrument to assess its acceptability and feasibility. This could be done informally, for example by inviting colleagues to fill it in and give feedback. In formal instrument development, researchers conduct a feasibility study to uncover potential problems in scale construction, preferably in a random sample representing the target audience. Researchers may use a pretesting method such as the Three-Step Test Interview to test and adjust the items (Hak, van der Veer, & Jansen, 2004):

- **Concurrent think-aloud**: Participants say their thoughts aloud while completing the instrument, to make the participants' thought processes observable (e.g., record pauses, reactions to scale items, fatigue, other behaviour).
- **Focused interview:** Researchers ask participants for direct feedback on their thought processes, to understand better what was going on for the participants.
- **Semi-structured interview:** Researchers ask for participants' reflections, opinions, and experiences of completing the scale, e.g., 'How was it to complete the scale?', 'What feelings were triggered, if any?', 'Can you give any feedback or recommendations?', 'Were the instructions clear?', 'Which items were unclear?'

8. Next studies

A pilot study tries out a questionnaire before it is tested on a larger scale, which can help to detect flaws, and identify its preliminary quality and effect sizes (Leon, Davis, & Kraemer, 2011). Subsequent studies may include different groups to establish norm groups and cut-off criteria for the scores; for example, clinical instruments which have been tested in clinical and non-clinical samples. Replication studies by other research groups can dismiss the criticism that the initial pilot/validation studies were biased as the original instrument developers conducted the study.

- **Ecologically valid sample:** Study in a random sample with diverse socio-demographic characteristics, representative of the target population, preferably in daily life contexts representative of the context in which the questionnaire will most likely be used.
- **Cross-cultural validity:** Study in culturally diverse samples in multiple countries to test the construct's presence, reliability, and validity across cultures. The translation should follow formal procedures (Harkness, Pennell, & Schoua-Glusberg, 2004).
- **Test internal reliability:** For example, test Cronbach's alpha for overall scale and scale if item deleted, calculate split-half reliability or Kuder-Richardson test for dichotomous items.
- **Test-retest reliability:** Participants fill in the questionnaires at different time-points; test correlations/prediction between measurements.
- **Intra-rater/inter-rater reliability:** Calculate reliability between and within multiple raters (if relevant).
- **Structural validity:** Test dimensional/factor structure with exploratory factor analysis (e.g., principal component analysis) in the feasibility study and confirmatory factor analysis in validation studies (e.g., SEM).
- **Concurrent validity:** Test correlations with other questionnaires measuring similar constructs (convergent validity) and dissimilar constructs (divergent validity).
- **Predictive validity/hypotheses testing:** Use repeated measures to test whether early scores predict later scores on this or other questionnaires (e.g., regression analysis or SEM).
- **Sensitivity:** Use the questionnaire to detect changes/differences within and between individuals (e.g., SD, outliers, effect size). Consider using a clear criterion/standard in the field as an anchor, e.g., a clinical interview to confirm observations.
- **IRT:** Gold standard in instrument development.

Step 7: Select a statistical test

Definition

This step helps you select a statistical test. Usually, each well-defined research objective requires one statistical test. For example, the objective 'testing the pre-post effects of CBT for cynophobia' may be tested with a t-test. Each test has a null hypothesis (H0), e.g., 'no significant effect' and one or more alternative hypothesis (Ha/H1), e.g., 'significant effect'.

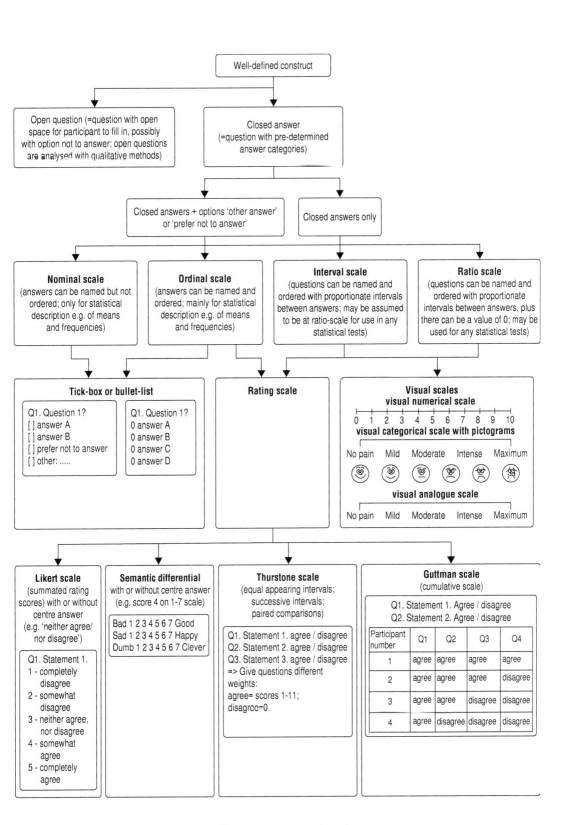

Figure 8.4 Steps in developing questions for a survey or questionnaire

Procedures

1. Identify your research objective
2. Identify the appropriate test

Use the decision-tree in Figure 8.5 to select the appropriate test, fitting your objective and variables. Note the differences between parametric and non-parametric tests, as Table 8.2 explains. Many tests use relatively similar procedures and mathematical calculations; choose the test with or model with the largest statistical power and/or the simplest test/model ('parsimony').

3. Read about the test's assumptions

Table 8.3 exemplifies some of the assumptions of common statistical tests (double check all assumptions, e.g. via statistics handbooks). For example, t-tests can only be done on normally distributed variables. A nominal variable does not have an order in the values (e.g., answer options male, 1, female, 2, non-binary, 3); an ordinal variable has values that can be ordered but their differences are unclear (e.g., 'primary school', 1, 'secondary school', 2, 'higher education', 3). Sometimes Likert with, Thrustone/Guttman scales and dichotomous dummy variables are treated as if they are interval/ratio/continuous variables with parametric tests. Learn when to select and how to interpret tests via handbooks, internet search, or the manual of statistical software (e.g., extensive help function in IBM-SPSS).

4. Do preparatory analyses (see Step 8)

For example, check the assumptions (e.g., normal distribution). If assumptions are not met, change the dataset (e.g., remove outliers, transform data) or select tests without these assumptions.

5. Do the test in statistical software

As IBM-SPSS is frequently used in therapy research, the next sections will refer to this, but other software can be used, e.g., R, SAS, Excel.

6. Interpret findings (see Step 9)

Examples

Describing a variable

Describe variables (e.g., median, mean, standard deviation, frequencies, skewness, kurtosis), and visualise variables (e.g., using bar charts, box plots, histograms, P-P plots for time series) (SPSS:analyze>descriptive-statistics>frequencies). If a questionnaire includes tick boxes with multiple answer options (e.g., 'tick all that apply'), describe the frequency of each answer option separately as a dichotomous dummy variable (SPSS:analyze>multiple-response). Examine author guidelines from journals and APA-JARS publication guidelines on what to report.

One sample case test

Test whether a score from one participant differs from the sample mean (SPSS:compare-means>means).

Compare sample with a criterion

Test whether your sample mean differs from a criterion, e.g., lower/larger than a clinical cut-off score (SPSS:compare-means>means).

Analyse clusters and similarities between answers

Imagine you have a set of variables describing participant characteristics and interests, and you want to predict which types of participants are interested in particular treatments. Use cluster analysis to create 'clusters' (i.e., groups) based on similarities between participants, and maximise distances between clusters. Hierarchical cluster analysis generates multiple solutions, K-means cluster analysis uses clusters pre-defined by the researcher, and two-step cluster analysis combines both (SPSS:analyze>classify). Multidimensional scaling analyses data on multiple dimensions, such as client preferences of therapy types and health centres; you may find an underlying dimension, e.g., the humanistic approach of their preferred therapies and centres (SPSS:analyze>scale>multidimensional). Discriminant analysis builds a predictive model for group membership, e.g., multiple variables predict whether participants have particular diagnoses (SPSS:analyze>classify>discriminate). Nearest neighbor analysis classifies cases based on their similarity to other cases (SPSS:analyze>scale>nearest-neighbour). Distances examine similarities/dissimilarities between variables or cases (SPSS: analyze>scale>distances).

Test psychometric instruments

Step 5 already described how to examine psychometric instruments, e.g., reliability analysis and IRT (SPSS:analyze>scale). Conduct explorative factor analysis for new scales (SPSS:analyze>data-reduction), and SEM for confirmative factor analysis for scales with known factors/subscales/dimensions. To compare diagnostic tests, ROC plots sensitivity versus specificity, with accuracy shown as the area under the curve (SPSS:analyze>classify>ROC).

Describing relationships between variables

Calculate correlations between two parametric variables with Pearson's Correlation (SPSS:analyze>correlate). Associations between non-parametric variables can be described and tested in multiple ways (SPSS:analyze>descriptives>crosstabs). Describe associations between nominal variables with Chi-Square, between ordinal variables with Spearman's Rank, and between dichotomous variables with McNemar's Test. Non-parametric associations may also be examined via optimal scaling (e.g., non-linear canonical correlations, PRINCALS, and HOMALS). Use Eta if one variable is categorical and one continuous, and Kappa to describe agreement between raters.

Predicting variables

Use one or more predictors, such as therapy characteristics ('independent variable') to predict one or more predicted variables, such as therapy outcomes ('dependent variable'): predictor/independent-variable → predicted/dependent-variable (SPSS:analyze>regression). Simple regression analysis uses one predictor to predict one outcome, and multiple regression analysis uses multiple variables. Hierarchical regression includes multiple predictors in blocks, e.g., to answer the question 'what is the effect of COVID-related stress on psychopathology, after controlling for age and gender?', the first block includes age and gender and the next psychopathology. Predictors can be inserted in regression analysis one at a time ('stepwise'; this is the most frequently used), entered all at once like a block ('enter'), removed in a single step from a block ('remove'), or all predictors are added like a block and subsequently the worst variables are deleted one-by-one ('backwards').

Regression analysis usually assumes a linear relationship between predictors and predicted variables, which can for example be examined via scatterplots. If there is a non-linear relationship, you may transform variables (see Step 9), or use alternatives, such as non-linear regression analysis or quantile-regression, to examine medians instead of means. To predict dichotomous or dummy variables (e.g., 0, no-suicide, 1, suicide) use binary logistic regression, such as predicting which personality characteristics are risk factors for suicide; use multinomial logistic regression for a set of predictors not restricted to two categories, such as personality characteristics predicting therapy preference. Ordinal variables can be used in ordinal logistic regression, and nominal variables in multinomial logistic regression or optimal scaling of categorical regression analysis. Survival analysis ('time-to-event analysis') examines the time it takes before an event occurs, e.g., death, failure (time on x-axis, survival probability on y-axis); Kaplan-Meier Curves compare independent groups on time to a dichotomous outcome, and Cox-Proportional Hazards control for demographic/clinical variables (SPSS:analyze>survival).

Frequency counts can be classified in multiple ways. General loglinear models analyse an Odd's Ratio of how frequency counts (continuous dependent variable) fall into categories (categorical independent variable), such as the relationship between number of people receiving therapy and whether a suicide was successful (SPSS:analyze>loglinear). Logit loglinear models analyse the relationship between a categorical dependent variable and a categorical independent variable, with possible continuous covariate variables, such as how does the clients' food type vary with their body weight and the types of rural/urban regions in which they live? Probit analysis can be used for dose-response analysis, analysing how effective a proportion/amount of an intervention/treatment is, e.g., number of therapy sessions.

There are regression analyses for special situations. If you do not have randomised control groups in a clinical trial, use a regression-discontinuity design: assign a cut-off/threshold above/below which an intervention is assigned, and calculate the average treatment effect by comparing observations close to either side of the threshold. If you have an observational study design without randomised control groups, consider propensity-score-matching to account for covariates predicting receiving treatment (e.g., predict receiving a diagnosis with multiple predictors). If the variance of a variable is not constant, such as cases high on an attribute varying more than cases low on that attribute, use weighted least-squares regression analysis. Use partial least-squares regression analysis if predictors are correlated or if there are more predictors than cases. Use two-stage least-squares regression if the errors of independent and dependent variables correlate. Use linear mixed models when variables exhibit correlated and non-constant variability. Use generalised estimating equations for repeated measurements or correlated/clustered observations. Use Kernel-Ridge regression analysis to model linear and non-linear relationships between dependent and independent variables. Use Tobit analysis, if scores on dependent variables are partially censored/truncated. Use ridge/lasso/linear-elastic-net analysis if independent variables correlate. Use Monte-Carlo to estimate possible outcomes of uncertain events, e.g., to predict/simulate long-term outcomes with multiple predictors.

Describing differences

Researchers may want to test differences between groups, such as an experimental group and control groups. Independent samples t-tests compare two groups with different individuals, e.g., depressed versus non-depressed individuals. Paired samples t-tests compare two pairs of observations in one group, such as baseline score and outcome score in the same individuals (SPSS:analyze>compare-means). Studies often include multiple measurement instruments. Doing multiple t-tests for each instrument increases the risk of a type I error. Therefore, select a test that can analyse multiple measurements at once, including their relations to each other, particularly if expecting correlations or interactions between measures.

One-way ANOVA analyses variances between two or more variables, such as differences between treatments (CBT, placebo, waiting list) in the incidence of depression (ANOVA assumes categorical independent variables, and normally distributed dependent variables) (SPSS:analyze>general-linear-model). Two-way/factorial ANOVA uses multiple categorical independent factors (e.g., effects of small/medium/large social contact, unemployed/employed/retired job status on depressive symptoms). MANOVA has multiple dependent variables, and ANCOVA/MANCOVA controls for possible covariates, which are nuisance/confounding variables you do not want to influence findings. Repeated-measures ANOVA (rANOVA) examines multiple measurement-moments.

To compare nominal variables, use Chi-Square (comparing two independent groups) or Cochran's Q-test (comparing two dependent groups) (SPSS:analyze>nonparametric). To compare two ordinal variables of two dependent groups, use Wilcoxon-Test. To compare two independent groups with ordinal variables, use Mann-Whitney-Test or the more powerful Kolmogorov-Smirnov-Test for continuous/ratio/interval variables. To compare three or more independent groups, use Kruskal-Wallis-Test. To compare three or more dependent groups, use Friedman's Test.

Testing nominal/ordinal variables: Optimal scaling

Some statistical tests cannot be conducted as the variables are nominal or ordinal, for example, with non-equal distances between answer categories (e.g., answer options 'male', 'female', and 'non-binary'). This section has already described many options, including optimal scaling, which is a group of statistical techniques deriving interval measures from nominal/ordinal variables, such as: non-linear canonical correlations for ordinal/nominal variables; multiple-regression analysis with categorical-regression analysis, analysis of factors/structure with non-linear principal components analysis (PRINCALS) and homogeneity analysis (HOMALS) or multiple-correspondence analysis for two categorical variables.

Assessing individual trajectories

Most clinical trials calculate effects by comparing measurements before the first and after the last therapy session. However, effects differ per session, and clients often change most during the beginning of therapy (Saxon, Firth, & Barkham, 2017). Therefore, it may be helpful to examine accumulative change-per-session or via critical-phase transitions. Furthermore, only reporting mean effects may hide the unique trajectories of individuals and sub-groups. Therefore, consider visualising and testing the trajectories of session-by-session scores of individuals or sub-groups. For example, assess growth via rANOVA (repeated-measures analysis of variance), possibly with a covariate to differentiate trajectories for different sub-groups, or use growth-curve multi-level analysis for nested data, latent-growth-curve-model to estimate growth in SEM, or Bayesian path analysis (Jung & Wickrama, 2008; Kahn & Schneider, 2013; Tschacher & Ramseyer, 2009).

Testing nested data

Many clinical trials include nested data: an individual client is embedded in the dyad/nest with one therapist, and the therapists are embedded in nests of different therapeutic modalities or therapy centres/locations. To account for nesting effects, conduct multi-level analysis (Kenny & Hoyt, 2014). Multi-level analysis may also be done in SEM or Bayesian statistics, and may require large sample sizes.

Testing mediators and/or moderators via the Baron & Kenny method

Whereas the first quantitative studies on psychological therapies tested whether therapy predicted outcomes (e.g., regression analysis: predictor → predicted; the arrow means causation), later studies included variables moderating these effects, such as client and therapist characteristics, and factors explaining or mediating the effects. Chapter 3 provides many examples of moderators and mediators.

A moderator is a factor affecting the relationship between two variables. For example, if therapy works better for women than men, gender is a moderator. For example, therapist competencies are important moderators, as 75% of clients recover with the most effective therapists and 43% in the most ineffective therapists (Saxon, Firth, & Barkham, 2017). Moderated mediation means that different mediators may work for different levels of the moderator, such as a strong therapeutic relationship may have larger effects on women than on men. Moderators may be included as a covariate in multivariate analyses, or examined via regression analysis or.

A mediator is a variable explaining the relationship between two variables such as between treatment allocation and outcomes. As described in Chapter 8, Step 5, researchers often have hypotheses about causality, such as allocating clients to a treatment (e.g., exposure therapy), predicting outcomes (decreased anxiety), via the use of particular therapeutic mechanisms (exposure), relationships and processes (e.g., good working alliance). It may be conceptually insufficient to merely report that allocating cynophobic clients to exposure therapy predicts decreased anxiety (exposure therapy → anxiety), as the therapist uses therapeutic mechanisms, relationships and processes (e.g., therapy allocation → exposure + relationship + processes → anxiety). Researchers may want to develop a conceptual framework of possible mediators and moderators (see Chapter 3) and test this to justify their inferences regarding causality (Kazdin, 2007, 2021).

A relatively simple strategy to analyse mediation and moderated mediation was proposed by Baron and Kenny (1986). First, regression analysis examines whether the independent variable predicts the dependent variable (exposure therapy → anxiety). Second, regression analysis examines whether the independent variable influences the mediator (exposure therapy → exposure). Third, regression analysis is conducted with both independent variable and mediator as predictors. Mediation is present when the mediator significantly predicts the outcome, and the independent variable is no longer a significant predictor (complete prediction) or has a smaller prediction effect or smaller significance level. This strategy seems to have sufficient statistical power for simple conceptual models, but researchers prefer SEM when many variables are included.

Testing models

Many recent therapy studies test complex conceptual models with multiple variables at several measurement-moments, via SEM or Bayesian networks. Complex models may do more justice to the complexity of therapeutic practice than simple statistical tests, and stand in line with complexity science, chaos theory, field theory, and network approaches. SEM is a powerful technique, as it examines multiple variables and their relationships at once (read more: Bowen & Guo, 2011; Hoyle, 2012; Schumacker & Lomax, 2004). However, complex models may require large sample sizes, and may be less suitable for inexperienced researchers.

SEM starts with building a conceptual model (see Chapter 3), which is subsequently tested in a dataset, and the goodness-of-fit may be assessed via multiple indices (e.g., root mean square error of approximation (RMSEA) < 0.06, $p(\chi2) > 0.05$, $\chi2/df < 2$, comparative fit index (CFI) > 0.95, Tucker-Lewis index (TLI) > 0.95); models can be modified to fit the data better, and a model may be considered better if $\chi2$ significantly improves. Complex models should not be formulated and tested for their own sake but follow logically from the underlying conceptual framework (see Chapter 3), problem or gap in the literature (see Chapter 5), and fit the research aims (see Chapter 6).

The following are examples to nudge advanced readers:

- **Paths:** Traditionally, therapy effects are tested on one outcome instrument at a time; however, in reality, clients may for example not only experience symptoms of depression but also anxiety, and changes in different symptoms/scales may interact. SEM models can include multiple 'paths', such as multiple variables, their relationships and interactions, including predictors, outcomes, mediators, and moderators at multiple measurement-moments. SEM can also model all possible measurement errors for each variable and each relationship.
- **Confirmatory factor analysis:** SEM can confirm a factor structure, for example of sub-scales in a psychometric instrument.
- **Latent variable:** SEM can be used when multiple instruments measure the same construct, and when there are latent-variables. For example, we cannot directly observe the latent variable 'IQ', but we may estimate this via observations of multiple manifest IQ test items.
- **Multi-level SEM:** SEM can conduct multi-level analysis with nested participants, such as clients within a therapist-client dyad with different therapeutic modalities within different locations. Furthermore, actor–partner interdependence models may help to assess mutual influences of individuals in dyadic relationships, such as therapists and clients.
- **Growth curve model:** SEM can model individual trajectories, such as session-by-session growth. Cross-lagged models or autoregressive-cross-lagged models can take into account that for example client scores after session 1 influence post-session-2 scores, etc.

Analysing networks

Traditional psychometric tests seem to assume that a latent variable, such as 'depression', causes the scores on items about specific depression symptoms, such as negative mood and suicidal ideation. However, network analysts argue that the symptoms/questionnaire items influence each other and interact with symptoms from other experiences (Fonsesca-Pedrero, 2018). Network analysis can increase our understanding of the internal structure of complex phenomena such as a psychological diagnosis, psychopathology, clinical phenomena, and the relative importance of symptoms and criteria. Similarly, social network analysis may help understand the therapeutic dyad and social networks (Prell, 2012). Networks may, for example, be analysed via SEM or Bayesian networks.

Analysing without assumptions of classical statistics

Bayesian statistics has not frequently been used in therapy research (Bolstad & Curran, 2016; Cleophas & Zwinderman, 2018). Yet increasing numbers of software programs and

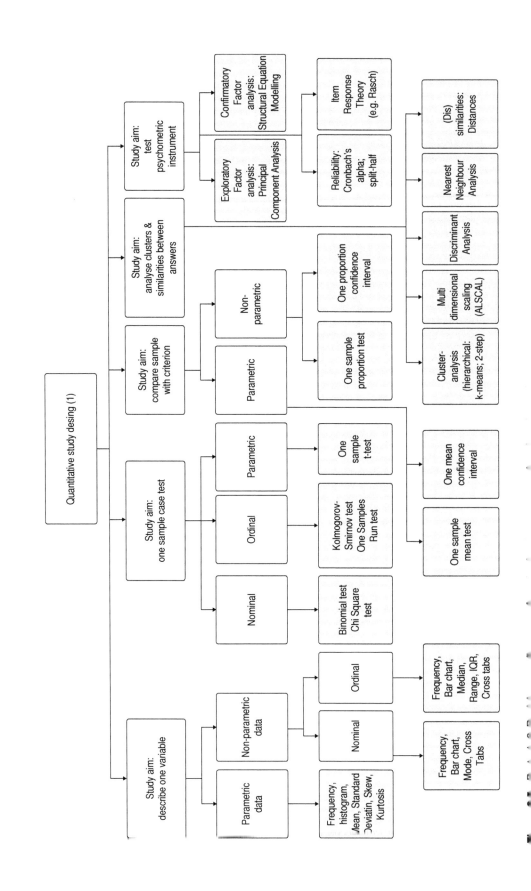

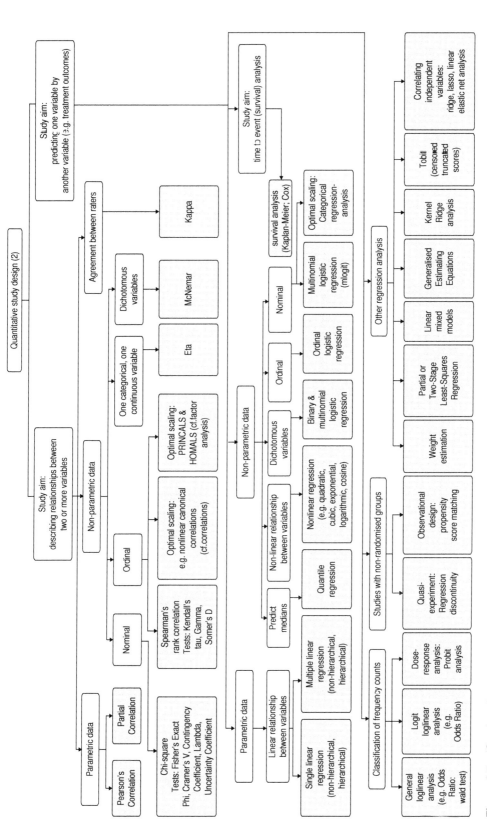

Figure 8.5 (Continued)

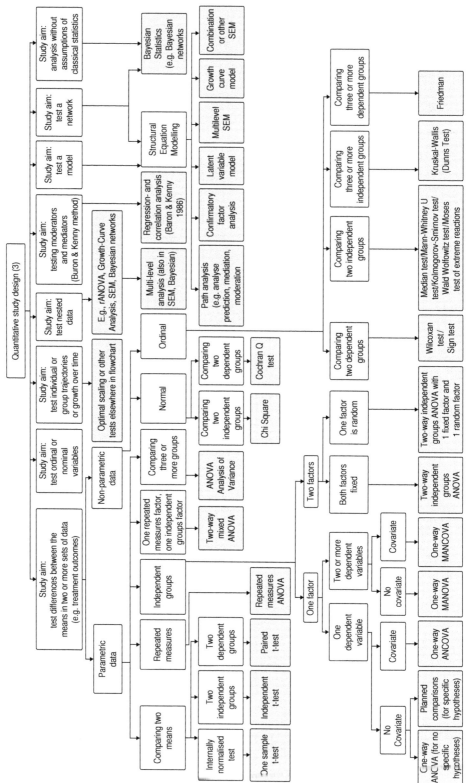

Figure 9.5 (Continued)

Table 8.2 Parametric versus non-parametric tests

	Parametric	**Non-parametric**
Statistical power	Powerful	Less powerful
Interpretability	Relatively easy	Sometimes more difficult
Condition 1: Level of measurement (scale)	Interval or ratio (e.g., numbers, semantic-differential, visual-numerical scale; often scales are treated as interval/ratio whereas they are not, e.g., Likert/Thurstone/Guttman scales)	Any scale
Condition 2: Distribution	Normal (Step 8 explains how to test distributions and standardise non-normal distributions)	Normal and non-normal
Condition 3: Sample size	Works well in larger sample sizes (e.g., N > 25), even if slightly non-normally distributed	
Examples	T-test, ANOVA	Wilcoxon, Kruskal-Wallis, Mann-Whitney

researchers use Bayesian statistics. Advocates argue that Bayesian statistics offer an alternative to flawed assumptions in classical statistics, is less prone to misinterpretations, and yields reliable results fast, even for small effects and small samples. Whereas classical statisticians formulate an H0 hypothesis that they do not update when getting new data, Bayesian researchers assume that we upgrade our beliefs by introducing new data. Instead of thinking about probability as fixed parameters, they think about these as distributions. Various Bayesian procedures have been developed which can answer research questions similar to classical statistics and more complex models, e.g., Bayesian hierarchical modelling and neural networks (SPSS:analyze>Bayesian).

Bootstrapping

Bootstrapping can be used in conjunction with many tests. Researchers may use bootstrapping to develop more accurate estimates. Bootstrapping may be unnecessary for informal or student research, but may be useful if findings can have substantial real-world consequences or when assumptions of tests are violated (e.g., small samples, skewness, kurtosis). In traditional tests, you use your sample to derive conclusions about a parameter in the general population (sample → population) ('parameters' tell you something about the general population, whereas 'statistics' tell you something about your sample). As we do not know the total population, we also do not know the true error of the parameter, which makes our estimations less robust. Bootstrapping tries to solve this problem by pretending that your sample is the population; this is helpful because you know the true value of your sample's error. Bootstrapping randomly re-samples your sample data and derives conclusions about your sample from this re-sampled data (re-sampled → sample). Re-sampling means taking the original dataset and samples from it to form a new sample. The more often you re-sample, the more accurate is your estimation (usually, 1000 or 5000 rounds of re-sampling). Many tests in statistical software offer bootstrapping options.

Step 8: Conduct preparatory analyses

Definition

A raw dataset includes all initial scores from the participants, such as the database from an online survey or inserted data from paper-and-pencil questionnaires. Often, raw data are not ready for analysis: they need several preparatory steps. A research report/thesis/article should describe these preparatory analyses. Not all steps are required for all studies.

Procedures

1. Compute sub-scales

Often, instruments have one or multiple sub-scales. Use the instrument developer's instructions to calculate a sum score or average score. Test whether your dataset justifies calculating these sub-scales, for example, via confirmatory factor analysis (testing the assumption that the scale has multiple factors/dimensions/sub-scales). Reliability analysis can be conducted for each scale; a scale's reliability may be improved by removing items (e.g., check 'Cronbach's alpha if item deleted'). Exploratory factor analysis may identify unexpected factors to reduce the number of variables. Test-development studies may include IRT. If you use multiple instruments to measure the same underlying/latent construct, consider using data-reduction techniques, such as SEM, in which a new aggregate variable is estimated via multiple instruments.

2. Analyse missing values

Research participants may not fill in every questionnaire and may not answer every question, creating so-called missing values (Parent, 2013). When inserting data into the statistical database, differentiate reasons why a value is missing; software may automatically do this, or replace missing values for a code (e.g., 999 = system-missing, such as questionnaire lost or not inserted; 888 = participant did not answer; 777 = value deleted as outlier).

Examine why values are missing. For example, are women more likely to skip particular questions? Statistical software often has standardised missing-value analysis. Alternatively, you may use regression analysis to predict the missing values, for example with a dummy variable with the values '0' for missing and '1' for not missing. Use any data to predict missing values; at least use socio-demographic data or non-missing baseline scores. Missing-value analysis may indicate whether values are random-missing or system-missing, which is important when interpreting the findings.

You may examine why you are missing single values, a full questionnaire, or a full measurement-moment. Some researchers exclude participants who have filled in less than 90% of all items or who have filled in less than 90% of all measurement-moments, and they exclude questionnaires in which less than 90% of all items are filled in (there are no hard guidelines for this). If you decide to exclude cases, scales, or items, examine whether the findings would be different if you would have kept them in your dataset, and reflect on this in the discussion of your research report/thesis/article.

3. Analyse dropouts

Research participants may drop out at different stages of therapy. Individuals may have many reasons to drop out, as studies have shown, such as: ethnic background, education, income, living situation, comorbid disorders, treatment duration, motivation, self-efficacy, impulsivity, control groups, therapist's experience and training, therapeutic relationship, and matching client preferences (Cooper & Conklin, 2015; Roos & Werbart, 2013). Describe the number of dropouts at each stage. Like missing values, examine possible predictors of dropout via baseline measurement and changes in scores in the sessions before dropout, e.g., via regression analyses. In clinical trials, researchers may examine the data they have without dropouts ('completer analysis'), reducing the sample size. Instead, researchers may do an intent-to-treat analysis, i.e., the effects for all clients who started treatment with the latest available data before they dropped out ('last-observation-carried-forward'), which may have more accurate but smaller effects. Researchers may also impute the missing data based on available data (multiple imputation), which may give artificially specific and less accurate effects.

4. Impute missing values

Missing values and dropout limit the number of participants you can include in statistical tests. Therefore, researchers often estimate what the possible answer could have been and replace the missing value with this. Several imputation techniques exist, such as the frequently used multiple-imputations-by-regression, i.e., using scores on other items to predict a missing value. Always double check whether you would have made different conclusions with/without data-imputation: thus, do the analyses twice and compare findings. If only a few questions are missing in a larger questionnaire, data may be imputed, except if this variable cannot be estimated, such as socio-demographics or a key question. The more estimations you do, the larger the likelihood that your final findings are inaccurate (increased risk of statistical error); therefore, you may only want to impute a small amount of missing data, and correct for the number of estimations (e.g., Bonferroni correction). Do not impute data if your study has weak statistical power, a small dataset, or many non-parametric variables (Scheffer, 2002). As data-imputation makes a scale look better than it is, examine a scale's reliability or factor structure with and without data-imputation.

5. Identify and cope with outliers

Use boxplots to identify possible outliers, which are extreme answers/scores. No strict guidelines exist, although any score of more than two standard deviations from the mean is usually considered an outlier. Examine possible causes of outliers, to rule out a procedural error of the researcher, such as errors in data entry or scoring. Try to explain outliers with other variables (Aggarwal, 2017). Outliers are part of the data and should ideally be kept in the analyses. However, outliers can disproportionally influence the findings in a study, particularly in small samples. Therefore, researchers may make the scores less extreme (e.g., 'Winsorising') or delete individual values, variables, or participants. The removal of extreme scores means a loss of data and makes the standard deviation smaller so the findings look more specific than they are; therefore, consider comparing findings with and without outliers (Aggarwal, 2017).

6. Check the assumptions of the statistical tests

Table 8.3 summarises the assumptions of some statistical tests. Use handbooks, internet searches, and the help function of your statistical software to find assumptions of statistical tests.

6.1 Measurement level

Parametric tests assume that variables are interval or ratio variables. Some scales, such as Likert scales and dummy variables, may be treated as interval/ratio scales even if they are not.

6.2 Check normal distribution

If a variable has a normal distribution, this means that there is an approximately equal number of individuals with scores larger than the mean as individuals with scores lower than the mean. This is often visualised as a bell curve in a histogram. However, most therapy samples are not normally distributed due to many individuals having extreme scores (Blanca et al., 2013). You may use the following practical rule of thumb to check the distribution (see Das & Imon, 2016, for tests of normality):

- **First:** Calculate skewness, i.e., symmetry of a distribution (rule of thumb: small skew is (-.05, 0.5), moderate (-1, -0.5) or (0.5, 1), large (-1 and beyond) or (1 and beyond)). Calculate kurtosis, i.e., how sharp/flat the peak of a curve is (rule of thumb: kurtosis for normal/mesokurtic distribution is about 3; leptokurtic kurtosis >3, platykurtic kurtosis <3).
- **Second:** Visualise the distribution with a histogram showing the distribution of scores in your sample; software can impose a hypothetical normal distribution to visually compare your sample with an ideal (SPSS:analyze>descriptive-statistics>frequencies, select 'variable', in the statistics-box select 'mean', 'Standard-Deviation', 'Kurtosis', 'Skewness' and in the charts-box select 'histogram with normal-distribution'; alternatively, use 'Q-Q plots' to check distribution; to check outliers, also select 'boxplots').
- **Third:** Although unnecessary for most research purposes, you may test normality with Shapiro-Wilk-Test, or alternatively Kolmogorov-Smirnov-Normality-Test or D'Agostino-Pearson-Test. Large samples (N>25) are more likely to be normally distributed, and you may be less worried about non-normal distribution. There are many possible solutions if a variable is not normally distributed (Pek, Wong, & Wong, 2018):

  o **Solution 1**: Check whether an extreme score causes the non-normal distribution (scores outside the 95% confidence interval are often considered outliers, checked visually in boxplots) and whether removal of outliers makes the distribution normal.
  o **Solution 2:** If you cannot make the distribution normal via outlier-removal, use a statistical function to normalise the variable, which can be done automatically in software (SPSS:transform>prepare-data-for-modelling>automatic, e.g., tick the popular option 'Box-Cox'). If the distribution is positively skewed (right peak), use logarithmic transformation (compute new variable with the logarithm of the old variable: ln(oldvar) or lg10(oldvar)) or hyperbolic arcsine in statistical software (ln(oldvar+sqrt(oldvar**2+1))). If the variable is negatively skewed (left peak), use power transformation (oldvar**3). If the variable is moderately positively skewed, residuals show positive heteroscedasticity, and the variable contains frequency counts, use square-root transformation (square-root of old variable: sqrt(oldvar) or oldvar**(1/3)). If the variable has a platykurtic distribution (flat peak), use inverse-transformation (1/oldvariable). If the variable contains proportions, use arcsine (arsin(oldvar)). Optimal binning transforms a numeric/continuous variable into a discrete variable with limited score options. Note that transformed variables can no longer be interpreted with the original scales and some transformations cannot cope with value '0' or negative values.

o **Solution 3:** If you cannot normalise the variable, check whether you could still use your non-transformed data, as some statistical tests are relatively robust for small violations of normality.
o **Solution 4:** Consider bootstrapping (see Step 7).
o **Solution 5:** Select another statistical test not requiring normal distribution.

6.3 Similar variances

To examine that groups have similar variances ('homoscedacity', i.e., scatter similarly), visually inspect boxplots or scatterplots with residual and predicted values (SPSS:analyze>descriptive-statistics). Less common is to use a similarity-of-variance test (e.g., Bartlett, BoxM, Brown-Forsythe, Fmax, or Levene). One-way ANOVA is relatively robust if variances are slightly dissimilar.

6.4 Randomness and independence of groups

This cannot be tested statistically. Check the study design.

6.5 Linearity of data

Check the scatterplot (SPSS:graph).

6.6 No extreme outliers

See above.

6.7 Reasonably large sample size

What is considered 'reasonable' depends on the population and topic, but usually N>30 is considered reasonably large.

6.8 Multicollinearity

This means that two variables are significantly correlated (SPSS:analyze>correlate).

7. Explore correlations

Explore how variables/scales correlate with each other to get an initial indication of the con-current validity of instruments. Examine unexpected correlations to understand their possible underlying cause; rule out that the correlation happened by mere chance, for example due to insufficient statistical power.

8. Decide to use instruments

Based on the previous seven preparatory steps, decide whether your instruments are sufficiently reliable and valid for use in your study (see Step 5).

9. Check *a posteriori* statistical power

Calculate if your study has sufficient statistical power to detect effects when testing hypotheses, for instance, in clinical trials. Statistical power is often assumed satisfying if larger than .70 and good if larger than .80. Power analyses need to be conducted on the standardised effect sizes for the primary outcomes in the final sample size after exclusion from outliers (for example, use online power-calculation tools, such as danielsoper.com, G*power).

Table 8.3 Assumptions of frequently used parametric tests

		Tests			
		Pearson's Correlations	T-test	One-way ANOVA	Linear regression
Assumptions	Level of measurement (scale)	Interval or ratio	Interval, ratio or ordinal	Interval or ratio	
	Approximate normal distribution	Yes	Yes	Yes	Yes
	All groups have similar variances ('homoscedasticity')	No	Yes	Yes	Yes
	Data/groups are random and independent	No	dependent and independent t-tests available	Yes	Yes
	Linearity of data	No	No	No	Yes
	No extreme outliers	Yes	Yes	Yes	Yes
	Reasonably large sample size	Yes	Yes	No	Yes
	Other			At least one participant per group; more participants than number of estimated coefficients	No autocorrelation; no or little multicollinearity

Step 9: Interpret and present quantitative findings

Definition

What does a score of '22' on the PHQ-9 scale mean? You will need some steps to interpret this.

Procedures

1. Interpret with cut-off points and compare with norm groups/benchmarks

Some instruments provide cut-off points, such as PHQ-9-scores of 12 and larger imply depression. Cut-off points have been established by comparing scores in a sample with depression with a sample without depression. Consider comparing scores with other studies as norm groups/benchmarks, such as national-health-service databases (Minami et al., 2007).

2. Test significance

You may first want to check your research findings are not due to mere chance. This is usually done by checking that the significance level/p-value is lower than .05 ($p < .05$). You may want to reduce the significance level if you do many estimations, such as doing many statistical tests. The reason is that in fishing-expeditions with many tests and many variables (i.e., 'many estimations'), you are likely to find false-positives. Therefore, you may only report findings with a lower p-value, e.g. < .001. Several types of correction exist, with Bonferroni correction the most frequently used (i.e., dividing p-value of 0.05 by the number of statistical tests). However, smaller p-values reduce the power to detect any real effects in small samples. You may consider a larger p-value for explorative research aims, which seems to prefer false-positives over false-negatives. You may also consider adjusting the p-values because your hypothesis is one-tailed instead of the standard two-tailed statistical tests (i.e., you know the direction of the effects: positive or negative). Given a large-enough sample size, any effect will become statistically significant, regardless of any significance level, and therefore effects in large samples should be interpreted carefully. If you do not find a significant effect, rule out that this may be due to carrying out the intervention in unintended ways, loosely adhered procedures, external variables influencing the findings, or instruments not being reliable, valid, or sensitive, or having a crude answer scale (e.g., yes/no answer options instead of a seven-point Likert scale). Negative effects can still be clinically important and contribute to the field.

3. Calculate and interpret standardised effect sizes

Usually, it is insufficient to conclude that a finding is significant; you will also need to say how large this finding is. For example, it is clinically crucial to know whether a treatment causes small or large changes in clients. Imagine you test the difference between two groups and find $t = 2.1$, $p = .002$. What does this mean? This test is significant because $p = .002$ is less than the significance criterion of $p < .05$. To interpret t-values, you will need to transform these into standardised-effect sizes, which is often calculated automatically in statistical software. Table 8.4 offers common effect sizes and their conventional interpretations, which should be mentioned in methodology sections (Cronbach, 1951). Do not ignore small effects, which may accumulate/add to the therapeutic effects (Wampold & Imel, 2015).

Table 8.4 Interpretation of frequently used standardised-effect sizes

Effect size	Small	Medium	Large
Cohen's D (derived from t-test)	.20	.50	.80
F in ANOVA	.10	.25	.40
e^2	.01	.06	.14
F in regression	.02	.15	.35
r	.10	.30	.50
R^2	.01	.06	.14
Cross-table: 2 × 2 Odd's Ratio	1.5	3.5	9
Chi-Squared	.10	.30	.50

4. Examine variation

Nobody is the same. Therefore, describe the range of scores with a 95% confidence interval (CI), average score (e.g., mean, medium, or mode), and the variation around the mean (standard deviation (SD), or standard error (SE)). Report skewness, kurtosis, outliers, and missing values for each scale. Consider possible ceiling effects in your data for individuals near the ceiling of the range of a measure (the opposite are called floor effects). For example, clients with high baseline scores show larger improvements than clients with low baseline scores, because they have more opportunities to change. For example, clients with PHQ-9 baseline scores of 22 and outcome scores of 4 change 18 points; clients with a baseline score of 5 and outcome score of 4 change only 1 point. Therefore, when you only include clients with the worst psychological symptoms, you will most likely get large effects. For example, British national mental health services have been accused of creating overly positive service evaluations by focusing their studies on clients with the worst baseline scores (Vos, Roberts, & Davies, 2019).

5. Transform data into clinically meaningful findings

It is insufficient to report the statistical significance and effect sizes of a clinical trial because you also want to know the effects are also clinically significant/meaningful (Carrozzino et al., 2021; Kraemer, Frank, & Kupfer, 2011). Table 8.5 shows popular ways to transform data into clinically interpretable findings.

6. Examine differences and/or associations

This is a reminder that a correlation is not the same as a difference or lack thereof. When examining the differences between two instruments, ensure instruments can be compared, for example with similar rating scales and scoring (if they use different scales/scoring, make them comparable by standardisation, e.g., to Z-scores or data recoding/computation; SPSS:transform>compute).

7. Examine correlations and causations

A significant correlation does not automatically imply causation. It is easy to conflate correlations and causations. Check the criteria of causality in Chapter 7, step 6. Causation may, for example, be examined with relevant statistical tests, such as repeated measures, combined with a well-defined cause of change (e.g., treatment) in a prospective/longitudinal, experimental study design. Your language should reflect whether your findings are correlations ('x was correlated with y') or causations ('x predicted y').

8. Present in figures

Visual figures can help to understand/present the inclusion/exclusion of participants at different research stages and relationships between variables. Figure 8.6 illustrates a frequently used flowchart in clinical trials.

9. Present in tables

Tables are usually added to a report/thesis/article for a quick overview of findings (tables should not replace texts).

10. Reflect on the validity, reliability, and trustworthiness of the study

In the discussion section, and preferably throughout all stages of research, reflect on the quality of your study, such as the instruments, study design, possible response shift, and trustworthiness,

Table 8.5 Overview of popular methods to describe clinically relevant findings

Clinical effect	Interpretation	Reference
Clinical change	The number of clients under and above a clinical cut-off point. For example, no longer meeting clinical criteria, or disappearance of a problem (e.g., no panic attacks anymore)	
ED50/ED75	The number of sessions needed to produce the desired effect in respectively 50% and 75% of the population	Kopta et al., 1994
Reliable change	The number of clients who changed reliably, i.e., their change is unlikely to be caused by the unreliability of the measurement. This number is calculated with the number of clients under and above a criterion and is based on the standard-deviation and Cronbach's alpha of the instrument (i.e., preferably test-retest reliability or alpha-coefficient in your study, or alpha in another study)	Jacobson & Truax, 1991*
Clinically significant change	Clinically significant change describes the change required for a person to come from a score typical of a problematic, dysfunctional client or service-user group to a score typical of the normal population. This requires researchers to compare the mean and standard deviation of their sample with the mean and standard deviation of a normal population	Jacobson & Truax, 1991 (revisited: Speer, 1992; Tingey et al., 1996)*
Recovery	Recovery is any case with statistically reliable change and scores below the clinical threshold at the end of treatment	Gyani et al., 2013
Growth curve	Calculation of growth curves for multiwave data	Speer & Greenbaum, 1995
Number needed to treat	The number of clients who need to be treated to prevent one additional bad outcome (e.g., number of clients that need to be treated for one of them to benefit compared with a control group in a clinical trial)	Kraemer & Kupfer, 2006
The area under the receiver-operating characteristic curve (ROC)	Compare the treatment group and control group responses in a ROC plot (e.g., false-positive rate at x-axis, true-positive rate at y-axis)	Kraemer & Kupfer, 2006
Recovery	Functioning well in many domains of life, e.g., social life, work life, measures of existential well-being, quality of life, and meaning in life	
Social outcomes	Variables such as arrest, truancy, hospitalisation, death, disease, etc.	
Subjective evaluation	Interview or open questions about the size and importance of change (e.g., Client Change Interview)	

This gives conservative estimates with similar clinical conclusions to other procedures (Ronk et al., 2012). Calculate online: www.psyctc.org/psyctc/root/stats/rcsc/

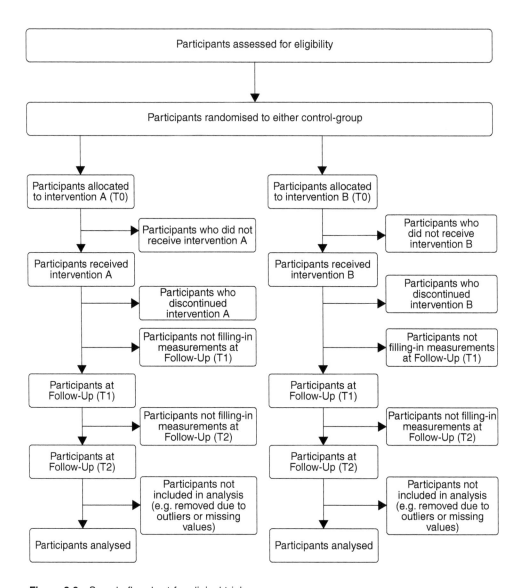

Figure 8.6 Sample flowchart for clinical trials

10.1 Quality of instruments

Step 5 described how you can reflect on the quality of your instruments, such as reliability, validity, sensitivity, specificity, interpretability/understandability, and IRT.

10.2 Quality of study design

Reflect on possible threats to your study's internal, external, construct, and measurement validity. Table 8.6 uses the definitions from Kazdin (2021; see his book for details). Internal validity refers to the extent to which researchers can derive valid conclusions from the study, because the effects seem to be caused by the intervention and not by external influences, such as maturation, attrition, or selection bias. External validity refers to the extent to which researchers can generalise the findings to different contexts and times. Construct validity refers to the extent to which an experiment's results can be attributed to the intervention and not to other factors, such as the researcher's expectations. Data-evaluation validity refers to the extent a relation is shown, demonstrated, or evident between an intervention and the outcome, and for example, not misled or obscured by the data and methods, such as statistical power, errors in data recording, and heterogeneity between participants.

10.3 Response shift

The effects in the analysis of repeated measures, such as session-by-session routine outcome monitoring, may have been caused by response shift (Sprangers & Schwartz, 1999). This means that if participants fill in the same questions several times, they may evaluate the same question differently because it has a different meaning to them due to having different internal standards (recalibration), values (reprioritisation), or redefinition (reconceptualisation). For example, participants mentioned the same problems as during a previous measurement-moment, but they interpreted these differently: 'in hindsight, I was more depressed than I thought'; 'by going through treatment, I started to understand that what I interpreted as absolutely crazy, actually is pretty normal. So I still experience it, but I am less bothered by it'; 'After treatment, I actually value it more to have a few good friends rather than the large amounts that I always longed for' (Truijens, 2022). Similarly, different populations have different standards, such as pain thresholds in individuals with chronic pain or self-harming behaviour.

Thus, response shift means that the observed change may not be explained by a real change but a change in the meaning of one's self-evaluation of the target concept/construct (Vanier et al., 2021). It has been estimated that approximately 70% of all clinical trials have clinically important response shift effects, which may obfuscate treatment benefits (Sprangers et al., 2023). Consequently, researchers and policy-makers should be careful when interpreting studies with repeated measurements such as most clinical trials. Researchers need to triangulate their findings via multiple data sources, such as using multiple questionnaires, cognitive and experiential interviews, sequential mixed methods (see Chapter 10), participants thinking aloud when filling in questionnaires, transparency of the underlying conceptual framework (see Chapter 3), and focusing less on *a priori* predictions and instead keeping an open mind for the direction and meaning of change (Truijens, 2022).

10.4 Trustworthiness

The above-mentioned reflective points are frequently applied in quantitative research. Additionally, researchers may want to use critical self-reflection and reflexivity throughout the research process, for example, via reflective research journals (see Chapter 4). They may also want to reflect on broader components of trustworthiness, as discussed in Step 8 in Chapter 9.

11. Other publication tips

Quantitative reports should contain enough details for others to replicate the study, e.g., describe all steps. When reporting findings, check the requirements from the journal or for example the APA guidelines (apastyle.apa.org/jars/quantitative). See more tips in Online Table 8.5.

Table 8.6 Validity of the study design (citations from Kazdin, 2021, Chapters 2–3)

Validity type	Description	Major threats to validity (name / description)	
Internal validity	'To what extent can the intervention rather than extraneous influences be considered to account for the results, changes, or differences among conditions (e.g., baseline, intervention)?'	History	'Any event (other than the intervention) occurring at the time of the experiment that could influence the results or account for the pattern of data otherwise attributed to the experimental manipulation. Historical events might include family crises; change in job, teacher, or spouse; power blackouts; or any other events.'
		Maturation	'Any change over time that may result from processes within the subject. Such processes may include growing older, stronger, healthier, smarter, and more tired or bored.'
		Testing	'Any change that may be attributed to the effects of repeated assessment. Testing constitutes an experience that, depending on the measure, may lead to systematic changes in performance.'
		Instrumentation	'Any change that takes place in the measuring instrument or assessment procedure over time. Such changes may result from the use of human observers whose judgments about the client or criteria for scoring behavior may change over time.'
		Statistical regression	'Any change from one assessment occasion to another that might be due to a reversion of scores toward the mean. If clients score at the extremes on one assessment occasion, their scores may change in the direction toward the mean on a second testing.'
		Selection biases	'Systematic differences between groups before any experimental manipulation or intervention. Any differences between groups (e.g., experimental and control) may be due to the differences that were already evident before they were exposed to the different conditions of the experiment.'
		Attrition	'Loss of subjects over the course of an experiment that can change the composition of groups in a way that leads to selection biases. Attrition affects other types of experimental validity as well.'
		Diffusion of treatment	'Diffusion of treatment can occur when the intervention is inadvertently provided during times when it should not be (e.g., return to baseline conditions) or to persons who should not yet receive the intervention at a particular point. The effects of the intervention will be underestimated if it is unwittingly administered in intervention and nonintervention phases.'

Validity type	Description	Major threats to validity (name / description)
External validity	'To what extent can the results be generalised or extended to people, settings, times, measures/ outcomes, and characteristics other than those included in this particular demonstration?'	**Sample characteristics** 'The extent to which the results can be extended to subjects or clients whose characteristics may differ from those included in the investigation.'
		Narrow stimulus sampling 'The extent to which the results might be restricted to a restricted range of sampling of materials (stimuli) or other features (experimenters) used in the experiment.'
		Reactivity of experimental arrangements 'The possibility that subjects may be influenced by their awareness that they are participating in an investigation or in a special program. The experimental manipulation effects may not extend to situations in which individuals are unaware of the arrangement.'
		Reactivity of assessment 'The extent to which subjects are aware that their behavior is being assessed and that this awareness may influence how they respond. Persons who are aware of assessment may respond differently from how they would if they were unaware of the assessment.'
		Test sensitization 'Measurement in the experiment may sensitise subjects to the experimental manipulation so that they are more or less responsive than they would have been had there been no initial assessment. This prospect is more likely if there is a pretest and that pretest is one that alerts awareness that assessment is going on and what the focus of that assessment is.'
		Multiple-treatment interference 'When the same subjects are exposed to more than one treatment, the conclusions reached about a particular treatment may be restricted. Specifically, the results may only apply to other persons who experience both of the treatments in the same way or in the same order.'
		Novelty effects 'The possibility that the effects of an experimental manipulation or intervention depend upon the innovativeness or novelty in the situation. The results attributed to the experimental manipulation may be restricted to the context in which that is novel or new in some way.'
		Generality across measures, setting, and time 'The extent to which the results extend to other measures, settings, or assessment occasions than those included in the study. There is a reason to expect that the relations on one set of measures will not carry over to others, or that the findings obtained in a particular setting would not transfer to other settings, or that the relations are restricted to a particular point in time or to a particular cohort—these would be threats to external validity.'

(Continued)

Table 8.6 Validity of the study design (citations from Kazdin, 2021, Chapters 2–3) *(Continued)*

Validity type	Description	Major threats to validity (name / description)
Construct validity	'Given that the experimental manipulation or intervention was responsible for change, what specific aspect of the manipulation was the mechanism, process, or causal agent? What is the conceptual basis (construct) underlying the effect?'	**Attention and contact accorded the client** 'The extent to which an increase of attention to the client/participant associated with the intervention could plausibly explain the effects attributed to the intervention.'
		Single operations and narrow stimulus sampling 'Sometimes a single set of stimuli, investigator, or other facet of the study that the investigator considers irrelevant may contribute to the impact of the experimental manipulation. For example, one experimenter or therapist may administer all conditions; at the end of the study, one cannot separate the manipulation from the person who implemented it. In general, two or more stimuli or experimenters allow one to evaluate whether it was the manipulation across different stimulus conditions.'
		Experimenter expectancies 'Unintentional effects the experimenter may have that influence the subject's responses in the experiment. The expectancies of the person running subjects may influence tone of voice, facial expressions, delivery of instructions, or other variations in the procedures that differentially influence subjects in different conditions.'
		Demand characteristics 'Cues of the experimental situation that are ancillary to what is being studied but may provide information that exerts direct influence on the results. The cues are incidental but "pull," promote, or prompt behavior in the subjects that could be mistaken for the impact of the independent variable of interest. *Post-experimental Inquiry*: Ask subjects at the end of an experiment about their perceptions about the purpose, what was expected, how they were "supposed" to perform. (If subjects identify responses that are consistent with expected performance (the hypothesised performance), this raises the possibility that demand characteristics may have contributed to the results.) *Pre-inquiry*: Subjects are exposed to the procedures (e.g., told what they are), see what subjects would do, hear the rationale and instructions, but not actually run through the study itself. They are then asked to respond to the measures (If subjects respond to the measures consistent with predicted or hypothesised performance, this raises the possibility that demand characteristics could contribute to the results.) *Simulators*: Subjects are asked to act as if they have received the procedures and then to deceive assessors (naïve experimenters) who do not know whether they have been exposed to the actual procedures. Similar to Preinquiry except that subjects actually go through that part of the experiment, if there is one, in which experimenters or assessors evaluate subject performance (If simulators can deceive a naive experimenter, i.e., make them believe they have actually been

Validity type	Description	Major threats to validity (name / description)	
Data-evaluation validity	'To what extent is a relation shown, demonstrated, or evident between the experimental manipulation or intervention and the outcome? What about the data and methods used for evaluation that could mislead or obscure demonstrating or failing to demonstrate an experimental effect?'	Low statistical power	'Power is the likelihood of demonstrating an effect or group difference when in fact there is a true effect in the world. Often studies have power that is too low to detect an experimental effect. Thus, no-difference finding could be due to the lack of a true effect or a study with too little power.'
		Subject heterogeneity	'Subjects recruited for a project will vary naturally in many ways. Yet, the extent of that variability can influence the conclusions that are drawn. If subjects can vary widely (in age, ethnicity, diagnoses, background, and so on), the variability (denominator in the effect size formula) also increases. As that variability increases, a given difference between groups (numerator in the effect size formula) becomes more difficult to detect. Generally it is advisable to specify the subject characteristics of interest and note inclusion and exclusion criteria so that variation is not unlimited.'
		Variability in the procedures	'How the study is executed can make a difference in whether a true effect is detected. If the procedures (e.g., in running a subject) are sloppy or inconsistent from subject to subject, unnecessary and undesirable variability is increased. And as with other threats related to variability that can interfere with detecting a difference when there is one.'
		Unreliability of the measures	'Error in the measurement procedures that introduces variability can obscure the results of a study. Measures that are not very reliable increase error in the assessment and as other sources of variability decrease the likelihood of showing group differences.'
		Restricted range of the measures	'A measure may have a very limited range (total score from high to low) and that may interfere with showing group differences. The scores cannot spread out all of the subjects because of the limited range. No differences in a finding might be the result of the restricted range of the measure that could not permit a large enough scale to differentiate groups.'
		Errors in data recording, analysis, and reporting	'Inaccuracies in data recording, analysis, and reporting refer to multiple steps in which inaccuracies enter into the data base or the data are used in a selective way where only some measures or analyses are reported. Errors and selective reporting obviously mislead, whether intentional or unintentional, and threaten the data-evaluation validity of the study.'
		Multiple comparisons and error rates	'When multiple statistical tests are completed within the same investigation, the likelihood of a "chance" finding is increased. This is a threat to data evaluation because false conclusions will be more likely unless some accommodation is made for the number of tests (e.g., by adjusting the p level across the many tests to take into account the number of tests).'
		Misreading or misinterpreting the data analysis	'The conclusions reached from the data analysis are not to which the investigator is entitled. Either the proper statistic was not run or the conclusion reached goes beyond the statistical test.'

Reflective questions

- Select three frequently cited clinical trials in your field. Reflect on the study design and how it could have been improved. Reflect on the reliability and validity of the instruments and study design. What is your overall assessment of this study's quality?
- Select three frequently cited studies on the development of questionnaires in your field. Reflect on the test development, reliability, and validity. Would you use this: why (not)?

Self-reflective or class-discussion exercise

Like all methods, quantitative methods have pros and cons. Reflect: do you agree/disagree with each statement; why/why not; what would a devil's advocate say?

Arguments pro-quantitative

- We must do quantitative research, as most therapy research is quantitative.
- Quantitative methods are pragmatic to communicate with medical sciences and policy-makers.
- Quantitative methods help to test hypotheses and generalise findings.
- If done correctly, quantitative research has a low risk of bias.

Arguments con-quantitative

- Therapeutic practice is often non-verbal, intuitive, embodied, and based on crystallised expert knowledge, which cannot be shown in-depth via quantitative methods.
- A realist-ontology and positivist-epistemology do not fit the lived experiences of clients/therapists.
- Therapists do not need good numbers but good practice.
- Pre-selected questionnaires may have fewer answer options than open questions or interviews.

9

How to Conduct Qualitative Research

Chapter aims

This chapter explains how to read, develop, and conduct qualitative research projects. A qualitative method helps to answer a qualitative research question, for example about the subjectively lived experiences of individuals. Qualitative research has become increasingly popular in psychotherapy research since the 1990s. Whereas Chapter 7 gave an overview of all methodological steps, this chapter zooms in on developing a qualitative mindset, selecting and conducting qualitative study designs such as interviews, conducting qualitative analysis, and reflecting on the study's trustworthiness. Chapter 10 explains how to mix qualitative with quantitative methods, and Chapters 11–12 how to conduct ethical research and discuss findings. (Recommended books on qualitative methods include Denzin & Lincoln, 2021; Marshall & Rossman, 2014; Silverman, 2021; Willig, 2022)

Steps in chapter

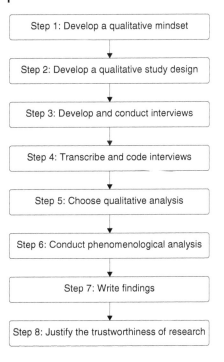

Step 1: Develop a qualitative mindset

Step 2: Develop a qualitative study design

Step 3: Develop and conduct interviews

Step 4: Transcribe and code interviews

Step 5: Choose qualitative analysis

Step 6: Conduct phenomenological analysis

Step 7: Write findings

Step 8: Justify the trustworthiness of research

Step 1: Develop a qualitative mindset

Definition

Qualitative research starts with developing a qualitative mindset, focusing on understanding and interpreting phenomena instead of explaining them, based on a qualitative ontological and epistemological position. A qualitative mindset may focus on lived experiences, construction processes, language, immersion, and interpreting-without-explaining. This qualitative mindset will guide researchers in their methodological decisions, analyses, and writing.

Components

Understanding, not explaining

The first research publications on human psychology were written during the Enlightenment, when humans were often seen as machines, acting rationally and predictably. For example, some medical doctors believe(d) that human behaviour could be explained with universal laws and distinct labels, such as universal diagnostic categories of mental health disorders, and that individuals could be treated with universally effective treatments (Vos, Roberts, & Davies, 2019).

This mechanistic worldview was criticised by philosophers such as Friedrich Nietzsche, who argued that humans have not only a rational, predictable side ('Apollonian') but also a dynamic, free, open side ('Dionysian'). This inspired early psychologists such as William James to conduct experiments that did not try to explain human experiences as distinct categories but understand the flow of our moment-to-moment experiences as a 'stream of consciousness'. These researchers stand in millennia-old traditions of what may be described as qualitative research methods *avant-la-lettre*, and have been influenced by theories such as phenomenology, existentialism, constructivism, hermeneutics, and idiographic and discursive psychology (Jovanović, 2011). Qualitative research has become 'a field in its own right. It crosscuts disciplines, fields and subject matters. A complex, interconnected family of terms, concepts and assumptions surround the term qualitative research or qualitative inquiry' (Denzin & Lincoln, 2021, p.2).

By the end of the 19th century, two distinctive research paradigms had emerged, as Wilhelm Dilthey (2010) described: the mechanistic approach which aims to 'explain' ('Erklären') human behaviour in objective, rational, universalising terms, and the new psychological approach which aims to 'understand' ('Verstehen') subjective dynamic human experiences. Bruner (1985) described this as research into daily life 'narratives' which he differentiated from 'scientific-paradigmatic research' (Bruner, 1985). This paradigmatic difference is also described as the difference between 'quantitative' and 'qualitative research methods'. Quantitative researchers often use deductivist hypothesis testing methods to directly tap into 'reality' to discover universal laws in human thoughts, feelings, and behaviours, preferably under controlled laboratory conditions. In contrast, qualitative researchers try to understand our unique idiosyncrasies and non-linear dynamic subjective daily life experiences that make us human. Qualitative researchers analyse how individuals experience and construct their understanding of themselves and their world via conversations, stories, rituals, meanings, memories, cultures, myths, and institutions. Qualitative research has, for example, deepened our understanding of how clients experience therapy processes and how therapists and clients construct their experiences and world together in unique ways that may not fit quantifiable universal laws.

Many qualitative researchers formulate research objectives but not research questions, possibly because they do not want to 'test' a hypothesis or ask a narrow research question, as they want to keep an open mind for whatever participants might share. For example, a qualitative study may aim to 'describe the participants' subjectively lived experiences' or 'describe how participants experience' a phenomenon. These examples shows how qualitative researchers try to understand human experiences in their totality, not only in laboratory studies or controlled experiments, but as they emerge in their life, including all dynamic, complex interactions (the awkward expression 'subjectively lived experiences' comes most likely from the modern German word for experiences, 'Erlebnis', which contains the word 'Leben', life, which contrasts with the more reductionist term 'Erfahrung' for emotions; Visser, 1998).

Qualitative ontological and epistemological position

Remember from Chapter 6 that positivist researchers believe that they can relatively directly measure reality like a thermometer directly measures body temperature. Most qualitative researchers do not believe in a positivist world that is directly measurable with universal laws and distinct variables. Individuals have their own experiences and perceptions of reality, and we cannot know reality without our subjective interpretations (relativist ontology). Consequently, qualitative researchers may not aim to create knowledge mirroring reality but instead systematically describe the subjective and intersubjective accounts of what individuals experience or construct as their reality (subjectivist epistemology). Many different non-positivist positions are possible, such as constructivism and critical realism. Always check which ontological/epistemological positions are consistent with a particular qualitative method.

Focus on construction processes

Merleau-Ponty (1964) wrote that researchers should not focus on the construction end result but on the construction process. He followed Husserl (1999), who differentiated 'noema', our experiences of something, from 'noesis', the experiencing process leading to the experience. The constructed/experienced result is not the same as the construction/experiencing process, just as a medal is not the same as swimming in a swimming contest. For example, instead of explaining with an MRI scan which brain region is activated in a depressed individual at a particular measurement-moment, qualitative researchers talk with individuals to understand how they experience their depression, how this has gradually evolved, and how this involves conscious, unconscious, embodied, and social processes. Therefore, qualitative researchers may ask not merely 'what' participants experience but also 'how' they experience a phenomenon (Vos, 2021a). For example, constructivists have described how medical narratives and public opinion influence how individuals construct their understanding of depression. Critical theorists have also analysed how social and political powers influence how we make sense of topics such as gender and identity.

Focus on language

Interviews and answers to open questions are often limited by language, for example because individuals cannot find precise words to describe their experiences. Their language is their transient expression of their experiences, which could be different when different interviewers or questions are used. We do not seem to be able to get around this: language is our 'house-of-Being' according to Heidegger (Wrathall, 2010). Therefore, qualitative researchers have examined how individuals use language and stories in social interactions. For example, how do therapists and clients linguistically shape their processes and relationships? How do therapists share a diagnosis, and how do clients interpret this?

When analysing language, qualitative researchers often go beyond what was factually said; for example, the sentence 'I love you' can be said lovingly or sarcastically. Ricoeur (1986) and Gergen and Gergen (1988) wrote that researchers need to interpret human actions and experiences like the clergy interpret holy texts. Researchers often develop their understanding of the underlying meanings by going back-and-forth between part and whole, such as interpreting a detail in the text which may help to understand the general meaning of the text (Rennie, 2007). Our interpretations are also embedded in our unique place and moment in time, where for example, traditions and paradigms influence our interpretations. This method of moving back-and-forward between part and whole is called hermeneutics, after Hermes, the messenger moving between humans and gods. Although researchers can develop a better understanding of the phenomenon in the hermeneutic process, Gadamer (2013) believed we cannot escape the hermeneutic circle in which knower, knowing, and known are intertwined.

Focus on immersion

The immersive mindset follows Dilthey's adage that we should develop an in-depth understanding and not theoretically explain individual experiences, processes, and meanings. This is like the phenomenological difference between being inside the hot, dynamic flow of experiencing the present (note the present tense) or cold outside observations or reflections from a position outside someone's flow-of-experiencing (Vos, 2017). For example, we get a different type of knowledge when we observe beach-goers from a distance in an airconned hotel room instead of when we take our towels and join them on the beach. Therefore, many qualitative researchers try to get as close as possible to their participants' experiences in their data collection, analyses, and interpretations.

Not explaining, but interpreting

Qualitative researchers aim to understand, not explain. Therefore, they temporarily put their theories and assumptions about the research topic to one side (or 'between brackets') to have open conversations with the participants and analyse their answers with an open mind. This is called 'phenomenological-bracketing'. Our theories and assumptions may still be in the back of our mind, but we use critical self-reflection and reflexivity to prevent these from disproportionately influencing our collection and analyses of information. When we immerse ourselves with an open mind into the experiences and stories of participants, we may initially feel lost, but after a while, we may become aware of a theme/meaning, like discovering a clearing in a forest (Wrathall, 2010). Peirce (1965) calls this abduction: a new meaning that was not there before shows itself. However, researchers may need some level of interpretation to understand underlying meanings. Interpreting-without-explaining means trying to describe the phenomena from the participant's perspective and what they experience as meaningful. Qualitative researchers seem to disagree on how much researchers need to interpret phenomena to understand their meaning (e.g., radical phenomenology versus hermeneutics/constructionism).

Popularity

A quick scoping review suggests that 10% to 20% of all publications on psychological therapies use qualitative methods. Qualitative methods seem to be particularly popular in humanistic psychotherapies and counselling psychology, possibly because they seem to share some epistemological values and criticisms of traditional paradigms in research and therapeutic practices. Furthermore, developing qualitative research skills, such as critical self-reflection and reflexivity, may benefit students' therapeutic competencies. some inexperienced researchers seem to select qualitative methods because they unrealistically expect these to be quick and simple; however, trustworthy qualitative research can be complex and time-consuming.

Qualitative lingo

If language is the 'house-of-Being', what does the linguistic house of qualitative research (sometimes called 'qualitative inquiry') look like? In contrast with quantitative researchers, qualitative researchers do not speak about 'data' but 'experiences', 'accounts', and 'stories'. Research participants are 'respondents', 'subjects' or 'co-researchers' (this chapter uses 'participants' and 'data' to be consistent with other for example researchers differ in their terminology to describe whether themes in texts 'emerge', 'are constructed', 'found', 'developed', 'discovered', 'generated', etc). Qualitative researchers may personalise texts with 'I' and 'we' where needed, and explicate critical self-reflection and reflexivity. Note that different qualitative methods may use different terms.

Step 2: Develop a qualitative study design

Definition

Many handbooks on qualitative methods skip how to develop the study design, possibly because qualitative study design and analytical methods are often intertwined (Marshall & Rossman, 2016). This step gives an overview of the most frequently used qualitative study designs. This should be read in conjunction with the steps in the methodology chapter. Whatever you choose, describe *what* study design you have selected, the rationale for *why* you have picked this, and the specific procedures for *how* you apply it. As Chapter 7 described, the qualitative study design follows logically from the research objectives and conceptual framework. See the decision flowchart in Figure 9.1.

Examples

Interview

Interviews aim to examine the lived experiences, processes, and meanings of individuals (Brinkmann, 2013; Roulston, 2010; Salmons, 2009). A range of different types of interviews exist (note that types may overlap):

- **Structured interviews:** All participants are asked the same pre-planned questions in the same order. These one-size-fits-all interview schedules may also include a list of probes (e.g., 'could you tell me more?') and prompts (e.g., closed/pre-coded/fixed answer options). Structured interviews reduce interviewer variability, and prevent questions being forgotten or formulated unclearly or biased. Structured interviews make coding and comparison of interviews more accurate and findings more trustworthy. Whereas its strengths seem to be its focus and specificity, structured

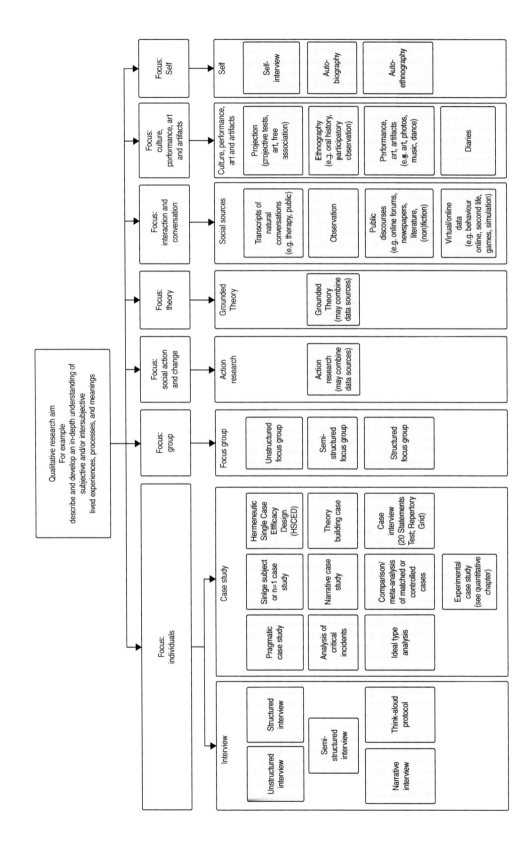

interviews may be slightly less sensitive to detect topics for which the interviewer has not prepared any questions. Feminist critiques highlight that structured interviews may epitomise the non-hierarchical relationship and power imbalance between interviewer and interviewee, as the interviewer aims to extract information from passive interviewees with relatively little reciprocity and empathy.

- **Unstructured interviews:** The interviewer does not ask pre-planned questions. Whereas structured interview questions may limit the topics and structure that participants may spontaneously share, unstructured interviews offer participants more free space to express their experiences, stories, feelings, and thoughts in their own way. For example, researchers may introduce the topic and study aims and invite participants to share any responses. The interview may ask follow-up questions in a free-flowing fashion tailored to the unique contributions of the participants. Examples include historical/biographical interviews, creative interviews and postmodern interviews (Fontana & Frey, 1994). This personalised approach may help participants feel at ease and result in a more natural, honest interview that can facilitate exploring new research fields. Although unstructured interviews may be sensitive to the participant's unique perspectives, they may not be sufficiently specific and relevant for the research aims, for example when the participant goes on a tangent or loses track of their thoughts. Consequently, unstructured interviews can be difficult to conduct and interpret in trustworthy ways, and more difficult to synthesise and compare between participants. There may be less transparency and consistency in the interviewer's questions, as interviewers may for example go on a tangent or ask suggestive questions; however, thorough interviewer training may reduce some interviewer bias. Unstructured interviews and interview coding may not be replicable (Morse in Denzin & Lincoln, 2021).
- **Semi-structured interviews:** Middle ground between fully structured and non-structured interviews. This usually includes a relatively small number of questions (three to nine) followed by pre-determined probes and non-directive follow-up questions. There is some comparability between research subjects as the main questions are the same, although variation will happen. This is the most frequently used interview method (Galletta, 2013).
- **Think-aloud protocols:** Participants are asked to say aloud any thoughts, for example when filling in a questionnaire (e.g., Hak, Van der Veer & Jansen, 2004). This could help with understanding moment-to-moment thoughts (Fonteyn, Kuipers, & Grobe, 1993).
- **Ethnographic interview:** Participants are stimulated to reveal their worldviews, and/or their perspectives/experiences on their culture. Ethnographic interviews may help to describe a topic, how participants structure their world, and differences between views (Spradley, 2016).
- **Narrative interview or life-history interview:** Participants are asked to tell a story (narrative) about their life (life-story or life-review interview) or specific periods or events (episode interview), for example chronologically, with beginning/middle/end, and particular rhetorical styles (Riessman, 2008).

- **Phenomenological interview:** Phenomenological interviews aim to develop an in-depth understanding of an individual's lived experiences of a phenomenon, while the researcher brackets their preconceptions.
- **Interviewing children:** When interviewing children, researchers adjust their interview style, tone, and topics, may use tools like puppets, and critically reflect on ethics and power issues (O'Reilly & Dogra, 2016).
- **Other interviews:** Recent developments in interviewing follow criticisms of the McDonaldisation and asymmetric, one-way, instrumental, manipulative, and researcher-monopoly nature of some interviews (Denzin & Lincoln, 2021). Recent authors also plea for more Socratic, Rogerian, and post-humanistic interviews, and have developed neopositivist, romantic, constructionist, and postmodern interviews.

Case studies

Case studies aim to develop an in-depth understanding of a specific individual ('case'), which may help to answer research questions about therapy outcomes, theory, clinical issues, client experiences, narratives, and organisational aspects of therapy (McLeod, 2010). Case study research is more than the study of case studies, as it requires developing an in-depth understanding of a case via rigorous study design and analysis. A case must have as rich a dataset as possible, for example with clinical records, diaries, questionnaires, clinical tests, and interviews with clients, therapist, friends, relatives, etc. Findings may be difficult to generalise and triangulate, which may be solved (partially) by using standardised procedures, outcome measures, comparison with other cases, time-series analysis, and critical self-reflection and reflexivity. McLeod (2010) describes different types of case study research:

- **Single-case experimental design:** Quantitative experimental design (see Chapter 8).
- **Pragmatic case study:** Gives a pragmatic overview of a case study, with as much information as possible and findings written in standardised/peer-reviewed ways.
- **Single-subject/n = 1 case study:** Examines, usually in time series, how an individual develops over time, for example to explore the effects of a new treatment on an exemplary/unique case.
- **Hermeneutic single-case efficacy design (HSCED):** Gives a rich-description and systematic analysis of case studies. HSCED uses a rich case record, including qualitative and quantitative data, analysed by a team of researchers with self-reflective affirmative and sceptic questions.
- **Narrative case study:** Describes a case from a narrative perspective and may include a narrative, life-history interview, diaries, autobiographical writing, psycho-history, and auto-ethnography.
- **Theory-building case study:** Uses a case to develop and explain clinical, aetiological, and/or therapeutic hypotheses. Early publications on psychological therapies often included case studies, but it has been proven challenging to avoid self-confirmation bias. To reduce bias, researchers may first formulate a detailed conceptual framework which they subsequently explore in the application to cases (Stiles, 2007).

Selecting a suitable case can be tricky (Lefebvre et al., 2019):

- **Single case study (also called 'intrinsic case study'):** This is a single case interesting in itself.
- **Critical incident/significant moments:** These cases are selected to understand incidents or important moments, e.g., in treatment.
- **Ideal-type case:** A composite case embodying key attributes of a set of similar cases. This can help to showcase relevant ideas for clinical practice, such as describing 'the overburdened type', 'the deviation type', 'the deficit type' of therapy clients.
- **Multiple case study design:** This may help generalise findings across cases. Cases can be matched or controlled cases, selected based on characteristics such as having received similar treatments.
- **Experimental case study design:** See Chapter 8.

Focus groups

Researchers may use focus groups to understand how a group of individuals experiences, socially constructs, and interprets a phenomenon (Carey & Asbury, 2016; Fern & Fern, 2001; Liamputtong, 2011). A focus group is not merely the sum of individual interviews and giving individual turns but facilitates social interaction and group dynamics. The facilitator stimulates synergy so the group generates new ideas beyond what an individual could come up with ('the whole is greater than the sum of the individuals'). Focus groups could be created for the research project or could be existing groups, e.g., therapy groups, hobby clubs, families, or friends. Several types of focus groups exist, such as:

- **Unstructured groups:** may facilitate group dynamics to emerge naturally but could take longer and be less focused
- **Structured groups:** may hinder group dynamics and synergy from evolving but could yield generalisable focused findings
- **Semi-structured groups:** middle ground between unstructured/structured groups
- **Nominal groups:** e.g., includes brainstorming techniques
- **Delphi groups:** e.g., researchers send key statements before group sessions
- **Co-operative inquiry groups:** participants are invited as co-researchers in the co-creation of the focus, content, and process
- **Interpersonal process recall:** e.g., therapists and clients watch and discuss session recordings together

Action research

Action research is sometimes divided into researchers aiming to make a change after completion of the research and researchers who aim to empower stakeholders and foster change through the study design (Herr & Anderson, 2014; McNiff, 2016). The latter may actively invite individuals whose voice is often oppressed in society as equal co-researchers who help shape the study design and data collection. This is often conducted in organisations, communities, and education. Participatory action research or co-operative inquiry is based on the idea that meaning is enacted through the participation of the human mind with their world and fellow humans; due to its dynamic and fluid method, researchers cannot predict what might emerge (Reason & Bradbury, 2001). The researcher is transparent about the aims and methods with co-researchers. Action researchers argue knowledge has to be practical and involves a willingness and capacity to analyse the powers in social systems constantly and critically, and stand on the side of oppressed individuals. Action research is influenced by critical pedagogues, such as Freire, and critical theorists, such as Habermas.

Grounded theory

Grounded theory aims to construct a new conceptual framework. Contrasting with other research methods, theory building is the primary aim and not secondary or a by-product. Grounded theory aims to develop a bottom-up theory based on one or multiple research methods, such as interviews and focused literature reviews. Grounded theory may be regarded as a study design and analytical method, and will therefore be elaborated in the next step.

Study designs using existing social sources (conversations, observations, interactions)

A researcher may examine naturally occurring or pre-existing data, such as observing individuals or naturally occurring conversations, interactions, discourses, and narratives. For example, a researcher may analyse therapy recordings, conversations, discourses, and narratives in the public domain, such as online forums, novels, newspapers, and literature. Researchers may analyse the content, but also the interactional style, micro-emotions/micro-aggressions, non-verbal physical behaviour, kinesics (body motion), proxemics (use of space), and intuitions (Finlay, 2006). Data may include internet/virtual ethnography, digital storytelling, behaviour in online forums or second-life games and simulations. This design's strength is that researchers do not influence the information, although it can be tricky to justify data selection. Without follow-up conversations, it may be challenging to understand what individuals precisely experienced or meant. Examples can be found in the next step.

Study designs using existing culture, performance, art, and artifacts

The following study designs may help to understand how individuals experience and construct their world via physical and cultural products. These study designs may be particularly helpful for topics that are less accessible for conscious reflection and verbal expression, for example due to psychological defence mechanisms or lack of linguistic skills.

- **Projection:** Instead of directly asking participants about their views/experiences, projective tests may reveal more unconscious processes, e.g., projective tests or free association (Steinman, 2009). This may involve arts-based and multimodal inquiry such as asking participants to draw, paint, make, or examine paintings or photos; asking interviewees about personally meaningful objects may also stimulate sharing other information (Bagnoli, 2009; Fraser & Al Sayah, 2011; Leavy, 2020; Rose, 2016).
- **Ethnographic methods:** Ethnography offers a broad range of study designs and data, e.g., research into oral histories and speaking with community elders (Gobo, 2008; Madison, 2011). This may include fieldwork and participatory observation, such as spending time in a community or hospital ward, systematically observing, listening, and talking with people. This may include analyses of physical surroundings, art, and indigenous/ethnic artifacts. This can give an in-depth understanding of how

individuals experience and interact with their physical and social context and how this context may influence their experiences.

- **Performance ethnography and ethnodrama/ethotheatre:** Research into art and drama therapies often includes a description and/or analysis of art and drama, e.g., arts-based inquiry (Hamera, 2006).
- **Reflective diaries or research journals:** Researchers may systematically analyse diaries or other researchers' research journals (Alaszewski, 2006).

Self-oriented study designs

- **Self-reflection:** Self-reflection is part of most qualitative methods (see Chapter 4). Sometimes, researchers conduct self-interviews before interviewing participants, e.g., to explore their own position and as an additional data source (Keightley, Pickering, & Allett, 2012).
- **Auto-ethnographic methods:** Through self-observation and analysis of various personal sources of data, auto-ethnographers aim to create personal stories and narratives about their life or experiences, assuming these resonate with the experiences of others (Jones, Adams, & Ellis, 2016). This may include self-interview, auto-biographic writing, diaries, digital/photo/video media, and cognitive mapping. Auto-ethnography can explore topics in which the researcher has unique experience or expertise, where it is challenging or unethical to recruit others or gain thick descriptions and deep self-insight. Auto-ethnography has been criticised for its thin line between fact and fiction, the difficulty to be rigorous in one's critical self-reflection, and the risk of intellectual navel-gazing and narcissistic self-indulgence. May be difficult to get published or get accepted for student research.

Step 3: Develop and conduct interviews

Definition

Interviews are the most frequently used qualitative study design. Therefore, this section gives key pointers on how to develop and conduct interviews (see Brinkmann, 2013; Roulston, 2010; Salmons, 2009).

Procedures

1. Define key concepts

Following the research aims and objectives (see Chapter 6), the interviewer needs to describe the topic and identify the specific concept, construct, or phenomenon they want to study. It is important to demarcate the concept to focus the interviews and avoid going off-topic. It can be helpful to develop a table with definitions of relatively similar but different concepts and to create a Venn diagram showing how concepts overlap and differ. Whereas a research publication may require academic terms and definitions (academic formulation), the researcher may translate this with easier synonyms and definitions for layman interviewees (public-friendly formulation). Researchers may use the following resources to define their key concepts:

- **Literature review:** Definitions from others, e.g., researchers, research participants, professional bodies and advocacy groups, and empirical evidence for definitions.
- **Invite stakeholders:** Definitions and experiences from invited research experts, experts-by-experience, and other stakeholders.
- **Critical self-reflection and reflexivity:** Changes in definitions, norms and meanings, controversies, and inconsistencies, reflection on social and political influences on how people understand this concept. Researchers write in a reflective research journal how they experience and define this concept, their biases, and preconceptions.

2. Consider pre-existing interview schedules

An interviewer may consider using or adjusting pre-existing interview schedules, which may avoid them reinventing the wheel, increase trustworthiness, and enable comparison. Interview schedules may be found via search engines and dedicated databases (e.g., PsycTests), and may include:

- **Clinical interviews:** Interviews to assess clinical phenomena, often about diagnostic categories (e.g., Structured Clinical Interview DSM, DSM Cultural Formulation Interview, Iowa Structured Psychiatric Interview, Present State Examination, Adult Attachment Interview).
- **Client helpfulness interviews**: Clients are asked what they find helpful or unhelpful in therapy, and their processes of change (Cooper, McLeod, & Ogden, 2015). Researchers ask about helpful experiences, and experiences that may be unhelpful, hindering, disappointing, harmful, or problematic. The Client Change Interview is the most frequently used mixed methods client helpfulness interview schedule (Elliott & Rodgers, 2008). This includes general questions ('What has therapy been like?') and changes ('What changes, if any, have you noticed since therapy started? Has anything changed for the worse? Is there anything you wanted to change that hasn't?'). Clients rate how expected, likely, and important each change is. Subsequent questions regard attributions ('What do you think caused these changes?'), resources and limitations ('What personal strengths/life situations have helped/limited you in making use of therapy to deal with your problems?'), helpful aspects ('Can you sum up what has been helpful about therapy?'), problematic aspects ('What kinds of things about therapy have been hindering, unhelpful, negative, or disappointing? Were there things in therapy which were difficult or painful but still OK or helpful? Has anything been missing?'). The Private-Theories Interview is a psychoanalytic interview schedule.
- **Template/hermeneutic aid:** These systematic questions and interpretational frameworks can be used to develop a holistic, in-depth understanding of a phenomenon. For example, an interviewer may ask how an interviewee experiences a phenomenon regarding seven fractions of their lifeworld: selfhood, sociality, embodiment, temporality, spatiality, project, and discourse (Sheffield School Template.

Ashworth, 2003). Interviewers may also ask interviewees how they experience a phenomenon in different dimensions of their life, such as their physical, personal, social, and spiritual worlds; by asking about their experiences, paradoxes and emotions in each world, the researchers develop a holistic understanding (structural existential analysis: Van Deurzen, 2014). These templates have been criticised for being subjective, non-systematic selections by the researchers. A systematic evidence-based alternative is Systematic Pragmatic Phenomenological Analysis, offering a template of ten questions/ perspectives for interview questions and analyses (see Step 6; Vos, 2021a).

- **Repertory grid:** This is a systematic approach to elicit how an individual experiences their social world via questions about ten elements (e.g., roles, for self or others, activities, careers) which they then compare with one another; these comparisons can lead to new constructs, and participants could be asked how they experience these constructs (Winter, 2003).

3. Develop unstructured interviews

Unstructured interviews do not have pre-determined interview schedules. Based on their clearly defined research aims, and academically formulated and public-friendly concepts, researchers prepare how they will describe the aim of the interview and how they will introduce the topic to the participant. They will also prepare instructions for the participants, such as inviting them to share whatever comes to their mind regarding the topic. Interviewers may flexibly use a pre-developed topic list to inspire their follow-up questions and to check whether the participant has discussed all potentially relevant topics; some researchers share this topic list with interviewees, although this may limit/bias them. To prepare themselves to keep the interviews as open/unbiased as possible (phenomenological-bracketing), interviewers engage in critical self-reflection and reflexivity, for example via a research journal, personal therapy, and self-interview.

4. Develop structured/semi-structured interview schedules

A schedule for structured and semi-structured interviews may include the following:

1 **Introduction/instructions:** How the interviewer will introduce themselves, express gratitude to the interviewees, introduce interview aims, describe the topic in public-friendly terms, and give instructions on what is expected from interviewees.
2 **Introductory interview questions:** Questions to set interviewees at ease, understand the context, gradually move to focused questions.
3 **Socio-demographic questions:** An interviewer often starts with simple questions to understand the life-situation of the participant, which may help to contextualise/ interpret the interviewee's answer, for example with a socio-demographic questionnaire (Online Table 7.3).
4 **Focused interview questions:** Stimulate interviewees to speak about the topic. It can be recommended to formulate questions in the following ways:
   i **Falsifiable:** Interviewees should be able to share experiences/opinions different from the researcher, e.g., 'what are your experiences about X' instead of 'what are your negative experiences about X?'
   ii **Non-leading:** Not suggestive/leading in a particular direction, e.g., 'do you also think...'

iii **Non-assumptive:** For example, 'how frequently do you use contraceptives?' assumes contraceptive usage.

iv **Clear and non-ambiguous.**

v **As simple as possible:** For example, no jargon, in words understandable for participants.

vi **Not double-barred:** For example, 'what is your opinion about X and Y?'

vii **Specific but open:** For example, instead of the double-barred question 'how often do you watch sad movies' ask multiple specific but open questions such as 'do you watch movies', 'how often do you watch movies', 'which feelings do you experience when watching movies'.

viii **Require little self-insight/self-awareness:** Preferably about topics the interviewee has reflected upon before.

ix **Consider memory bias:** As individuals may generalise when they talk about a period in their life and leave out much detail, researchers may want to ask very specific questions about specific life events instead of asking about periods in general. It can be difficult for individuals to remember what they were feeling and thinking at a particular point in time, and people often interpret the past through the lens of their current experiences and mood (e.g., 'mood congruent retrieval bias'). Therefore, researchers may want to interpret their participants' answers about the past as reconstructions and not as perfectly accurate accounts; thus, research objectives should be formulated as examining how individuals look back at their past (and not as examining true facts of their past). Instead of asking what individuals thought in the past, and how they think now, it may be easier for individuals to describe how they feel and think in the present, and describe whether and how this may have changed over time, e.g. 'What changes, if any, have you noticed in yourself since therapy started?' (cf. Client Change Interview: Elliott & Rodgers, 2008).

x **Ethical:** Sensitive and respectful about private, political, or controversial topics.

xi **Non-intrusive:** Avoid or be sensitive regarding emotionally loaded topics such as traumatic life experiences; unlikely to trigger disruptive emotions, particularly in vulnerable individuals.

xii **Not triggering of defence mechanisms or socially desirable answers:** Interviewees may not talk honestly about socially undesirable topics, such as crimes, (self-)harm, suicide.

xiii **Non-comparing:** Interviewees are not asked to evaluate or compare themselves with others as people often overestimate themselves (i.e., the Lake-Wobegon effect).

xiv **Correct words:** Interviewees may give different answers depending on whether you ask them to describe their 'feelings', 'thoughts', 'memories', 'interpretations' (Vos et al., 2008).

xv **Give the option of not answering**.

5 **Probes:** Probes stimulate interviewees to continue/elaborate. Probes are usually non-directive, e.g., 'mm' or 'can you say more about this?' Research/ethics proposals often include a list of possible probes.

6 **Prompts:** Prompts are more specific ways to stimulate interviewees, e.g., answer options on cards. May risk directivity and bias but may allow mixed methods analysis.

7 **Follow-up questions:** In unstructured interviews and some semi-structured interviews, the interviewer may ask spontaneous follow-up questions tailored to what the interviewee has said. This risks self-confirmation bias, tunnel-thinking,

and directivity. Halo bias means that previous answers bias subsequent questions, stereotyping/pigeon-holing interviewees, and not allowing counter-examples.

8   **Ending questions:** At the end, a reviewer may ask 'how did you experience this interview?', 'would you like to add/change anything?', 'do you have any recommendations?' Some researchers ask, 'what was the most important message or conclusion for you during this interview?' (Vos, 2021a).

9   **Question order:** Interview questions are usually placed in a logical order to stimulate flow, for example, from simple to complex questions, and broad to specific topics. In structured and often semi-structured interviews, interviewers stick to a pre-determined order.

10   **Sharing questions:** Some researchers send interviewees the interview schedule beforehand. This stimulates researcher transparency, decreases uncertainty and anxiety, and allows participants to prepare themselves and pre-reflect. Particularly helpful for interviewees who prefer structure/certainty, such as individuals on the autistic spectrum. However, this may reduce spontaneous answers.

5. Assess the quality of interview schedules

Researchers ask for feedback from experts/supervisors/stakeholders, assess the quality of the interview schedule and make adjustments where needed (e.g., reflective questions in Online Table 9.1).

6. Decide interview organisation procedures

Interviewers may consider several practical aspects:

- **Online/in-person:** reflect on pros/cons (Online Table 7.5)
- **Location:** e.g., easily accessible, quiet, safe space with other people nearby, protecting the privacy of interviewee and interviewer
- **Recorder:** e.g., reliable, tested, password-/data-protected, professional, back-up emergency recorder
- **Consent forms:** bring consent-forms to the interview (see Chapter 11)
- **Distress protocol:** procedures if interviewee shows distress (see Chapter 11)
- **Debrief protocol:** information for participants after the interview (see Chapter 11)

7. Conduct a self-interview

Researchers may conduct a self-interview before interviewing others to examine the feasibility of the interview schedule, understand what it is like to be interviewed, and facilitate critical self-reflection (Keightley, Pickering & Allett, 2012). A self-interview means for example that the researcher is interviewed by themselves or someone else, such as a supervisor or therapist. Self-interviews may improve the critical self-reflection and reflexibity and the study's trustworthiness. Ideally, the researcher reflects on the self-interview together with the interviewer or a research supervisor, particularly to identify the assumptions and blind spots which may be difficult to identify on their own. A self-interview may be described in a methodology chapter/section, but may also be included as a separate (sub)section in the findings chapter/section. This description of the self-interview may include the researcher's critical reflections about their experiences of being interviewed, assumptions about the topic (e.g. themes/subthemes or priorities that came up during their own interview), blind spots and biases, and the implications for how they will cope with their assumptions and blind spots during the interviews and analyses, and how they have possibly rephrased the interview or changed the research procedures in response to the self-interview.

8. Conduct a feasibility study

The interviewer may conduct a feasibility interview to develop their interviewing skills and identify flaws in the interview schedule/procedures. At the end of the interview, the interviewer may ask participants what it was like to be interviewed, their perception of the practicalities/organisation, interview introduction/instructions, which questions were easy/difficult, any emotions triggered, and any recommendations. A researcher may first conduct one interview case study, analyse this data and write a report to check the feasibility of the interview schedule and analytical procedures.

Step 4: Transcribe and code interviews

Definition

Interviews are usually transcribed before data analysis. Transcriptions can be trusted more than biased or incomplete notes taken during interviews.

Procedures

1. Transcribe

Most qualitative researchers transcribe interviews themselves to prevent ethical concerns with external transcription companies and transcription errors with transcription software. This also allows immersion in the interviews. Interview transcription is time-intensive and can require one/two days per interview hour. Interviews are transcribed as accurately as possible, both what was said and how it was said. For example, sentences are usually kept short, with commas for sub-clauses, quotation marks when citing others, and brackets for interruptions [interviewer: OK]. Emphases can be highlighted with question/exclamation marks and *italics*. Para-verbal communication can be placed between parentheses (laugh; inaudible; 6-sec silence). For confidentiality purposes, names such as [her sister] are replaced with brackets. Researchers check how they should transcribe/code the interviews for their qualitative analysis method. For example, conversation analysis entails a complex coding system containing transcribing phonetics, pauses, and non-verbal communication. Translations of interviews in other languages are often done after analysis as interpreters may influence the findings (See more tips: Azevedo et al., 2017; Easton, McComish, & Greenberg, 2000; MacLean, Meyer, & Estable, 2004).

2. Rate with multiple raters and observation schedules

The non-verbal behaviour/interactions in recordings may be coded by multiple assessors, for example with the help of an observation schedule defining aspects of behaviour/interactions and examples/anchors (e.g., 'self-stroking behaviour' with anchors 'small strokes' and 'large strokes'). Inter-rater agreement could be statistically calculated with Kappa, and disagreements may be discussed until agreement is achieved. Chapter 3, Step 9 gives examples of coding schemes.

3. Write in reflective research journal and memos

Transcribing and analysing may trigger feelings, thoughts, and associations, which can be valuable sources of information. Therefore, researchers jot down any responses in field notes and memos which they can save in their dataset or reflective research journals. Memos are reflections about codes and how they relate to data and other codes, and raising significant codes to categories. Memos are 'the narrated records of theorist's analytical conversations with [themselves] about the research data' (Lempert, 2007, p.132), and usually answer questions such as 'do I see a pattern?', 'how could this pattern be explained?', 'what is said and what is not said?', and 'what is my influence as interviewer/transcriber/analyser?' (Birks, Chapman, & Francis, 2008).

4. Insert in software

Depending on the type of qualitative analysis, researchers may want to insert interview transcripts into qualitative data analysis software such as NVivo or Atlas (Fisher, 2017; Friese, 2019; Jackson & Bazeley, 2019; see QADAS options in Online Table 7.4). Software may for instance help with systematically analysing rich qualitative data, and analysing the quantitative frequency of words. As shown in the following sections, many researchers insert interviews in tables in a text editor such as Word.

5. Identify meaning-units

After immersing themselves via interview transcription and reading whole transcripts, most qualitative researchers divide the text into different meaning-units. A meaning-unit is a part of a text, ranging from one word to some paragraphs conveying one idea/meaning. Often, researchers re-adjust the meaning-units after re-reading. Each meaning-unit is, for example, inserted into a different row in a table in a word processor for example, with the following columns:

- **Timestamp on recording**
- **Meaning-unit**
- **Non-verbal observation:** e.g., non-verbal observations for each meaning-unit
- **Initial interpretation:** e.g., researcher's initial interpretation of the meaning/theme of this meaning-unit
- **Researcher notes:** e.g., associations and self-reflective observations

6. Coding meaning-units

After identifying the initial meaning-units, qualitative researchers may compare the initial meanings of the different meaning-units to identify similarities and dissimilarities (Wicks, 2017). They may start seeing common themes across meaning-units. They continue developing new themes until they reach a point of saturation where no new themes are identified. One meaning-unit may be categorised/clustered into multiple themes (in some methodsdescribed as 'subordinate themes' or 'sub-themes'). Categorising/clustering is a creative process, which heavily relies on the researcher's ability to see patterns without disproportionally imposing their preconceptions. Subsequently, the researcher may examine connections between themes, and identify overarching/larger themes (sometimes known as 'superordinate themes'). Researchers may add three columns to a table in a word processor (see Table 9.1):

Table 9.1 Example interview transcript

Time	Text (divided into meaning-units)	Initial interpretation	Subordinate theme	Superordinate theme	Template dimensions	Researcher notes
01:04:02	I always feel sad (sigh).	Sadness, possible depression	Depression	Mental health problems	Types-of-meaning framework (Vos, 2022): Unfulfilled hedonistic meaning	Unsure whether 'sadness' refers to a clinical diagnosis

- **Theme:** The researcher's identification of the theme in this meaning-unit; after re-reading the transcripts, the researcher may revisit the initial interpretation/theme.
- **Overarching theme:** After re-reading the transcripts, the researcher may identify a cluster or superordinate theme across the themes.
- **Template/hermeneutic aid:** Some researchers add columns for the pre-defined dimensions/categories of a template/hermeneutic aid.
- **Researcher notes:** Researchers may add interpretations (e.g., inferences, meaning, explanations, lessons, ordering, alternative interpretations).

Step 5: Choose qualitative analysis

Definition

Qualitative information can be analysed in different ways. This section gives an overview of the most frequently used qualitative analyses in psychological therapies. As many phenomenological methods exist, these are described separately in the next step. The flowchart in Figure 9.2. is based on the most frequently used methods in therapy research, and therefore slightly deviates from other canonical typologies of qualitative research (e.g., Denzin & Lincoln, 2021).

Procedures

As this section will elaborate, researchers first determine their research aims and the collected data, and subsequently they select an analytical method that fits these aims and data best. This selection will also depend on their epistemological/ontological positions, competencies, and resources. Figure 9.2 offers a decision-tree for selecting a qualitative analysis.

1 **Decide qualitative research aim and qualitative study design.**
2 **Choose analysis according to data type:** Most analytical methods can be used with verbal data, such as interviews and focus groups. Other analytical methods may examine concepts, theories, culture, or ethnographic products.
3 **Choose analysis according to research aim:** Different analytical methods answer different research aims.
4 **Select analytical school:** Many analytical methods have multiple schools. For example, there are many different types of phenomenological analysis. Schools may

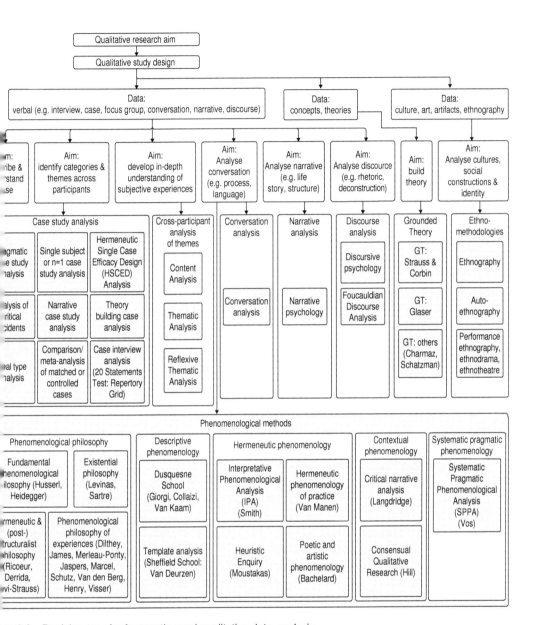

re 9.2 Decision-tree for frequently used qualitative data analysis

not be fundamentally different but be historical relics, grown out of paradigmatic thinking, personal tastes, self-promotion, politics, and cronyism (NB: the evolution of qualitative schools seems similar to quantitative schools).

5 **Read more:** To deepen their knowledge and position their research project, researchers search for and read handbooks/instruction texts on the chosen method, and examine the strengths and weaknesses of studies in which the method has been applied.

6 **Specify procedures/steps:** Researchers identify the specific analytical procedures/ steps for their research project.

Examples

Case study analysis

Data: Verbal, mixed.

Aim: Describe and understand cases.

Pros/cons: In-depth understanding of an individual; may be difficult to generalise and tri-angulate and may have ethical issues, which may be solved in the study design. Conducting case studies may also train clinical skills, e.g., analysing a client in-detail. Frequently applied on psychological therapies.

Schools: See case studies in Step 2 of this chapter (McLeod, 2010).

Content analysis and (reflexive) thematic analysis

Data: Verbal.

Aim: Identify generalisable categories and themes across participants. Researchers may want to identify commonalities across individuals by identifying common themes in the answers of multiple interviewees.

Pros/cons: Relatively straightforward. The implicit assumption that themes can be gener-alised has been criticised for being positivist, i.e., assuming universal laws in human experi-ences. Although these analytical methods allow findings to be generalised across study par-ticipants, they may not be generalised beyond small non-representative samples. Frequently applied in psychological therapies.

Schools:

- **Content analysis:** Aims to identify themes across subjects. Sometimes regarded as semi-quantitative and positivist, for example when reporting frequencies. Example procedures: researcher categorises all answers across participants question-per-question and subsequently reports how often each category is given as an answer to a question.
- **Thematic analysis:** Aims to identify themes. A theme is more than the content of a person's answer to a question and focuses on the meaning for the interviewee. A theme may be difficult to put into a few words, like a theme in music is a configuration of certain musical cues with a specific meaning for the listener. Various thematic analyses exist (Guest, MacQueen, & Namey, 2011). Example procedures: identify themes across participants and categorise themes into groups with a superordinate theme name.
- **Reflexive thematic analysis:** Frequently used in psychological therapies, adding critical self-reflection reflexivity to identifying themes. Clarke and Braun (2018) described seven steps:

    1   Transcription
    2   Reading and familiarisation
    3   Coding
    4   Searching for themes
    5   Reviewing themes

6   Defining and naming themes
7   Finalising analysis

Phenomenological analysis

Data: Verbal (mixed).

Aim: Develop in-depth understanding of subjective experiences. Whereas content and thematic analyses primarily aim to identify broad themes across research subjects, phenomenological analysis primarily aims to describe and develop an in-depth understanding of the lived experiences of one individual at a time. The comparison of individuals may come later after the analysis of each participant, but identifying cross-participant themes is usually only a secondary aim. Researchers use phenomenological-bracketing to temporarily set aside their presuppositions about the topic and participants. For example, they conduct and describe the interviews as closely as possible to the client's experiences (although hermeneutic phenomenologists attribute a larger role for researcher interpretations).

Pros/cons: This offers in-depth understanding of a phenomenon. Popular in psychological therapies. This often appeals to novice researchers for its apparent simplicity, but untrained researchers may unintentionally not apply 'phenomenology' but 'an analytical method *inspired by* phenomenology'. It can be difficult to phenomenologically bracket one's assumptions, particularly in hermeneutic-phenomenological methods, which could, for example, render a method such as 'interpretative phenomenological analysis' into 'interpretative analysis' with unfalsifiable interpretations and unethical misuse of participants to impose and allegedly 'confirm' one's assumptions (self-confirmation bias) (Zahavi, 2018). A lack of phenomenological-bracketing may be caused by researchers merely using simple self-reflection, which may be solved by systematic critical self-reflection and reflexivity. It may require training of researchers, rigour, and time-commitment.

Schools: See the next step in this chapter (e.g., Langdridge, 2007).

Conversation analysis

Data: Conversations and social interactions.

Aims: Develop an in-depth understanding of the content and processes of conversations. This is based on Wittgenstein's argument that our subjective and intersubjective reality is primarily constructed through language. For example, individuals, institutions, and societies may use particular 'language games'. Talk is more than empty signs, and may imply actions and unique meaning for individuals. For example, therapists within a mental health service may use the language of a DSM-diagnosis, but a diagnosis may have a different meaning for clients than for therapists. Sometimes applied in psychological therapies.

Pros/cons: Detailed understanding of conversational processes, language usage, social interactions, and the social construction of experiences. Due to the time-intensive data-transcription and analysis process, studies may be limited to a small number of textual passages, which may be difficult to generalise.

Schools: Whereas Wittgenstein's analyses remained relatively abstract, ethnomethodologists such as Goffman analysed micro-social processes of practical reasoning in daily life, and researchers such as Schelgoff and Sacks developed conversation analysis. The researcher selects specific passages from transcripts of conversations (although other texts may be used), such as therapy sessions from a few therapist–client dyads; this selection needs to be precise and justified. The texts are transcribed in more detail than in other methods, e.g., including phonetics. After analysing a passage, the researcher may search for other passages in the text confirming or rejecting analyses. Researchers may use principles/rules of thumb to identify patterns of how an institutional reality is constituted, such as the organisation of turn-taking in conversations, conversation sequences, lexical choice, and interactional asymmetries. (See Hutchby & Wooffitt, 2008; Stivers & Sidnell, 2012.)

Narrative analysis

Data: Verbal.

Aim: Understand how individuals make sense of their experiences and construct their reality via stories to themselves and others. Narratives help us order the often unorganised world and life events and construct a narrative identity for ourselves. Labov and Waletzky (1967) noticed people tend to organise stories with a beginning, middle, and end, a time-space orientation, complicating plot, climax, evaluation, result or resolution, and a coda/link to the present. Clients also often tell stories in therapy, which has inspired the emergence of narrative psychotherapy. Narrative analysis is more than an analysis of a narrative, as it tries to understand the subjective meaning of the story for the individual and the meaning for social interaction, for example by analysing how the story is structured, language use, and co-construction between speaker and listener. Researchers have found narratives can be described along the dimensions of stable/regressive/progressive and neutral/pessimistic/optimistic. Narrative analysis is sometimes applied in therapy research.

Pros/cons: In-depth understanding of the content, processes, and structures of how individuals construct their reality via stories. Often close to how individuals use stories in daily life social interactions. Some individuals may find it difficult to tell stories spontaneously, which may be ameliorated by good interview instructions/questions. Similar to the limitations of other methods, specific narratives may be difficult to generalise and may be biased.

Schools: There are many ways to conduct narrative interviews. Life-story or life-review interviews are used more often than episode interviews. Riessman (2008) describes how typical interviewees could be invited to tell stories which will be transcribed and analysed to identify exemplar narratives, which can subsequently be used to understand the interviewee's experiences. McLeod and Balamoutsou have developed a method for narrative analysis of therapy transcripts. The JAKOB method offers a psychoanalysis-inspired narrative analysis of therapy transcripts. Narratives can also be analysed via mixed methods, such as by using the Narrative Process Coding Scheme, Core Conflictual Relationship Theme, Narrative Coherence Rating, or the Scale to Assess Narrative Development (Herman & Vervaeck, 2019).

Discursive psychology and discourse analysis

Data: Any qualitative data.

Aims: Understand larger discourses, written or spoken debate, in a society or community about a topic. Discourse analysis shares many ideas from conversation analysis, influenced by social psychology, semiotics, and psychoanalysis. Whereas conversation analysis seems to focus more on language use and the interaction in text passages, discourse analysis tries to identify hidden meanings in often large texts or debates. Discourse analysis often focuses on marginalised populations, with the long-term aim of social change. Discourse analysts, for example, Frankfurt-school-like critiques of dominant discourses, ideologies and paradigms in therapeutic practice, research and society, or they may use post-structuralist critiques of structural linguistics. Discourse analysis has become more popular in social psychology since the turn of the millennium.

Pros/cons: Findings can critique dominant discourses and inspire reflexive conversations about this. However, this may be biased due to the important interpretive role of the researcher and sometimes lack of detailed procedures, although this may be reduced via critical self-reflection/reflexivity. Sometimes applied in therapy research.

Schools: There are multiple schools and not one overarching methodology (Boréus & Bergström, 2017; Wodak & Meyer, 2015), but all share the ideal of being solid, comprehensive, and transparent (Jørgensen & Phillips, 2002).

- **Discursive social psychology:** Discourse analysis has sometimes been described as an attitude or analytic mentality rather than a method with step-by-step procedures. There are many ways to analyse discourses (Avdi & Georgaca, 2007; Potter, 2013). Potter, Wetherell, and Edwards have focused their analyses on naturally occurring talk. Billig (2009) developed an analytical approach to rhetoric to understand how individuals position themselves regarding discourses.
- **Foucauldian discourse analysis (FDA):** According to Michel Foucault, discourses facilitate and limit, enable and constrain what can be said by whom, where, and when (Parker, 2014). FDA focuses on discursive sources within a culture, particularly how the social distribution of power and oppression evolves in discourse. FDA can be applied to broad trends and concepts. Several systems have been proposed (Arribas-Ayllon & Walkerdine in Willig, 2019; Kendall & Wickham, 2004). Parker (2014) proposed 20 steps, from selecting texts (1–2) and systematically identifying subjects and objects (3–12), to identifying discourses that structure the text and reproduce power dynamics (13–20). Willig (in Smith, 2015 identified six FDA steps:

1 **Discursive construction:** Identify how the discursive phenomenon is constructed in the text (e.g., a cancer patient refers to cancer as 'it').
2 **Discourses:** Locate how the discursive phenomenon is located in broader discourses (e.g., biomedical discourses).
3 **Action orientation:** Detailed analysis of how the discursive phenomenon fits in the broader discourse (e.g., goals, functions, impact).
4 **Positionings:** Identify subject positions within a discourse (e.g., rights, duties).
5 **Practice:** Explore how the discursive constructions and positionings open up and/or close down opportunities for action, e.g., what can be said and done in the community/society.
6 **Subjectivity:** Explore participants' experiences, feelings, and thoughts.

Grounded theory

Data: Concepts/theories, mixed-data.

Aims: Construct a new conceptual/theoretical framework of social phenomena via mixed data, as unbiased as possible. Grounded theory started with Glaser and Strauss' seminal text *The Discovery of Grounded Theory* (2017). They aimed to build a theoretical/conceptual framework of social phenomena grounded in the data rather than being imposed upon it.

Pros/cons: Theory building is the primary aim, in contrast with other analytical methods, where this is often a secondary aim or by-product. Grounded theory can be challenging for novice researchers due to its complex procedures and required rigour, but may offer freedom for creativity and new ideas. Risks induction bias, although this could be prevented by a rigorous study design, including systematic reviews, selection of expert interviewees, and critical self-reflection and reflexivity. Common in sociology and anthropology, sometimes applied in therapy research. Note that in grounded theory studies, researchers may edit or extend the literature review that they may have done at an earlier stage in their research project (they may wait with conducting a literature review until they have conducted interviews, but often, research, ethics or grant committees require researchers to conduct a literature review at an early stage of research); if they make any changes in their literature review after interviews, they are transparent in the chapter/section on the literature review what they have changed and why they have changed this.

Schools: There are three leading schools. Strauss and Corbin (1990) stressed systematic procedures to discover concepts. Glaser (1978) told researchers to wait patiently to let concepts emerge. Others include, for example, Charmaz (2015), Corbin and Strauss (2014), and Glaser (1978) give clear step-by-step guides:

1. **Formulate broad, open research questions:** For example, 'how do women manage a pregnancy complicated by mental health problems?' Research questions emphasise activities and social processes.
2. **Interview in purposive sample:** Data collection stops when the category system or theory is saturated, i.e., each extra participant adds few new categories (often 8–20 participants).
3. **Conduct a focused literature review:** Review literature for further information, examples, and counter-examples. To keep an open mind, grounded theory researchers do not conduct a focused literature review before interviews (if research committees require a prior literature review, researchers conduct a broad scoping review).
4. **Open coding:** Soon after data collection, the researcher generates as many categories as possible via open coding, which is process of identifying and naming data by breaking down, examining, comparing, conceptualising, and categorising data: 'each line, sentence, paragraph etc. is read in search of the answer to the repeated question: "what is this about? What is being referenced here?"' (Borgatti, 2023, p.8). Where possible, categories are formulated as activities and processes.
5. **Identify higher-order clusters of categories from the initial categories.**
6. **Axial coding:** Compare the clusters/categories in relationship to one other, frequently searching for causal explanations and interactions. For example, categories, higher-order clusters, and axial codes are compared within and across cases, leading to further refining. The researcher may use memos and diagrams.
7. **Identify main category.**

Ethnographic methodologies

Data: Ethnographic information, e.g., participant observations, interviews, art, culture, artifacts, media-coverage. Auto-ethnography describes one's own life/life events as participant researcher.

Aims: Understanding cultures, actions, interactions, and conduct in daily life contexts.

Pros/cons: Contextual understanding and rich information about behaviour and actions. Helpful for topics participants may be reluctant about, unaware of, unable to articulate, or find irrelevant. It may be time-consuming, sacrifice breadth for depth, and quality depends on the researcher's skills. Rarely applied in therapy research.

Schools:

- **Ethnography:** Since the foundational publications by Mead, Malinowski, and Evans-Pritchard, many ethnographic methods have emerged (Atkinson, 2007; Fetterman, 2019; Gobo, 2008; Siddique, 2011). Typical steps include:

  1 **Development of observation guide based on literature**: what will be observed (e.g., setting, activities, interactions, participants, verbal/non-verbal)
  2 **Initial broad field notes:** thick description, e.g., chronology, spoken keywords/ phrases, non-verbal, diagrams, timing
  3 **Focused in-depth field notes:** after multiple observations, the researcher is more familiarised, has built rapport, and has deconstructed assumptions
  4 **Confirmation:** testing hypotheses/interpretations
  5 **Analysis:** e.g., coding; other analytical methods may be used (e.g., content/ thematic analysis)

- **Auto-ethnography:** The researcher focuses on their own experiences and life story via a broad range of data-collection and reflective methods (see Step 4).
- **Performance ethnography, ethnodrama/ethnotheatre:** These research methods are more common in arts and humanities research than in therapy research, except for drama or arts therapies, which may include examination of performance and art (see Step 4).

Step 6: Conduct phenomenological analysis

Definition

This section gives an overview of phenomenological methods, which generally aim to develop an in-depth understanding of subjective experiences.

Examples

Philosophical start: Phenomenology originated with philosophers such as Brentano, Husserl, Heidegger, Gadamer, and Merleau-Ponty (Moran, 2002; Stanghellini et al., 2019; Zahavi, 2018). Phenomenology is the understanding/meaning/study ('logos') of phenomena. *Phainó-menon* means 'that which shows itself'. Heidegger explains this with the Ancient Greek word for truth, *a-letheia*, dis-covery: we remove the covers we have put over the phenomena to let them show themselves (Wrathall, 2010). Phenomenology describes this process of removing covers, like removing the outer layers from a mango so its core can show itself to us, or like unpeeling the layers of an onion where there may not be a core but at least we have removed superficial or less-meaningful layers (Vos, 2017, 2021a). How do phenomenologists try to uncover phenomena to let them show themselves?

First, phenomenologists remove superficial covers. They put their assumptions and pre-conceptions temporarily between brackets (called 'phenomenological-bracketing' or 'epoché'). For example, we decide not to use DSM-criteria and clinical theories to understand our participant's experiences of depression. This also means that phenomenologists try not to focus on theoretical concepts and abstractions but on 'the reality of lived experiences in the here-and-now', which refers to 'the totality of our senses, all relationships to the world and ourselves, including past, present and future potential' (Vos, 2021a, p.2). This may also include looking at the phenomenon from different angles so we can differentiate superficial/less-meaningful perspectives from deeper/more-meaningful perspectives ('imaginative free variation').

Second, instead of explaining the phenomenon with our preconceived ideas, we try to describe it as close as possible to how it shows itself. For example, instead of listening to an interviewee through the filters of our psychological theories, we try to listen with a natural attitude or mundane reasoning.

Third, we do not place any initial hierarchies of significance or importance on the participant's experiences. Although as researchers we may have our preconceptions about what is important, we need to let these hierarchies emerge from the participant's experiences and stories. For example, a participant may share topics A and B; we set our interest in topic A aside to hear the client describe topic B as the most meaningful.

In this stage, some themes may spontaneously show themselves, and some categories and hierarchies amongst themes may become visible (e.g., lower-order/sub-ordinate/lower/sub-themes and larger-order/super-ordinate/larger themes). Phenomenologists differ in opinion on whether it is possible to identify universal 'essences' underlying the unique experiences of individual participants ('eidetic reduction'). Some believe a systematic phenomenological process can dis-cover essences, like unpeeling the outer layers can show the core of a mango; others believe our experiences do not have a core, just as unpeeling an onion will not lead to a core (Vos, 2017, 2021a). Argued from a pragmatic perspective, interviews with some participants may show clearer hierarchies than others, and for some individuals, researchers may be able to identify clearer themes and hierarchies than others. The possibility that themes and sub-themes reveal themselves also depends on the researcher's ability to phenomenologically bracket themselves. For example, a researcher who merely uses simple self-reflection may implicitly impose their preferences when identifying themes; thus, critical self-reflection and reflexivity may (partially) prevent being biased and swayed-away.

Applied phenomenology: By the end of the 20th century, phenomenological philosophy seems to have been replaced by several 'new schools' of applied phenomenology (Crotty, 1996; Langdridge, 2007). These phenomenological methods can be relatively easily applied to empirical phenomena, for example to understand the lived experiences of clients and therapists via interviews (see example in Online Table 9.2). Applied phenomenological analysis often consists of the following steps: reading an entire transcript while phenomenologically bracketing the researcher's presuppositions, letting meaningful units/themes show themselves, categorising these units/themes into groups with overarching higher-order names, and writing the findings with a focus on the overarching themes/story.

Applied phenomenology schools: These applied-phenomenological approaches may be organised into four very loose schools, as elaborated below (Vos, 2021a; Dowling, 2007). Descriptive phenomenology describes the phenomenon as close as possible to the lived phenomenon, such as in the Duquesne-School and template analysis. Hermeneutic phenomenology integrates hermeneutic philosophy (e.g., Gadamer, Ricoeur) and semiotics (e.g., De Saussure, Peirce), such as in interpretative phenomenological analysis, hermeneutic phenomenology of practice, heuristic enquiry, and poetic phenomenology. Contextual phenomenologists include analysis of the social construction process via narratives or teams of researchers, such as critical narrative analysis and consensual qualitative research. Responding to criticisms about insufficient rigour and reflexivity in these schools (Vos, 2021a; Crotty, 1996), systematic pragmatic phenomenological analysis was developed to offer detailed procedural steps to analyse and develop a systematic in-depth understanding of qualitative, quantitative, or mixed data (Vos, 2021a). In sum, these applied-phenome-nological schools seem to differ on seven dimensions: essentialist/existentialist ontology, researcher-oriented/participant-oriented, non-systematic/systematic, hermeneutic-con-structivism/critical realism, sensitive/specific interviews, simple-self-reflection/critical-self-reflection-and-reflexivity, no-guidance/guidance (explained in Online Table 9.3; Vos, 2021a).

Read more: Online Table 9.4 explains key phenomenological concepts, and Online Table 9.5 the three fundamental steps in phenomenology. Spinelli (2005) gives an accessible introduction to phenomenological ideas, and Moran (2002) gives a comprehensive overview of philosophical phenomenology. Langdridge (2007) provides an accessible introduction to applied phenomenology.

Phenomenological philosophy

Aims: Phenomenological philosophers ask fundamental questions about the essential conditions under which phenomena appear in the ways they do; for example, we need an eye (condition) before we can see something (appearances of phenomena). In other words, phenomenological philosophers often focus on how humans experience and interpret phenomena in general but they seem less interested in the specific experience of specific individuals of particular phenomena.

Pros/cons: Provides a fundamental understanding of human processes of experiencing and understanding in general. These texts can be challenging to read for untrained readers. The analysis is often theoretical, based on auto-ethnographic self-analysis or ideal-case studies. . Whereas phenomenological philosophers often focus on the totality of our human potential and our general structures/mechanisms, applied-phenomenological researchers focus on how individual(s) actualise particular possibilities in their unique time and place. For example, whereas Merleau-Ponty examined how humans perceive phenomena in general, an applied study examines how particular individual(s) perceive(s) a specific phenomenon.

Schools: Key phenomenological philosophers include Brentano, Husserl, and Heidegger. Hermeneutic philosophy evolved partially from Heidegger's examinations of how our unique position in time and space determines how we experience and understand phenomena, and Gadamer (2013), who elaborated on the researcher's hermeneutic-interpretative role. This subsequently influenced the emergence of hermeneutic and (post-)structuralist philosophers, such as Ricoeur, Derrida, and Levi-Strauss. In line with Heidegger's attention to existential themes – e.g., death awareness as a penultimate gateway to developing an understanding of Being – existential philosophy and psychology evolved, initially with a German-French school with thinkers such as Sartre and Levinas (Vos, 2018, 2019). Several phenomenological philosophers bridged phenomenological philosophy and applied phenomenology by studying the general processes of human experiencing. For example, Merleau-Ponty (1969) examined how phenomena can be perceived and embodied. Others phenomenologically explored specific fields (e.g., Jaspers – psychiatry; Schutz – sociology; van den Berg – psychology). Phenomenological philosophers also inspired existential therapists (Vos, 2019).

Descriptive phenomenology

Aims: Descriptive phenomenology describes a phenomenon as close as possible to the participants' subjectively lived experiences. Compared to hermeneutic phenomenology, descriptive phenomenologists pay relatively less attention to the researcher's interpretative role. Thus they seem to stand more in Husserlian traditions than in hermeneutic traditions, and they seem less contextual and systematic than contextual and systematic-pragmatic-phenomenological schools.

Pros/cons: Uses the researcher's creativity and intuitions, which may help to identify meanings that may be difficult to grasp via rigid analytical procedures. Some analytical methods may be difficult for novice researchers due to a lack of systematic rigour and formalised procedural guidance. This method requires much critical self-reflection and reflexivity. Sometimes applied in therapy research.

Schools:

- **Duquesne School:** The Duquesne School at Pittsburgh University has several influential applied phenomenologists, such as Giorgi, Colaizzi, and Van Kaam. Their research often aims to elucidate the essence of a phenomenon in the participant's lived experiences. For example, Giorgi's method integrates psychological concepts and has been used in therapy research. Following Husserl, Giorgi (2009; Giorgi & Giorgi, 2003) maintains that the object of phenomenological description can solely be achieved through a direct intuitive grasping of the essential structure, like developing a creative insight. Consequently, Giorg idoes not provide a rigid step-by-step system but describes ways to develop a phenomenological attitude to intuitively grasp phenomenological essences. Rivera's (2006) conceptual encounter includes a dynamic interplay between the researcher's and participants' accounts. This may include the practice of bracketing-off assumptions, not treating any assumptions as more important than others, searching for the most meaningful among participant experiences, and engaging in imaginative variation to distinguish more-meaningful from less-meaningful interpretations (Colaizzi, 1978; Wertz, 1984). Despite few formal guidelines, several Duquesne researchers seem to follow these steps (McLeod, 2011):

  1 Collect texts/transcripts
  2 Read the text/transcript to get a sense of the whole
  3 Identify significant statements
  4 Discard irrelevant repetition and non-revelatory statements
  5 Identify central themes or meanings implicit in statements
  6 Integrate themes into a single exhaustive description of the phenomenon (Polkinghorne, 1989)
  7 Member-checking: asking participants how the researcher's description matches their experiences (Colaizzi, 1978)

- **Template analysis:** This chapter's Step 2 introduced how researchers may use 'templates' or 'hermeneutic tools' both for interview questions and interview analysis. The Sheffield School Template recommends examining seven fractions of our lifeworld (selfhood, sociality, embodiment, temporality, spatiality, project, discourse). Structural existential analysis examines our experiences, paradoxes, and emotions regarding our physical, personal, social, and spiritual worlds. Systematic pragmatic phenomenological analysis offers systematic guidance with ten evidence-based questions/perspectives. These templates help develop a more holistic understanding of phenomena but may bias the interviews, particularly when using less-systematic and non-evidence-based templates (Vos, 2021a).

Hermeneutic phenomenology

Aims: Develop an idiographic understanding of the individual's lived experiences via phenomenological and hermeneutic analyses. Contrasting with other applied-phenomenological schools, hermeneutic phenomenology highlights the role of researchers as active interpreters of phenomena.

Pros/cons: Due to the researchers' active-interpretative role, hermeneutic-phenomenological methods may risk bias. Lack of self-reflection can undermine the study's trustworthiness, so researchers should use critical self-reflection and reflexivity. Zahavi (2018) critiques hermeneutic-phenomenological applications for misinterpreting phenomenological concepts such as bracketing/epoché and natural-attitude. Hermeneutic-phenomenological methods are some of the most frequently applied qualitative methods in therapy research.

Schools:

- **Interpretative phenomenological analysis (IPA):** IPA uses transcribed interview data to identify sub-ordinate themes, which may be subsequently grouped into super-ordinate themes (Smith & Fieldsend, 2021). Contrasting other phenomenological approaches, IPA researchers interpret the meaning of the interview content as psychological constructs they may have already identified in a systematic literature review before the interviews. 'Without open coding', researchers apply a series of interpretative readings of the text. The interpretation is done line-by-line and focuses on identifying what it might mean for the participant to have these experiences in this context. The interpretations should be made sensitively and reflexively to avoid the researcher imposing subjective perceptions. One of the possible reasons for the popularity of IPA is the availability of clear procedural steps:

  1 **Read and re-read text:** e.g., immerse oneself into the participant's world
  2 **Initial notes:** e.g., written in the middle column of a page, with descriptive comments on the content of meaning, linguistic comments on language use, and conceptual comments on emerging questions or possibilities
  3 **Develop general themes** (sub-ordinate themes)
  4 **Search for connections across emergent themes** (super-ordinate themes)
  5 **Commonalities between idiographic accounts of multiple participants may (or may not) be identified:** In contrast with thematic analysis, IPA does not primarily aim to identify common themes across participants but understand the subjective meanings for each individual. Some IPA studies only report themes for each participant, whereas others report commonalities.

- **Hermeneutic phenomenology of practice:** The Canadian phenomenologist Van Manen focuses on practice and action. Although he follows Husserl's emphasis on describing the pre-reflective lifeworld, he also pays attention to the researcher's interpretations, because 'if we simply try to forget or ignore what we already know, we might find that the presupposition persistently creeps back into our reflections' (van Manen, 2016, p.47). Consequently, van Manen focuses less on phenomenological-bracketing, and gives researchers some interpretative and pedagogical space. Van Manen's method has also been used in conjunction with templates in therapy research.
- **Heuristic enquiry:** Moustakas (1990) developed a method for systematic Husserlian self-exploration of existential topics (Sultan, 2018). The researcher's passionate involvement may help reach analytical depth that cannot be achieved via other methods. This may be particularly relevant when others cannot be interviewed or the researcher has unique experience. Heuristic enquiry emphasises the personal meanings with significance for the individual so the individual remains visible in their wholeness. Procedural steps include initial engagement with the topic, immersion in the topic, incubation time to stand back and give space for implicit meanings to emerge, illumination of breakthroughs or new insights, explication and critical examination, creative synthesis, and validation by others.
- **Poetic/artistic phenomenology:** Some researchers use poetry or other art forms in data collection, analyses, and/or presentation. For example, poems may do more justice to complex subjective experiences than interviews, and researchers may ask participants to write poems and/or present the findings in poems, for example via Bachelard's poetic phenomenology (Butlin, 2016).

Contextual phenomenology

Aims: Develop a critical and reflexive understanding of how individuals experience and construct their experiences, identities, and perceptions in their social context. Combines phenomenology with other qualitative methods.

Pros/cons: Include a more critical and contextual understanding of phenomena than other phenomenological methods. This may help to do justice to societal and political pressures on individual experiences. Consensual qualitative research increases the study's trustworthiness by the team-based approach but may be more challenging to organise.

Schools:

- **Critical narrative analysis (CNA):** CNA draws upon the work of Ricoeur, phenomenology, and hermeneutics. CNA is a form of narrative analysis 'in which disparate components are philosophically grounded and practically combined into one analytical approach' (Langdridge, 2007, p.129). CNA understands experiences and meanings as context specific, interpretative, and co-created. The researcher draws on broader discourses constraining the participants' narratives, via their empathic understanding of topics such as gender and sexual orientation as hermeneutic. CNA data analysis may be complex and time-consuming, and includes six steps: critiquing illusions of subjectivity; identifying narratives, narrative tone, and rhetorical function;

exploring identities and identity work; systematically using thematic priorities and relationships; destabilising narratives; synthesis.

- **Consensual qualitative research:** This team-based method combines grounded theory, comprehensive process analysis, descriptive phenomenology, and feminist critique. A group of 4 to 12 researchers collect and analyse data, including an independent external auditor. Each researcher identifies dimensions and summarises core ideas in the qualitative data for each case. Subsequently, cross-analysis helps identify categories within domains across cases (Hill et al., 2005).

Systematic-pragmatic-phenomenological analysis

Aims: Systematic Pragmatic Phenomenological Analysis (SPPA) systematically aims to examine the lived experiences and meanings of a phenomenon for one or more individuals. Many quantitative studies focus on the single question 'what is a phenomenon', and many qualitative studies on the single question 'how does an individual experience this phenomenon'. In contrast, SPPA provides a holistic perspective on a phenomenon with ten possible research objectives (researchers may decide to focus on all ten or fewer objectives): the ontological status of the phenomenon, what type of meaning the individual experiences, how the individual approaches meaning, where the individual is in relation to society, when the individual experiences the phenomenon, how the phenomenon relates to who the individual is, how much freedom the participant has, why the individual experiences what they experience (existential question), and what impact the experience may have on daily life.

Pros/cons: Systematic, pragmatic, clear procedural guide available. Broader applicability than other phenomenological methods, as SPPA can be used on any qualitative, quantitative, or mixed data. Few published studies (Vos, 2019, 2020, 2021a, 2022a).

School: SPPA was developed in response to criticisms about insufficient rigour and reflexivity in applied-phenomenological schools (Crotty, 1996; Vos, 2021a) and to return to the rigour of fundamental-phenomenological philosophers (Vos, 2021a). SPPA is based on critical-realist and pluralist epistemology. Contrasting with other methods, SPPA offers systematic guidance for each part of the research process. For example, researchers are stimulated to carefully develop their research objectives and interview questions with the help of the ten research objectives. Interviews consist of two parts which are analysed separately: broad questions ('how do you experience topic X?') followed by questions operationalising each research question; this strategy makes interviews both sensitive and specific. Researchers engage in systematic critical self-reflection and reflexivity, as described in Chapter 4. Instead of only researchers interpreting data after the interviews, interviewees are also asked at the end of the interview to share their conclusions. Data are analysed via reflexive sub-steps. The researcher starts with a round of open analysis of the data without the research objectives in mind, followed by a second round of analysis for each research objective. First, themes are synthesised per participant and subsequently across participants.

Step 7: Write findings

Definition

This step includes generic tips and tricks on writing qualitative studies. Always double check author guidelines from journals or the APA (apastyle.apa.org/jars/qualitative). See Ponterotto and Grieger (2007) for more advice.

Tips

Include all steps described in this chapter

For example, describe the method, justify why this helps to achieve the research objectives, and describe how you have applied this. The latter means explicating in detail analytical procedures (e.g., interview schedule, transcription, coding, analysis of themes).

Self-reflection

Be transparent about the training of the coders, as this influences trustworthiness. Describe the procedures to engage in critical self-reflection and reflexivity, such as a reflective research journal, memos, and self-interview. Convince the reader you do not only know in theory but have actually been reflective: show throughout the text that you are critically self-reflective and reflexive. For example, use a reflective word-choice that shows humility about your position, explicate methodological decisions, mention alternative interpretations, and unexpected findings that may contradict your preconceptions. If allowed in the analytical method, show a personalised discursive style in portraying your involvement in the analyses.

Language

Use language coherent with your research method (see Step 1).

Balance

Qualitative publications often have longer findings sections than quantitative studies due to thick data-description. The main challenge will be balancing detailed, thick data-description and preventing the reader from feeling overwhelmed by details. Qualitative research often benefits from clear, explicated textual structures (see Chapter 2), such as many summaries and a clear central theme or storyline. It may be helpful to limit the findings to a maximum of five themes and seven sub-themes, as research indicates that our working memory can usually simultaneously grasp between five and nine concepts.

Naming themes/sub-themes

The naming of themes and sub-themes should be done very carefully so the name applies to all the examples falling under it; some researchers prefer to use words or sentences from the participants. It needs to be clear what the differences are between themes or sub-themes, why they are not combined, and why they are not further separated into more themes or sub-themes. What are the relationships between themes/sub-themes; are they mutually exclusive or overlapping?

Justify your interpretations

Support your interpretation of qualitative findings, for example by citing participants (e.g., at least one citation per sub-theme).

Describe sample

Describe the socio-demographic/life situation of each participant to contextualise the findings (Online Table 9.1).

Clear referencing

It needs to be clear what was said by the participants and what is the interpretation from the researcher. Some qualitative studies have different sections/chapters/parts for 'findings' and 'interpretations', where the latter includes more direct involvement of the researcher's voice. Some methods allow or require qualitative researchers to cite references in the findings sections; otherwise, literature should be excluded from the findings section.

Presentation aids

Add tables and figures to give an overview of the findings, if possible (Tables 9.2–9.3, Figure 9.3). Some researchers report the number of times that themes/sub-themes are cited to be transparent about how common themes are across the participants (Table 9.3), although others have criticised this for being reductionist, and giving the false impression of generalisability. Qualitative researchers seem to have more freedom than quantitative researchers to be creative in how they synthesise and present findings, as long as they follow relevant publication guidelines (Denzin & Lincoln, 2021).

Table 9.2 Example socio-demographic table

	Case 1	Case 2
Pseudonym	John	Maria
Age	23	25
Gender	Male	Female
Other relevant characteristics		

Table 9.3 Example table for qualitative findings

Between-participant theme	Between-participant sub-theme
Theme 1 (N=…)	Sub-theme 1 (N=…)
	Sub-theme 2 (N=…)
	Sub-theme 3 (N=…)
Theme 2 (N=…)	Sub-theme 1 (N=…)
	Sub-theme 2 (N=…)
	Sub-theme 3 (N=…)
	Sub-theme 4 (N=…)
Theme 3 (N=…)	Sub-theme 1 (N=…)
	Sub-theme 2 (N=…)
	Sub-theme 3 (N=…)
	Sub-theme 4 (N=…)
	Sub-theme 5 (N=…)

Note: there are no strict guidelines for the number of themes/sub-themes; however, it may be recommended to have between three and seven themes, and within each theme between three and seven subthemes, in line with the 'magic number seven plus or minus two' (Saaty & Ozdemir, 2003). N = number of participants mentioning this (sub)theme.

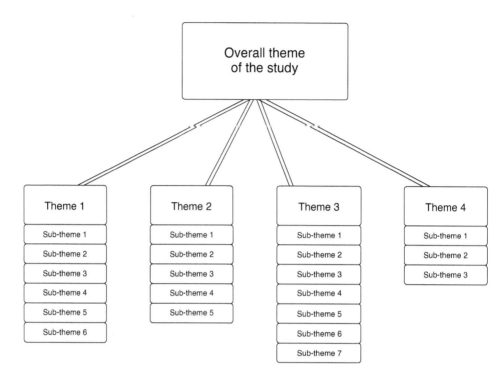

Figure 9.3 Example figure for qualitative findings

Step 8: Justify the trustworthiness of research

Definition

How can we trust a study? To answer this question, quantitative researchers describe validity and reliability. However, these concepts are based on positivist assumptions, such as the probability that our observed values adequately mirror 'true values' in 'reality'. Qualitative researchers have developed alternative ways to describe the extent to which a study can be trusted. Trustworthiness does not aim to prove how our study corresponds with reality but aims to show that we can trust the researcher's steps in the research process. This chapter discusses several criteria and frameworks that have been suggested to describe the trustworthiness of a study (impatient readers may jump to the procedures section).

Explanation

Some researchers advocate for universal criteria and standards on trustworthiness (Elliott, Fischer, & Rennie, 1999; Morrow, 2005; Morse et al., 2002; Shenton, 2004). However, what does it mean to say a research project is 'trustworthy'? How do we know what is 'trustworthy'? Constructivists argue that trustworthiness is a social construct, not a universal, timeless truth. All our ideas about trustworthiness are created by us, reflected and unreflected habits, theories and assumptions about how we do research. What is the consensus? There does not seem to be one overarching qualitative theory, and qualitative researchers seem to differ on many points, even as fundamental as their ontological and epistemological position (Hunt, 2011; Yardley, 2015). Formulated with the philosopher Thomas Kuhn (1970), it seems as if qualitative research is still in a pre-paradigmatic stage with relatively little consensus about some fundamental aspects of their.

Therefore, we may not want to search for a universal trustworthiness framework that applies to all qualitative methods. Instead, we may focus on whatever trustworthiness framework is used in our specific research field or 'research cell'. This means that researchers may examine how other researchers around them and authorities in their field describe trustworthiness. Many qualitative methods are associated with specific practices, consensus, and guidelines about trustworthiness (Madill, Jordan, & Shirley, 2000; Reicher, 2000). However, a radical relativist may also criticise this approach: the trustworthiness framework that others use may not apply to a unique research project.

I propose a pragmatic approach. Regardless of whether it is fundamentally possible to develop universal trustworthiness frameworks, we can be inspired by seeing how others argue their research's trustworthiness. A trustworthiness framework may not be regarded as a rigid universal checklist but as a summary of best-practice examples. A trustworthiness framework can be a source for critical self-reflection and reflexivity, alongside other sources of inspiration, but cannot replace our reflexive practices (see Chapter 3). Using terms that others frequently use may also pragmatically stimulate our professional communication and possibly the co-construction of some understandable, transparent, and coherent narratives within our research cell and neighbours. Therefore, researchers may want to familiarise themselves with the most cited trustworthiness frameworks.

Examples

APA's fidelity-and-utility framework

A milestone is the publication of the APA's trustworthiness framework, recommending researchers reflect on the fidelity and utility of each research step (Levitt et al., 2017). For example, reflect on the following for each step in this book (Table 9.4):

- **Fidelity to the subject-matter:** The researcher's intimate and authentic connection with the topic, such as immersion, thick data-description, multiple expressions, or portrayals of phenomena. To what extent and how do you do justice to the topic?
- **Utility in achieving research aims:** The effectiveness of the study design and methodology in achieving the research aims/objectives/questions/hypotheses. Is the method useful, and to what end?

Yardley's reflective dimensions

Cecilia Yardley (2015) is one of the most cited authors on trustworthiness in therapy research. At each step, researchers may want to reflect on her five reflective dimensions (slightly reformulated):

- **Sensitivity to context:** The researcher is aware of and appropriately responds to the unique context, such as the socio-cultural setting, participants' perspectives, ethical issues, empirical data, critical literature review.

- **Commitment and rigour:** The researcher is committed to conducting the research rigorously, e.g., via thorough data collection and deep/broad analysis.
- **Methodological competencies and skills:** The researcher has competencies required to conduct this research project and applies skills in ways/levels considered standard/norm in the field; e.g., in-depth engagement with the topic, rigorous analysis, and researcher training.
- **Coherence and transparency:** The research project is coherent, with a transparent coherence/structure; e.g., the research steps follow each other logically, methods and data are written clearly, the conceptual/theoretical framework and methodological applications are logically connected, all methodological decisions are explicated and justified, with critical self-reflection and reflexivity.
- **Impact and importance:** The research project addresses an important topic, with the potential to contribute to the field with implications for practice, theory, research, and/or society.

Common components of trustworthiness

Many handbooks on qualitative methods recommend researchers reflect on six common components of trustworthiness: credibility, dependability, transferability, confirmability, triangulation, and authenticity, as Table 9.5 explains (Lincoln & Guba, 1985; Denzin & Lincoln, 2021). Qualitative therapy research often includes these six components of trustworthiness (Online Tables 9.6–9.7). Similarly, researchers may want to reflect on whether these components of trustworthiness may be relevant and how their research project addresses these.

Procedures

1. Identify trustworthiness guidelines for your method, topic, and field.
2. Explore how other researchers discuss trustworthiness.
3. Critically reflect on how trustworthily you have conducted each step in the research (e.g., ask the seven questions in Table 9.4).
4. Critically reflect how your research fulfils the common components of trustworthiness (e.g., ask questions in Table 9.5).
5. Write in a reflective research journal.
6. Summarise your reflections in your academic texts (e.g., add a section/sub-section on 'trustworthiness' in your research proposal/report/thesis/article). Consider using common terms that readers understand.

Instructions for using Table 9.4: Ask the following seven questions about each major step in this book. Use as inspiration for reflection, not as a rigid checklist; not every question may be relevant.

1. How does this step do justice to the research topic (fidelity to subject matter)?
2. How does this step help you achieve the research goals (utility in achieving research goals)?
3. How are you aware of and respond to the unique context of this step (sensitivity to context)?

Table 9.4 Reflective questions for the trustworthiness of each research step

Research step (Relevant book chapters)	1. Fidelity	2. Utility	3. Sensitivity to context	4. Commitment and rigour	5. Competencies and skills	6. Coherence and transparency	7. Impact and importance
Definition of topic (Chapter 4)							
Critical self-reflection and reflexivity (Chapter 4)							
Literature review (Chapter 5)							
Research aims, objectives, questions, hypotheses (Chapter 6)							
Ontological and epistemological position (Chapter 7)							
Study-design (Chapters 7/9)							
Sample/recruitment (Chapter 7)							
Data-collection/ interviews (Chapters 7/9)							
Practical organisation (Chapter 7)							
Data-analysis (Chapter 9)							
Transcription and coding (Chapter 9)							
Writing-up (Chapter 9)							
Ethics (Chapter 11)							
Discussion and dissemination of findings (Chapter 11)							

4. How are you committed and rigorous in this step (commitment and rigour)?
5. How do you have the required competencies and apply your research skills competently in this step (methodological competencies and skills)?
6. How coherent is this step in itself and in relationship to other steps? How transparent are you about this coherence, and how do you justify yourself (coherence and transparency)?
7. How important is this step for the field, and how could it benefit the field (impact and importance)?

Table 9.5   Reflective questions for common components of trustworthiness

Credibility

Definition:

Research findings mirror the views of the people under study (cf. quantitative content validity).

Examples:
Triangulation; transparent/systematic records; researcher competencies; peer debriefing/supervision; well-established methods; relevant/justified sampling; participants' freedom of expression; thick data-description; logical arguments; participant input on findings (e.g., member-checking).

Dependability

Definition:

Findings are consistent and repeatable in different times/conditions (cf. quantitative reliability).
Examples:
All methodological/analytical steps are documented, described, and justified clearly so that others could hypothetically repeat the study. Coding recoding: taking time off after initial data coding to recode later with fresh eyes. Multiple (co)researchers/external auditors collect/analyse data.

Transferability

Definition:

Evidence that study findings could (hypothetically) be applicable/generalised to other individuals/samples/situations (cf. quantitative construct validity).

Examples:
Transferability of data-collection (e.g., tools/interview schedule, sample recruitment), data analysis (e.g., thick data-description, i.e., robust/detailed account of data), context (e.g., location, culture), participants (e.g., socio-demographic), researcher (e.g., training), research tools (e.g., interview schedule).

Confirmability

Definition:
The study findings/analyses/interpretations are based on participant narratives and words rather than potential researcher biases (cf. quantitative objectivity).

Examples:
A clearly documented audit trail, critical self-reflection and reflexivity: describe how this was done (e.g., reflective journal, supervision) and show throughout the research process and written documents.

(Continued)

Table 9.5 Reflective questions for common components of trustworthiness (*Continued*)

Triangulation

Definition:

Research data comes from different sources to develop a comprehensive understanding of the research topic, and multiple perspectives help to converge and corroborate findings (cf. quantitative criterion validity).

Examples:
Triangulation of data (multiple data sources), investigators (multiple (co)researchers/supervisors), methodologies (multiple methods), theories (multiple perspectives/interpretations) (Denzin, 1978). Sometimes called 'crystallisation' to refer to the process whereby the data, reflective memos, and field notes all crystallize into a full and balanced representation of findings (Ellingson, 2009).

Authenticity

Definition:

Giving explicit voice to researchers and participants, to address power, multiple values, empowerment, representation, and accountability (Lincoln & Guba, 1985; not in quantitative research).

Examples:
Fair/ethical procedures, critical self-reflection/reflexivity, recruitment procedures, ontological authenticity (unique meanings), educative authenticity (learning potential), catalytic authenticity (action potential for social justice agendas), tactical authenticity (change potential; Amin et al., 2020).

Instructions for Table 9.5: Reflect on which common components of trustworthiness are relevant for your research project and reflect on how your research meets them.

━━━ Reflective questions ━━━

- Select three frequently cited articles with different qualitative methods in your field. Reflect on their study design and data analysis; what could have been done differently? Reflect their trustworthiness. What skills can you learn? Would you cite this study: why (not)?
- Conducting reflexive-thematic analysis (RTA) can be a good exercise for learning qualitative research competencies shared by many qualitative methods. Search for three texts in the public domain, such as newspapers or interviews, related to your research topic, and apply the seven RTA steps from Clarke and Braun (2018).
- Select three interview studies in your field. Critically reflect on their interview schedules; how could you improve this, and what questions/formulations would you use?

10

How to Conduct Mixed Methods Research

Chapter aims

This chapter explains how to read, develop, and conduct mixed method (MM) research projects. MM is more than simply using quantitative and qualitative methods as described in previous chapters: multi-methods are not mixed methods. Whereas Chapter 7 gave an overview of all methodological steps, this chapter zooms in on developing aims, study design, sample, and analyses with an MM mindset. Chapters 11–12 explain how to conduct MM research ethically and discuss its findings. (Recommended introductions include Clark & Ivankova, 2015; Creswell, 2021; Creswell & Clark, 2017; Tashakkori & Teddlie, 2021.)

Steps in chapter

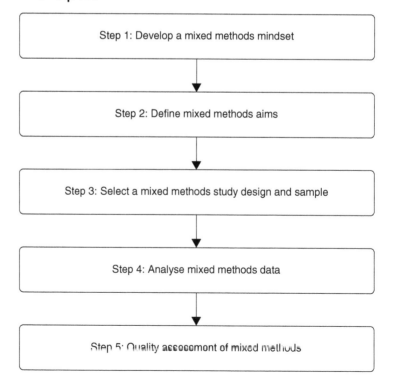

Step 1: Develop a mixed methods mindset

Step 2: Define mixed methods aims

Step 3: Select a mixed methods study design and sample

Step 4: Analyse mixed methods data

Step 5: Quality assessment of mixed methods

Step 1: Develop a mixed methods mindset

Definition

Conducting MM research starts with developing an MM mindset and distinguishing this from a multi-methods mindset. MM requires an ontological and epistemological position underpinning both quantitative and qualitative methods. Similar to other methods, MM researchers often use their own MM lingo. This MM mindset will guide researchers in their methodological decisions, analyses, and writing.

Components

Mixed methods, not multi-methods

Mixed methods does not merely mean using multiple research methods. Mixed methods have three ingredients: quantitative, qualitative, and mixing both. The whole is more than the sum of its parts, just as a good glass of wine is more than putting some grapes together – it also involves processes such as fermentation and ripening. This does not mean multi-methods research cannot be helpful; it just means MM is more than for example adding some open questions to a multiple-choice questionnaire.

Mixed methods epistemology

Previous chapters have shown how methodological purists may divide the research field of psychological research between quantitative and qualitative methods (Teddlie & Tashakkori, 2006). This divide seems grounded in different epistemological positions that may appear incommensurable. Quantitative approaches emphasise commonalities, certainties, and objectivity under controlled conditions. Qualitative approaches embrace the diversity of individual lived experiences in ever-changing socio-cultural contexts. These epistemological differences often lead to different methodological decisions, such as experimental versus non-experimental study designs with questionnaires versus interviews.

MM researchers recognise the differences between quantitative and qualitative methods but label these as complementary rather than competing. This relationship has been described as 'augmentation': researchers from one methodological approach do not seek complementary perspectives to confirm their vision but to provide a more comprehensive, complex, and dynamic picture of the research topic (Landrum & Garza, 2015).

MM researchers may cope with the potential ontological/epistemological differences in two ways. Parallel ontological/epistemological positions mean that a researcher switches their position when they conduct the quantitative or qualitative parts of the study, or the study may be performed by two researchers with two different positions (e.g., positivist and constructivist positions). This seems to imply a 'dialectical engagement' in MM: 'an ongoing and recursive process of trying to understand another [whereby] our own beliefs and assumptions are disclosed, and these assumptions themselves can become objects of examinations and critique' (Carter & Gradin, 2001, p.4). This dialogical nature of mixing methods with different ontological/epistemological positions seems to require a willingness and capability of researchers to engage in critical self-reflection and reflexivity; this is sometimes described as 'reflexive mixed methods research' (Hesse-Biber, 2015). However, most MM studies also include, at least in the synthesis stage, an ontological/epistemological middle ground that allows both qualitative and quantitative methods, such as critical realism. It is common for MM publications to reflect explicitly on their ontological/epistemological foundations.

Popularity

MM seems increasingly popular amongst researchers on psychological therapies:

> Psychotherapy is a notoriously complex and ever-developing field, and our growing sense has been that mixed methods research can contribute to more complete – both broad and deep – knowledge and understanding... For a multifaceted disci pline to develop and survive, we need to move beyond the qualitative quantitative divisive chasm between scientific [i.e., quantitative] and humanistic [i.e., qualitative] knowledge. (Bager-Charleson, McBeath, & Vostanis, 2021, p.48)

Mixed methods lingo

As a young field, there is still some variety in MM terminologies (Clark & Ivankova, 2015). MM researchers may use both quantitative and qualitative language. Older MM publications call the methodology differently (e.g., mixed methodology, methodological triangulation, multi-method, integrated research, combined research, mixed research). MM researchers may publish their study's quantitative and qualitative parts in different journals – each with different quantitative/qualitative lingo – or publish in an MM journal with MM language. Whatever terminology you use, be consistent and check which terms are required by the research institution or publisher.

Step 2: Define mixed methods aims

Definition

This step describes how to develop the aim of an MM study. Authors should explicitly state MM in the title, abstract, and introduction.

Procedures

Rationale

Researchers may decide to use MM because they feel they would be limited if they only used a quantitative or qualitative method. For example, qualitative research usually only includes a small non-representative sample, due to which findings cannot be generalised, and it may be difficult to test hypotheses or show the prevalence of a phenomenon as qualitative research usually does not include numbers. Qualitative methods may allow researchers to capture an in-depth understanding of participants' voices, sketch the personal and social context of stories, and may appeal more to the reader's imagination than numbers. On the flipside, qualitative research may have a larger risk of subjective bias, although this may be ameliorated by critical self-reflection and reflexivity. In contrast, quantitative research has systematic methods to argue its validity and reliability. MM may support triangulation by obtaining two datasets with different methods. In sum, mixing methods may help amplify the combined strengths and let methods compensate for/offset the weaknesses of each other (Rossman & Wilson, 1985). MM offers a more comprehensive-complementary view, a combination of qualitative exploration and quantitative validation/generalisation, a more detailed understanding of quantitative findings, and, most of all, examining opportunities for development (Creswell, 2021). In sum, MM may do more justice to a multifaceted research topic.

One research aim

Although it is possible to develop three separate quantitative, qualitative, and MM aims, it can be helpful to develop one overarching MM aim, showing how quantitative and qualitative methods are connected. However, it can be challenging to develop an overarching MM aim. An example is: 'this study aims to use anxiety questionnaires to test the effects of CBT for cynophobia, the results of which will be further explored via in-depth interviews to understand how clients experience the helpfulness of CBT for cynophobia'. This aim uses quantitative terms (e.g., 'tests', 'effects') and qualitative (e.g., 'experience', 'understand', 'helpfulness').

Three research objectives

MM will most likely have at least three research objectives, regarding quantitative methods and qualitative methods and how they are mixed.

Step 3: Select a mixed methods study design and sample

Definition

The quality of MM research stands or falls by its study design. Therefore, describe and justify the study design and show the procedures for applying this. (Researchers may want to consult Clark & Ivankova, 2015; Creswell & Clark, 2017; Hanson et al., 2005; Tashakkori & Teddlie, 2021.)

Explanation

The key question is what you mean by 'mixing' methods and at which research stage. Figure 10.1 provides an overview of the most frequently used MM study designs, visualised with diagrams. MM researchers often visualise the study design in diagrams and keywords describing the relationship between different study parts (Morse, 2016). For example, uppercase (QUAN/QUAL) indicate prioritised methods, lowercase letters lesser priority (quant, qual), '+' convergent methods, '→' sequential methods. Boxes present data collection/analysis for each method; a circle shows the interpretation phase. Bullet points could give information on methodological procedures (e.g., sample size, variable names, data cleaning, data imputing, interview transcription, identifying themes, describing results) and research products (e.g., article, book). Arrows show the sequence of procedures.

An MM study may collect one sample from which both quantitative data and qualitative data will be derived. You still need similar considerations for sample characteristics and size (e.g., quantitative *a priori* sample size calculation, qualitative purposive/homogeneous sampling). The decision about your sample follows logically from your study design. For example, in clinical trials, you may interview 10% with the largest effects, 10% with medium effects, and 10% with the smallest effects. Many studies consist of two separate databases, and synthesis only happens after analysis, indicating they are actually multi-methods and not mixed methods. Therefore, consider how and at which research stage you will integrate databases (Bryman, 2006).

Examples

Convergent design

Quant-data and qual-data are collected and analysed separately, and results from both are merged to compare or confirm/validate results; e.g., from the start of a clinical trial, researchers use interviews and questionnaires at several stages of the intervention.

Explanatory-sequential design

After quant-data are collected, qual-data are collected to explain quant-data in more detail. For example, the effects of a clinical trial are tested with questionnaires, and subsequent interviews with clients with the largest or smallest change may help understand the treatment effects.

Exploratory design

First, qualitative research identifies particular needs/experiences in the population, such as the need for treatment. Second, a quantitative survey confirms these findings with generalisable data or a clinical trial shows how to fill these therapeutic needs.

Intervention design

This overlaps with previous examples, but researchers collect qualitative data before, during, or after the trial – e.g., a case study or interviews with a sub-group of clients – to understand the research findings in more detail.

Multistage-evaluation design

This is an extended intervention design. Step 3 in Chapter 8 described that new treatments are often developed in multiple studies, where quantitative and qualitative methods play different roles at different research stages.

Social justice or transformative design

Quantitative research has been criticised for not doing justice to participants' lived experiences, and interviews have been criticised for the potential power imbalance between interviewer and interviewee. Mixing methods could help do more justice to the participants throughout the research process, for example via community based participatory research. Ensure your research aim explains how your study design will help to do justice.

Complex mixed methods design

This design includes aspects of previous study designs; researchers may be creative in their design.

Step 4: Analyse mixed methods data

Definition

Often, quantitative and qualitative data are analysed independently. Some quantitative findings may influence the interpretation of qualitative data (e.g., in grounded theory or

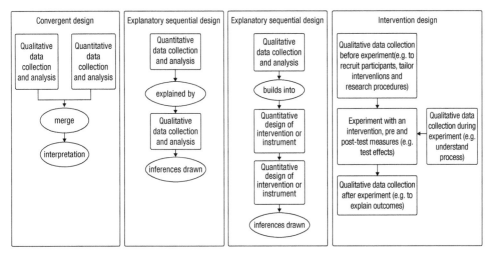

Figure 10.1. Frequently applied examples of MM study designs

hermeneutic phenomenology where the researcher does not rigidly phenomenologically bracket-off their preconceptions). At the stage of reaching conclusions and discussing the data in relation to each other, mixing may become more important. There are no specific guidelines for MM analyses and MM discussion (Clark & Ivankova, 2015). Whatever procedures you use, explain what, why, and how you do this.

Step 5: Quality assessment of mixed methods

Definition

MM researchers can reflect on the quality of the quantitative and qualitative research parts separately, but they can also explicitly reflect on the quality of the mixed methods.

Examples

Separate quality assessment: Quantitative researchers usually describe the research quality in terms of validity and reliability, and qualitative researchers in terms of trustworthiness. MM researchers do both. In an MM study design, the strengths of one method may offset some weaknesses of another.

MM-specific quality assessment: In addition to reflecting on validity, reliability, and trustworthiness, some researchers reflect explicitly on quality criteria of MM research, often referred to as 'inferential quality' and 'inference transferability'. The following criteria have been suggested (Creswell & Clark, 2017; Creswell & Tashakkori, 2007; Creswell et al., 2011):

- Mixed methods, not merely multi-methods
- Conceptual framework in terms of MM
- Explication and justification of MM research aims
- Explication and justification of MM study design
- Justified type, research stage and procedures of merging/connecting data

- Sampling, data collection and analyses explained in MM terms
- Offsetting strengths and weaknesses of quant/qual methods
- Commensurability and multiple validities of methods/data
- Consistently using MM
- Discussing strengths and limitations of MM
- Contribution to MM literature
- Critical self reflection and reflexivity, including ontological/epistemological reflexivity

■■■■ Reflective questions ■■■■

- Select three frequently cited MM studies in your field. Examine how they describe and justify the methodology; what could they have done differently? How trustworthy, valid, and reliable is the study? What skills can you learn?
- Reflect on your feelings and preferences regarding quantitative and qualitative methods. Have you always felt this, or have you changed? How have your feelings been influenced by life experiences, methodological paradigms of your education/research institute and public discourses? What would you need to do to look beyond your usual methodological preferences?

11

How to Conduct Ethical Research

Chapter aims

This chapter describes how to develop an ethical mindset, conduct ethical research, and develop an ethics proposal. An ethical mindset is more than ticking the checkboxes on the forms of ethics committees. An ethical self-reflective attitude means continuous self-reflection about the ethical dimensions of your research and acting ethically throughout all research stages. General introductions to ethics include Singer (2011), Copp (2005) (philosophical ethics), Sieber (2012) (ethics in quantitative research), Wiles (2012) (qualitative research), Emanuel et al. (2008) (general human research); Bond (2015), Pope and Vasquez (2016) (psychological therapies). Check ethics guidelines from professional bodies such as the APA and BPS (apa.org/ethics/code; bps.org.uk; Knapp et al., 2012; Young, 2017).

Steps in chapter

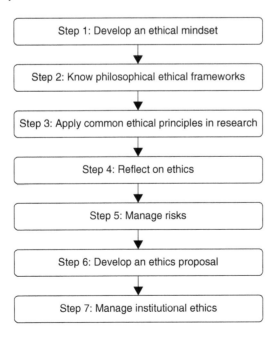

Step 1: Develop an ethical mindset

Step 2: Know philosophical ethical frameworks

Step 3: Apply common ethical principles in research

Step 4: Reflect on ethics

Step 5: Manage risks

Step 6: Develop an ethics proposal

Step 7: Manage institutional ethics

Template

G. Ethics proposal

Step 1: Develop an ethical mindset

Definition

An ethical mindset describes a self-reflective ethical attitude, not blind conformism to norms or guidelines. An ethical researcher is aware of relevant laws and ethical guidelines.

Components

Self-reflective ethical attitude, not moral conformism

Traditionally, many researchers seem to have assumed an ethics of entitlement, giving them the right to research and know the other (Glesne, 2007). Other researchers have followed a communitarian ethics, through which they socially negotiated values and moral commitments with other stakeholders (Denzin & Lincoln, 2021). Other researchers have simply relegated ethics to regulatory bodies such as institutional ethics review committees.

However, therapy researchers seem to increasingly describe ethics as a reflexive process. This seems to refer to the etymology of the word 'ethics' which comes from the Ancient Greek 'ethikos', referring to an individual's way of being or attitude. Ethics should not be confused with conforming to moral and legal conventions or merely ticking the boxes on ethics application forms required by ethics committees. An ethical individual reflects critically on ethical conventions and requirements, considers the most ethical options, and translates this into concrete ethical behaviour: an ethical way of being (Etherington, 2004). A recent trend in research ethics involves reflexive research praxis, which may only secondarily be reflected in documents such as ethics applications. Research is not merely about collecting impersonal data, but affects real humans. Consequently, not all research aims justify all means –most researchers nowadays, for example, regard Zimbardo's prison experiment and Milgram's shock experiment as ethically unjustifiable.

Modern educational and research institutions may not be conducive to developing a self-reflective and reflexive ethical attitude, for example due to peer pressure, time pressure, and lack of resources. Researchers may feel hindered by the formalisation and legalisation of ethical procedures, such as the forms required by research and ethics committees. This seems to reflect the broader trend of legalisation and bureaucratisation of society, which is gradually replacing critical ethical debates with tick boxes (Moyn, 2018). This trend may also be found in mental health care, where the question 'what is going on with my client, and how can I help them best?' seems more often replaced with 'what risks does the client pose to themselves and others, and how could I legally prove I have followed the rules if anything goes wrong?' (Vos, Roberts, & Davies, 2019). Be critical of this reductionist trend and recognise the ethical needs underlying bureaucratic forms and procedures. A reflexive ethical attitude requires critical self-development and sensitising yourself to ethical issues. This chapter gives some pointers, but you may want to read more about ethical frameworks, research ethics, and practice ethical reflection.

Act within legal and ethical guidelines

During World War II, Nazi doctors experimented on concentration camp prisoners. After World War II, the world concluded 'never unethical research again'. Therefore, the Nuremberg and Helsinki Medical Codes lay out how research participants should always be fully informed about the intervention, should not be harmed, and should give informed consent to participation. In the spirit of these codes, governments have developed legal frameworks and guidelines for ethicalresearch and data protection and safeguard academic integrity. Step 7 in Chapter 2 already invited you to identify relevant research and ethics guidelines from your professional bodies.

Step 2: Know philosophical ethical frameworks

Definition

Researchers should familiarise themselves with the main philosophical ethical frameworks to develop their self-reflective ethical attitude. This step in the book merely gives a brief, almost stereotyping, introduction, and readers are recommended to read more (e.g., Singer, 2011; Copp, 2005).

Components

Moral relativism and subjectivism

Some relativist or subjectivist philosophers have argued that there is no absolute right and wrong (moral nihilism) and/or that we cannot know this (epistemological moral scepticism). Proponents include Pyrrho, Hume, Nietzsche, and some postmodernists.

Divine command theory

Some religious thinkers identify clear differences between Good and Evil, for example decreed by Holy Books. Humans can understand the difference by following Scriptures and enlightened people. Examples include religious authors.

Stoicism

Epictetus argued that the greatest good was contentment and serenity. Self-mastery, conquering one's will, and detaching from material wealth lead to peace of mind, *apatheia*. Allowing others to disturb your mental equilibrium is like offering yourself in slavery; similarly, disturbing others' equilibrium is putting them in slavery. Things that cannot be changed should not be fought.

Virtue ethics

Ancient Greek philosophers such as Socrates and Aristotle argued that self-knowledge might help individuals act virtuously. People naturally do what is good if they know what is right; evil/wrong actions result from ignorance. Aristotle elaborated a system of virtues, including moderation. Epicurus wrote that the greatest good was prudence, exercised through moderation, caution, and avoidance of pain. Modern virtue ethics proponents include MacIntyre and Nussbaum.

Natural law theory

People have inherent inalienable rights, not merely given by law, but by God, nature, or reason. Proponents include Cicero, Aquinas, and the European Convention on Human Rights. This is often also combined with social contract theory, which states that by living in a society, individuals surrender some freedoms to an authority – a ruler or ruling majority – in exchange for protection of their remaining rights and social order.

Utilitarianism

The ethical course of action maximises a positive outcome, such as happiness and well-being, reducing its opposites of pain and suffering. Bentham and Mill introduced this consequentialist theory.

Kantian deontology

According to Kant, people act out of duty (deontology). It is not the consequences of actions that make an action moral but the motivations of the acting individual. Kant's three formulations of the categorical imperative are: Act only according to that maxim/ principle by which you can also will that it would become a universal law; Act in such a way that you always treat humanity, whether in your person or the person of any other, never simply as a means, but always at the same time as an end; Every person must act as if they were, through their maxim, always a legislating member in a universal kingdom-of-ends. Simply formulated, ask yourself whether it would be good if everyone made the same decision.

Critical theory ethics

Critical theorists have argued that the dominant ethical frameworks in research are for example based on colonial, Western, white, ethnic-majority, paternalistic, patriarchic, heterosexual, and binary gender norms and values, which oppress a diversity of values, such as an ethics of care and relational ethics. Examine how ethical frameworks and research paradigms may have evolved via structural power imbalances and unequal privileges, and have muted oppressed voices (Denzin & Lincoln, 2021).

Evolutionary ethics

Authors such as Kropotkin argue that ethics is evolutionary, as a social instinct that may benefit the survival of the human species. The popularity and survival value of particular ethical norms and values should be seen in the context where they became dominant – without claiming universality (Vos, 2020).

Psychology of ethics

Psychologists have studied how individuals develop their ethical standpoints. For example, Kohlberg identified the stages of pre-conventional morality (acting according to punishment, obedience, individualism, and self-oriented exchange), conventional morality (maintaining good relationships and social order), and post-conventional morality (following social contract, individual rights, universal principles). Kohlberg has been criticised for conflating moral development with following explicit social norms, excluding principles such as authentic care (Killen & Smetana, 2013)

Step 3: Apply common ethical principles in research

Definition

Whereas Step 2 reviewed the major philosophical-ethical frameworks, this section reviews how researchers may translate these into applied research principles.

Examples

- **Voluntary participation:** Participants are not coerced but free to join a study or not, stop their participation at any time, and withdraw their contributions/interview/ questionnaire data within a pre-given time limit. Their decision to participate or not does not influence any other services/treatments they receive. For example, clients still obtain treatment if they refuse a mental health service to use their data for routine outcome monitoring or service audits.
- **Transparent communication and informed consent:** Participants should know what they are saying 'yes' to. The information needs to be understandable, e.g., avoid jargon and complex language. Researchers cannot deceive participants and must share the study's aims and procedures. Participants should be able to ask questions and talk with an independent researcher (e.g., supervisor, independent therapist, department head). In rare situations, researchers may withhold some details or conduct covert research, requiring careful ethical considerations, and informing participants afterwards. Before the study starts, participants sign an informed consent form confirming they understand the study aims, procedures, and opportunities to ask questions and withdraw. It is unethical and illegal to include participants who are insufficiently able to understand what they are consenting to, such as minors or individuals with severe cognitive impairment; usually, researchers exclude them or ask consent from a legally responsible person on their behalf. In sum, the cornerstones of informed consent are competence, knowledge, and volition of participants.
- **Non-maleficence:** Do no harm: there should not be a realistic likelihood that participants will get harmed. If participants seem to be getting harmed, such as emotional distress during an interview, empathic support and care should be delivered, and they should be reminded of the opportunity to stop. Researchers should not conflate their researcher role with a therapist role, as this may create a sense of coercion and research bias. At the end of questionnaires/interviews, participants receive a debriefing sheet telling them what to do if they experience distress afterwards.
- **Beneficence:** The research ideally benefits the participants.
- **Fidelity and responsibility:** Researchers treat everyone in a fair, just manner.
- **Anonymity and confidentiality:** Individuals have the right to privacy. For example, all questions in an interview/questionnaire should be relevant and justified: a researcher cannot ask about topics such as sexual orientation, religion, or income without justification. Researchers should keep the file with identifiable data – e.g., name, contact details – separate from other data files (e.g., interview transcripts, questionnaires), and identifiable information should be removed or replaced with pseudonyms. Data should be saved in a locked safe or password protected file accessible

only to researchers. The participants' contribution can only be used for the agreed research purposes. Research institutes often have data protection policies, following (inter)national data-protection laws and guidelines.

- **Limitations to privacy:** Researchers need to explain to ethics committees and participants when they may limit privacy. For example, when a participant reveals a serious risk of harming themselves or others, the researcher may be ethically and legally obliged to inform authorities.
- **Sensitivity for individual rights, dignity, and differences:** Different individuals have different needs that researchers need to consider. For example, researchers should use non-offensive and non-reifying/non-labelling language and tailor language to individuals. Researchers should not use gendered language and not assume a person's gender but explicitly ask for their pronouns. Different (sub-)cultures may have different values/norms about what they experience as ethical behaviour and appropriate language. It is not the duty of participants to explain their (sub-)culture or religion to the researcher, as this may create unethical pressure and an experience of 'othering'. Researchers must do their homework to understand their participants' (sub-)cultural and religious norms and values. Researchers should train themselves in asking questions sensitive to (sub-)cultural, religious, sexual, and socio-economic diversity, for example via class exercises or research supervision. Researchers should develop self-awareness about their biases and privileges, including ingroup/outgroup bias and stereotypes. Data analyses should be similarly sensitive, and grounded in ethical self-reflection and reflexivity (Etherington, 2004).
- **Integrity:** Scientific integrity includes, amongst other things: transparency, honesty, accountability, and accuracy and truthfulness in all academic activities. Researchers disclose potential conflicts of interest and focus on the public interest. This may include sharing and auditing datasets for verification and crediting co-authors. This implies not cheating, stealing, plagiarising, or committing fraud. This also means that researchers do not selectively report findings (e.g., only positive findings), delete participants/outliers without reporting this, selectively report sub-scales and experimental conditions, manipulate, make up, or do not report data. Researchers should be direct and not roundabout or obscuring in their reporting.
- **Ability to consult:** Researchers should develop a network they can consult to help them in ethical reflections. This includes actively asking for and openly welcoming advice from peers, supervisors, examiners, and ethical/research committees.
- **Ethically appropriate responsiveness:** Ethical researchers respond sensitively to ethical issues arising in their research. Researchers proactively identify possible ethical issues throughout the research process and respond to this according to the unique situation.

Step 4: Reflect on ethics

Definition

This step reminds researchers to engage in ethical self-reflection actively and take responsibility for their ethical learning process (Etherington, 2004).

Components

In line with research on stages in moral development (Killen & Smetana, 2013), it may be argued that researchers differ in their level of 'ethical maturity', i.e., their ability in critical ethical self-reflection (Carroll & Shaw, 2012). Authors seem to agree on three components of becoming an ethical researcher:

1. Reading key ethical frameworks, professional and legal guidelines.
2. Engaging in critical ethical self-reflection and reflexivity, e.g., via research journals, exercises, conversations with peers/supervisors.
3. Explicating ethical components of the research project, e.g., in an ethics proposal.

Step 5: Manage risks

Definition

An important aspect of ethical self-reflection is imagining and reducing potential risks that the research project may hold for all stakeholders (Reeves, 2015). The key questions involve: what are possible risks, how likely is each risk, how severe is the impact of anything going wrong, what procedures will be used to prevent the risks, and what procedures/protocols will be followed if anything may go wrong?

Examples

Researchers assess potential hazards and risk, how these could be prevented, and what could be done if the worst were to happen.

- Names and contact details of emergency contact persons
- Potential physical hazards of the site, travel, work procedures, knowing emergency procedures and exit routes, political unrest, risk of catching/spreading viruses/bacteria
- Interpersonal risks, such as aggression from participants
- Participants with a risk of self-harm/suicidal ideation (see Step 6)

Step 6: Develop an ethics proposal

Definition

Researchers often write an ethics proposal after they have written a research proposal and before data collection, as Chapter 7 described. An ethics proposal stimulates researchers to consider ethical aspects and explicitly reflect on legal and ethical guidelines and best practices. Template G gives an example of an ethics proposal template that researchers may use as a basis for their ethics proposal.

Components

Many research institutions provide researchers with an ethical documents pack with ethical forms, templates, and guidelines. This ethical documents pack may contain the following.

Ethics application form

See Template G for suggestions on what may be included, e.g., detailed step-by-step procedures (e.g., in a flowchart) of how individuals are recruited, and steps in research participation. This also includes detailed inclusion/exclusion criteria and how these will be checked, by whom, with minimum discrimination and researcher bias.

Participant Information form

All research participants receive a sheet with essential information about the research project:

- Title
- Names and professional/institutional contact details of researchers, research supervisor, funder, and independent contact person (no private accounts for privacy protection)
- Solicitation of participation: e.g., the person is 'invited' to participate
- How to tell researchers they want to participate (e.g., email, call)
- Description of participation procedures (e.g., filling in one ten-minute questionnaire)
- Advantages of participation (e.g., sharing feelings, contributing to research which may benefit similar individuals)
- Disadvantages, risks, costs, inconveniences (e.g., time, energy, travel, emotions)
- Compensation for participation/costs/damage and compensation procedures
- How data is handled anonymously and confidentially (e.g., anonymisation, access only given to researchers)
- Selective refusal (e.g., the participant can decide not to answer a question)
- Opportunity to ask questions to researchers and independent contact persons (e.g., supervisor, manager)
- Opportunity to withdraw (explicate until when and how)
- Signature lines, date, names, formal stamp or authorisation of approval

Risk form

Many research institutes have a form asking researchers to identify potential hazards/risks and how these could be prevented/minimised and managed if they do happen (see Step 5).

Recruitment material

Posters, leaflets, social media posts, and emails should be added to the ethics proposal so the ethics committee can check whether the research is presented in transparent, non-deceiving, non-coercive ways.

Data protection form

Many research projects include a leaflet detailing how data protection is managed according to national and international laws and guidelines (e.g., EU GDPR, UK Data Protection Act). This may include, amongst others, where and how information is stored in a protective way, how long data is saved (personally identifiable data, such as name/date of birth, deleted after one year, interviews/questionnaires deleted after ten years), and publishing only non-identifiable information in an aggregate form with pseudonyms.

Informed consent form

This form is a summary of the participant information form and is signed by researchers and participants. This may include: title; research aim/questions/objectives/hypotheses; summary of participation procedures; possible risks; voluntary participation; compensation for participation and/or in case harm were to happen; opportunity to ask questions; opportunity to withdraw; agreement with audio/video recording if applicable; agreement with anonymised publications.

Participant debrief form

As a reminder and post-participation support, participants receive a debrief form after the interview/questionnaire. This may include: research title; research aim/questions/objectives/ hypotheses; statement and justification of deception, if applicable; confidentiality of data analyses; contact details of researchers; resources in case participants experience negative emotions after participation (e.g., contact GP or therapist, Befrienders, Samaritans, nearest hospital Accident & Emergency); promise that findings will be shared with the participant.

Distress protocol

Procedures if interviewee shows distress (e.g., empathic support, offer to pause/stop interview, external/professional help such as nearby people, hospital Accident & Emergency). Do not conflate therapist and researcher roles.

Suicidal risk protocol

As suicidal risks may pose significant ethical and legal risks, researchers may want to develop suicide protocols for when they suspect a participant may be considering self-harm/suicide. Researchers should be professionally trained to work with participants at risk of self-harm and/or suicidal ideation. Always take signs seriously, respond empathically and sensitively without labelling, further assess risks and protective factors, consult experienced colleagues/ supervisors, and know which authorities to contact in an emergency (e.g., participant's GP/ therapist, emergency phone numbers). Check for self-harm and suicidal-ideation guidelines in your research institution or mental health service.

Step 7: Manage institutional ethics

Definition

An ethically reflexive attitude reaches beyond a researcher's own research project and recognises ethical challenges in the broader context of the research project.

Components

Critical theorists and action researchers argue that all research should contribute to social justice (Chapman & Schwartz, 2012). A 'critical research ethics would value and recognise the need to expose the diversity of realities, engage with the webs of interaction that construct problems in ways that lead to power/privilege for particular groups, reposition problems and decisions toward social justice, and join in solidarity with the traditionally oppressed to create new ways of functioning' (Denzin & Lincoln, 2021, p.172). For example, researchers identify vulnerable groups in society, social problems these groups are confronted with, the institutions that deal with these problems, and the use(fullness) of research, relevance, implementation, and accessibility of interventions for these groups (Denzin & Lincoln, 2021). Social justice is a critical-theoretical lens that influences all research steps, from conceptual framework to research aims, methodologies, and publications.

Researchers have published approximately 50,000 studies on psychological aspects of social justice (Vos, 2022b) on six mutually reinforcing dimensions: unjust context (e.g., inequality, privilege, structural injustice, traumatic events), unjust actions by others (e.g., micro-aggressions, discrimination, institutional discrimination/victimisation), transactional dynamics (e.g., transactional drama triangle, co-dependency, *folie-a-deux*), internalisation of social injustice (e.g., shame, guilt, PTSD), denial of injustice (e.g., terror management theory), and victim's actions contributing to the cycle of injustice (e.g., moral injury, intergenerational patterns, trauma bonding). Research has shown that psychological therapies and community projects can break the vicious cycles of structural injustice, such as treating underlying traumas and helping clients develop skills and build social connections (Vos, Roberts, & Davies, 2019).

Thus, psychological research may contribute to developing a better understanding of social justice and how to stimulate this, but some authors question the structural integrity of our academic activities and institutions (Bretag, 2016; Jussim, Krosnick, & Stevens, 2022; Roberts, 2018). Critical theorists have highlighted structural unethical practices, power dynamics, paradigms, and output-obsessed ethics in academia. Feminist and queer theorists have critiqued oppressive structures, glass ceilings, narcissistic academic leaders, and discriminatory and paternalistic/patriarchal practices, for example regarding the allocation of positions and grants. Some authors have also argued that the ethical values, independence, and credibility of academic research are under fire in neoliberal countries, for example due to funders such as Big Pharma and Big Tech disproportionately influencing research. For example, some funders require access to raw data, editing articles or vetoing publication of unfavourable findings, due to which for example one in two medical studies cannot be trusted completely (Vos, 2021). Consequently, universities have been criticised for becoming more focused on money than on providing the best education possible and making a difference in society via research that matters (Roberts, 2018; Vos, 2020; Vos, Roberts, & Davies, 2019). This continuous battle-of-the-fittest-academic may lay the groundwork for plagiarism, fake data, corruption, bullying, and coercing participants into research.

What will be your ethical response?

━━━━ Reflective questions ━━━━

Learn key ethical frameworks

- Read ethics guidelines from relevant professional bodies.
- Identify two ethical dilemmas you have faced in therapy or research. For each ethical framework, reflect on and summarise possible responses (read more on ethical frameworks if needed).
- Consider how your research may contribute to social justice.
- Examine which unethical practices may be happening around you. When do you feel pressured to act unethically? Can your conscience ignore unethical activities? How will future generations judge you? Imagine you are looking back on your deathbed, will you be proud of how you acted?

Ethical reflection exercise

Reflecting on the below ten ethical dilemmas,

a   identify the main ethical problem
b   consider relevant ethical perspectives (use ethical frameworks, ethical research principles)
c   consider relevant law/professional guidelines
d   what would you do
e   reflect how your actions may reflect your history, social position, and privileges
f   imagine what a devil's advocate with different ethical principles would do.

1   A client in your six-session clinical trial says after session three that they are considering withdrawing.
2   Your position as researcher depends on publications in high-impact journals. Fraudulently changing numbers in your article may stimulate better publications.
3   An interviewee becomes emotional during the interview.
4   A participant mentions suicidal thoughts in a survey.
5   When randomising clients to experimental treatment 'A' or control group 'B', a researcher learns that a client believes they would benefit from 'A' but not 'B'.
6   A researcher finds crucial information in an interview that could make the participant identifiable.
7   Several websites offer participants money to fill in their online survey, but payment could bias answers and coerce participation.
8   You are interested in the lived experience of tenants in social housing. How would you formulate recruitment posters sensitively and non-discriminatorily?
9   You know that your manager has published an article with partially fake data.
10 A funder only gives money if you agree not to publish unfavourable findings.

12

How to Discuss and Disseminate Research

Chapter aims

This chapter describes how to discuss research findings in a publication and write your final research report or thesis. This chapter also introduces how to disseminate your findings via publications and presentations.

Steps in chapter

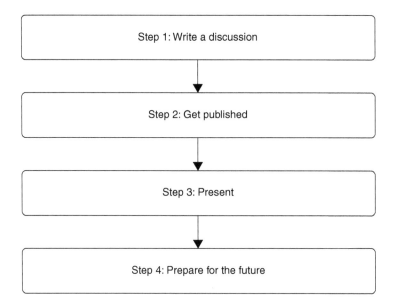

Templates

H. Final thesis

I. Article

Thesis checklist (online)

Thesis presentation (online)

Step 1: Write a discussion

Definition

A discussion, section or chapter in a research report/thesis/article aims to interpret and describe the meaning and significance of your findings in light of what was already known in the field. The discussion also highlights and explains new findings and understandings.

Tips

- **Connections:** The discussion highlights the logical connections with previous parts of your research project, with a clear textual flow and logical arguments (see Chapter 2). The reader is reminded how the study aims (see Chapter 6) were developed to answer a problem in the field and a gap in the literature (see Chapter 5). The discussion highlights key findings, and conceptualises and contextualises their meaning, importance, and innovation in the broader field, which may reach beyond the already-discussed literature review (see Chapter 3). The discussion shows how your methodological decisions have helped answer your research questions and achieve objectives and how hypotheses have been confirmed/rejected (see Chapter 7). The discussion critically reflects on the study's reliability, validity, and/or trustworthiness (see Chapters 8–10). The researcher critically reflects on the research strengths and weaknesses (see Chapter 3), including ethical considerations (see Chapter 11). This leads the researcher to final conclusions and recommendations for researchers, practitioners, and society.
- **No repetition:** The discussion is not a repetition of the findings section but highlights and interprets findings from a big-picture perspective. Readers have already read your findings but want to understand their meaning and significance.
- **No new findings:** Discussion cannot discuss new findings.
- **Realistic:** Do not speculate, overinterpret, overgeneralise, or use induction bias.
- **Understandable:** The discussion needs to be understandable for readers who have not read or understood the findings section.
- **Competent:** The discussion can demonstrate research competencies, e.g., self-reflection, logical synthesis, conceptualisation, contextualisation, and deep understanding of the topic.
- **Writing style:** Remember basic academic skills (see Chapter 2). Researchers often use first-person, present tense, past tense for previous research, and if possible sub-headings.

Components

Key message

Briefly reiterate the research aims as an introduction to showing how the findings answer these (see Chapter 6). Briefly summarise findings for each objective/question/hypothesis. If you have many findings, focus on the primary research aims/questions/objectives and the most significant/innovative findings: what is the key message? In quantitative research, this may include a systematic discussion of how the findings support/reject the hypotheses, the main findings, and variation/errors.

Contextualising key findings

Describe similarities and differences between your findings and previous studies. Describe how findings challenge, elaborate, support, and contribute to the research field.

Interpreting and conceptualising key findings

Highlight surprising, contradictory, and innovative findings. Hypothesise possible but realistic explanations, and consider alternative explanations based on other research. This should not merely include studies already mentioned in your literature review (see Chapter 5) but also the broader field (see Chapter 3), which may require scoping the literature for extra publications (use this as an opportunity to update your previous literature review).

Limitations

All discussions lead to a statement such as 'This research is limited by…', followed by self-reflections on potential weaknesses. This includes critically discussing methodological decisions such as: method, number of measurements, study duration, recruitment procedures, instruments (e.g., reliability/validity/sensitivity/precision, interview bias), data collection, organisational procedures (see Chapter 7). This also includes reflection on instrument reliability and validity, validity of study design, response shift (see Chapter 8, Step 8), and trustworthiness (see Chapter 9, Step 8). The researcher critically reflects on sample size and characteristics (e.g., ecological validity, random/representative sample, quantitative *a posteriori* power, missing values and data-imputation, significance level and correction for the number of tests/estimations, qualitative homogeneity); this may lead to reflection on the potential generalisability/transferability of the findings beyond the study sample. Qualitative researchers may want to re-read their reflective research journal to identify how their reasoning and thinking about the topic may have evolved, and to critically reflect on their relationships with the participants, topic and social context (see Online Table 4.2). Revisit ethical dilemmas encountered. Reflect on personal or professional conflicts of interest, and roles of funders.

Implications/recommendations

Considering the limitations, discuss realistic implications and recommendations for researchers, research programmes, research field, research population/clients, practitioners, and other stakeholders such as advocacy groups, policy-makers, and society. Be realistic and share possible strategies to create change, e.g., dissemination and lobbying strategies.

Step 2: Get published

Definition

Many researchers conduct research because they hope to make a difference in their research field and the real world. They cannot achieve this aim if their research is not shared with others, and their report/thesis merely collects dust in a drawer. Therefore, researchers must develop a realistic dissemination plan, be proactive, insistent, and persevere in getting published.

Examples

Thesis

Template H offers two examples of student thesis structures; check the required format, length, and style with your institution. Do not forget to send a copy to your institution's library or research depository.

Article in research journals

- **Common steps:** Select journal; write article according to journal's author instructions; submit; receive review (e.g., rejection/minor revisions/major revisions/acceptance); rewrite; resubmit; possible new round of review/rewriting; acceptance; feedback from copyeditor; submission of final manuscript; e-pub ahead of print; printed.
- **Length:** Journal articles are short, usually 6000 words, implying you need to leave out details. Consider adding: 'further research details may be requested from the authors'.
- **Proofreading:** Consider using tools like Grammarly, although this never replaces human proofreaders. Particularly if English is not your native language, consider hiring a proofreader.
- **Target the right journal:** For example, check title, mission statement, word limit, published topics and methods, author instructions, and editorial board, and ask colleagues. Some journals publish rejection rates (www.apa.org/pubs/journals/statistics). Some institutions are subscribed to the Cabelis database describing which journals may be reputable and which predatory. Online Table 12.1 provides an overview of therapy journals ranked in order of impact. Check your reference list for relevant journals.
- **Pre-registration:** Some journals only accept clinical trials registered before data collection.
- **Dataset:** Some journals require submission or publication of datasets.
- **Consider impact factors:** Impact factors tell how frequently an average article in this journal is cited. To increase your impact, consider submitting to higher impact journals first (but be realistic).
- **Open access:** Ideally, you want everyone to access your article, including those not subscribed to a journal. Some journals offer the opportunity to pay for immediate open access and sometimes free open access in the long term.
- **Author instructions:** Follow the journal's author instructions to prevent rejection.
- **Letter to the editor:** The letter aims to explain why the editor should consider publishing your article and may include: key message, research aims, relevance for their readers, and similar publications in their journal. Without explicitly saying it, argue why your article may get cited and increase the journal's impact factor. Be ambitious but realistic in underlining your work's innovative and important character and contributions to the field.
- **Submit to one journal at a time:** Bear in mind the time review may take; reviewers are often unpaid volunteers with large workloads.
- **Cope with feedback/rejection:** Undoubtedly, you will receive feedback and rejections that may feel challenging. Leave the feedback aside for some days, calm down, and look at it with some distance. Remember that reviewers/editors are not aiming to destroy you (do consider possible political/paradigmatic reasons behind their

decision). Use the pointers for emotional coping strategies in Step 1 in Chapter 2. Write in your reflective journal.

- **Revise:** Most manuscripts get rejected. You may be asked to resubmit with minor/major revisions if lucky. Do not forget resubmission deadlines. A revision consists of the revised manuscript (usually with visible track changes) and a letter that may contain gratitude to the reviewers/editor and a step-by-step discussion of how you address each point of feedback (e.g., copy their feedback in **bold** letters, followed by how and where in the revised manuscript you address this). Follow their requirements and recommendations to increase your likelihood of acceptance; however, if you disagree, state your reasons in detailed, well-argued, sensitive, and non-offensive ways. Critically reflect on whether your disagreement may be due to your biases; ask colleagues for a third opinion. If reviewers are inconsistent, ask the editor for advice. Gain experience by asking colleagues or supervisors to become a ghost reviewer/co-reviewer.
- **Learn more:** Ask your supervisors and peers for feedback. Learn from frequently cited articles. See more in Silvia (2015).

Magazines, journals, newspapers

Professional bodies may have newsletters or magazines which may accept articles, although these usually focus on the discipline or organisation (e.g., *Therapy Today, Counselling Psychologist, American Psychologist, The Psychologist*). Journals and newspapers for the general audience rarely accept articles from outsiders. You may send a press release, letter to the editor, and emails to journalists/editors (as news desks usually ignore unsolicited press releases, use personal connections).

Academic websites

If you own the copyright (e.g., your article is not published in a journal), you can make it publicly available on your research profiles (e.g., ResearchGate, Academia.edu, FigShare, ORCID, ImpactStory, LinkedIn, scholar.google.com).

Social media/forums

You will know best how to find these in your field. Do not forget the website or social media of your research institute.

Book publisher

Writing books and getting published is fun (guess what I am doing now?). Ask advice from published authors and follow workshops or training on writing books and book proposals. Search for publishers dedicated to your field. You will need to send a book proposal to a publisher; often, publishers provide templates. Look at your book from the publisher's eyes, not from what you want: would your book sell well?

Self-publication

Better self-published than not published. Online self-publication may be fast, but without a marketing campaign, readers may not find you. Examples include KDP/Amazon, Apple Books, Barnes & Noble Press, Kobo,

Step 3: Present

Definition

Giving research presentations is an essential academic skill that requires practice and feedback. Watch some of the countless online instruction videos, follow workshops, or read instructional guides (Nicol & Pexman, 2003; Wempen, 2010).

Examples

Structure

Presentations apply all basic academic skills (see Chapter 2). Structuring your presentation is crucial: break it into parts/chapters and sub-parts/sections. Apply the tell-tell-and-tell principle: start the presentation with study aims, key message/conclusions, and an overview of the structure, follow this with detailing your methodology and findings, and end with a discussion (see Step 1). An overview of a presentation structure can be found online in PowerPoint Template N. You may want to adjust your tone/structure/template for non-academic audiences.

Format

PowerPoint is the most frequently used software for presentations; alternatives include Google Slides, Prezi, Visme, and Keynote. Choose a readable, professional font, sans serif, size at least 20 points. Include only keywords and key sentences; maximum 30 words per slide if you expect the audience to read. Approximately one slide per minute; tables and figures with more information can be presented, but the font needs to be big enough, and tables explained. Keep time for the Question and Answer section at the end. Use professional academic designs with relevant and professional pictures. Have a professional tone. Practice-practice-practice in front of the mirror, friends, and peers. Search for academic PowerPoint presentations online (search terms: topic AND .ppt).

Conference presentations

Conferences can help you share your research and build professional networks. Find relevant conferences on websites from professional bodies and ask colleagues. You usually need to be invited to give a keynote. You must submit an abstract to present via a non-keynote lecture or workshop. Usually, presenters also pay conference fees (except keynote speakers).

Lectures at institutions

Many universities, research institutions, mental health services, and placement providers organise research seminars. Ask colleagues where, when, and what happens, and how you could contribute.

Public lectures

Many organisations and charities organise in-person and online events. Consider video-recording a lecture and sharing this online via YouTube/Vimeo (e.g., https://joelvos.com/videos).

Step 4: Prepare for the future

Research does not automatically make an impact: most lecturers and practitioners only use research as one of many resources (Safran et al., 2011). Therefore, it may also not be enough to have written a research/report/thesis, published an article, and presented your research to relevant audiences. You may need to proactively bring your research to your target audience, such as creating practical step-by-step recommendations and offering workshops. If you are more ambitious, ask yourself which strategy you need to influence policy-makers (Knapp, McDaid, & Mossialos, 2006; Purtle et al., 2020). How can you ensure that your research ends up on the desk of power-holders? Who can lobby for you? How does social change in your field work? Creating social change also means that you can show the meaning and practical implications of your research without academic jargon and distracting details. Reflect on how realistic it is that influential individuals and policy-makers will read and use your work.

Finally: celebrate, be proud, and take time to recover before your next research adventure! Take time to reflect. What have you learned about doing research, your field, and yourself? How could you improve your research skills? How could you help improve the research field and therapeutic practices? Where are opportunities for further research? What would you need to make this happen, such as applying for research grants or researcher vacancies?

It has been my honour to walk alongside you, step-by-step in your research project. Enjoy your research journey!

━━━━ Reflective questions ━━━━

- Select three frequently cited articles in your field. Examine their discussion; what would you change? What lessons can you learn?
- Look at your reference list. Where did these authors publish? Could you publish there?
- Reflect: what do you want to happen with your research findings? What would you do if you had a magic wand? What practical steps/resources could make this happen?
- Based on your study: suggest three follow-up research projects, three therapeutic applications or implications, three policy changes, three newspaper headlines, and a one-paragraph press release.
- Who would be interested in your findings? How could you reach them? How could you lobby relevant policy-makers?

APPENDIX: TEMPLATES

Instructions

- Printable, editable templates can be downloaded from https://joelvos.com/doingresearch
- Templates can be used by researchers to structure their research texts. Templates can be shared for educational purposes but must contain a reference to this book.
- Disclaimer: templates require tailoring to your situation and do not guarantee success. For example, templates may contain more details or numbers than needed. Remove or add numbers and sections/sub-sections depending on your situation.
- Templates assume that previous research templates have been used.
- Frontpages may include: title, name, student number, address/faculty, contact details.
- Abstracts may be unstructured or include the sub-headings: background, aim, method, findings, discussion.
- The introduction of each section summarises in several sentences: the aim of this section, main message, how this section builds on previous sections, how this fits in the broader text and helps achieve its overall aim, method, overview of parts/sub-sections (see Chapter 2).
- The discussions of each section summarise in several sentences: the conclusions or main findings, how these findings fit in the overall text and may help achieve its overall aims, self-reflection on limitations, remaining questions, link to next section (see Chapter 2).
- Templates refer to chapters in this book.

A Preliminary interest statement

Frontpage

Abstract

1   Introduction (½ A4)
    1.1. Appealining
    1.2. Essay aims or key message

1.3. Definitions/criteria of central concepts

1.4. Chapter overview

2 Personal background (1–2 A4)

(Chapter 4)

2.1. Introduction

2.2. Method of self-reflection

2.3. Personal motivation about topic

2.4. Personal experiences and beliefs about topic

2.5. Critical-theoretical framework (if relevant) (Chapter 3)

2.6. Strengths and weaknesses of using personal experiences

2.7. Discussion

3 Research background (1–2 A4)

(Sketch preliminary conceptual framework via scoping mini-reviews; Chapter 3)

3.1. Introduction

3.2. Main clinical/psychological concepts

3.3. Aetiological concepts

3.4. Outcomes-related concepts

3.5. Therapeutic-mechanisms-related concepts

3.6. Client-related concepts

3.7. Therapist-related concepts

3.8. Therapeutic-mechanism-related concepts

3.9. Process-related concepts

3.10. Competencies-related concepts

3.11. Discussion

4 Preliminary focus (1 A4)

(Chapter 5)

4.1. Introduction

4.2. Preliminary gap in literature

4.3. Preliminary research aim

4.4. Preliminary relevance and innovation

4.5. Preliminary contribution to field

4.6. Discussion

5 Preliminary methodology (1 A4)

(Chapter 6)

5.1. Introduction

5.2. Preliminary methodology ideas

5.3. Relevant guidelines from professional bodies

5.4. Practical organisation

5.5. Learning plan

5.6. Timeline

5.7. Discussion

6 Discussion (½–1 A4)

6.1. Conclusion/key message

6.2. Self-reflection/limitations

6.3. Implications/next research steps

B Literature review plan

Frontpage

Abstract

1 Introduction (½–1 A4)

1.1. Appealing opening

1.2. Essay aims or key message

1.3. Personal background (e.g., summarise interest statement, motivation, preliminary research aim, critical-theoretical framework; Chapter 4)

1.4. Research background (e.g., trends, preliminary conceptual framework; Chapter 3)

1.5. Definitions/criteria of central concepts

1.6. Chapter overview

2 Review aims (½ A4)

(Chapter 5; this may include multiple objectives/questions, such as multiple non-systematic scoping mini-reviews to sketch the research background and conceptual framework, and a systematic major-review of studies similar to this research project)

2.1. Overall aim

2.2. Objectives/questions

3 Review method (1–2 A4)

(Chapter 5)

3.1. Review type

3.2. Eligibility criteria

3.3. Search engines

3.4. Draft search terms

3.5. Search strategy

3.6. Recording procedures

3.7. Quality assessment

3.8. Synthesis

4 Discussion (½ A4)

4.1. Conclusion/summary

4.2. Self-reflection/limitations

4.3. Implications/recommendations/next research steps

C Systematic literature review

Frontpage

Abstract

1   Introduction (½–1 A4)

1.1. Appealing opening
1.2. Essay aims or key message
1.3. Personal background (e.g., summarise interest statement, motivation, preliminary research aim, critical-theoretical framework; Chapter 4)
1.4. Research background (e.g., trends, preliminary conceptual framework; Chapter 3)
1.5. Definitions/criteria of central concepts
1.6. Chapter overview

2   Review aims (½ A4)

(Chapter 3)
2.1. Overall aim
2.2. Objectives/questions

3   Review method (1 A4)

(Chapter 3)
3.1. Review type
3.2. Eligibility criteria
3.3. Search engines
3.4. Draft search terms
3.5. Search strategy
3.6. Recording procedures
3.7. Quality assessment
3.8. Synthesis

4   Mini literature reviews of research background (1–2 A4)

(Chapter 3; describe conceptual framework via multiple non-systematic scoping mini-reviews of clinical, aetiological, outcomes-related, mechanism-related, client-related, therapist-related, relationship-related, process-related, and competences-related models; findings can be structured via themes, chronology, narratives, or Chapter 3's nine conceptual models)
4.1. Introduction
4.2. Findings
4.3. Discussion

5   Major literature review of similar studies (1–2 A4)

(Chapter 3; describe studies similar to your research project via a systematic review; findings may be structured via themes, chronology, narratives, or Chapter 3's nine conceptual models)

5.1. Introduction

5.2. Findings

5.3. Discussion

6 Discussion (1 A4)

6.1. Conclusion/key message

6.2. Contextualise key findings

6.3. Interpret and conceptualise key findings

6.4. Self-reflection/limitations

6.5. Implications/recommendations/next research steps

D Essay on methodology

Frontpage

Abstract

1 Introduction (½ A4)

1.1. Appealing opening

1.2. Essay aims or key message

1.3. Definitions/criteria of central concepts

1.4. Chapter overview

2 Research overview (1 A4)

(Chapter 5; summarise literature review)

2.1. Introduction

2.2. Mini literature reviews of research background

2.3. Major literature review of similar studies

2.4. Gap in the literature

2.5. Research aim

2.6. Research objectives, questions, hypotheses (Chapter 6)

3 Epistemological and ontological position (1 A4)

(Chapter 7)

3.1. Introduction

3.2. Self-reflection methods

3.3. Epistemological position

3.4. Ontological position

3.5. Discussion

4 Methodology (1 A4)

(Chapter 7; explain, justify, and specify)

4.1. Introduction

4.2. Type of method

4.3. Experimental status
4.4. Number of measurement-moments/contacts
4.5. Period

5 Sampling (1 A4)

(Chapter 7; explain, justify, and specify)
5.1. Introduction
5.2. Inclusion/exclusion criteria
5.3. Sample size
5.4. Recruitment strategy
5.5. Worst-case scenario alternatives

6 Data collection (1–3 A4)

(cf. Chapters 8–10)
6.1. Introduction
6.2. Data-collection tools
6.3. Data-collection procedures
6.4. Alternatives considered

7 Data analysis (1–3 A4)

(Chapters 8–10; explain, justify, and specify)
7.1. Introduction
7.2. Analysis preparation (e.g., transcription, software, coding, scoring, preparatory analysis)
7.3. Data analysis
7.4. Detailed data-analysis steps/procedures
7.5. Alternatives considered

8 Ethics (½–1 A4)

(Chapter 11; elaborated in ethics proposal)
8.1. Ethics guidelines and principles
8.2. Preliminary ethics of sampling, Data collection, and risks
8.3. Preliminary ethics of data analysis and research integrity
8.4. Preliminary ethical reflections

9 Research quality (½–1 A4)

(Chapters 8–10)
9.1. Introduction
9.2. Reliability and validity and/or trustworthiness
9.3. Discussion

10 Discussion (½–1 A4)

10.1. Conclusion/key message
10.2. Self-reflection/limitations
10.3. Implications/recommendations/next research steps

Appendices

- Recruitment material
- Questionnaires/interview schedule
- Treatment manual/experiment protocol
- Scoring/coding schemes

E Essay on critical self-reflection and reflexivity

Frontpage

Abstract

1 Introduction (½–1 A4)

1.1. Appealing opening
1.2. Essay aims or key message
1.3. Chapter overview

2 Theoretical context

(Chapter 4)
2.1. Introduction
2.2. Theory: what are self-reflection and reflexivity?
2.3. Relevance: why are self-reflection and reflexivity important?
2.4. Definitions/criteria of central concepts
2.5. Discussion

3 Personal self-reflection (1–2 A4)

(Chapter 4; may summarise/replace previous essays)
3.1. Introduction
3.2. Personal motivation
3.3. Personal experiences and beliefs
3.4. Critical-theoretical framework (Chapter 3)
3.5. Strengths and weaknesses of using personal experiences
3.6. Self-reflection method during research (e.g., reflective research journal)
3.7. Discussion

4 Ontological and epistemological self-reflection (1–2 A4)

(Chapter 7; may summarise/replace previous essays)
4.1. Introduction
4.2. Epistemological position

4.3. Ontological position

4.4. Discussion

5 Methodological self-reflection and reflexivity (1–2 A4)

(Chapter 7)

5.1. Introduction

5.2. Study design

5.3. Sample

5.4. Data collection

5.5. Data analysis

5.6. Validity and reliability, and/or trustworthiness (Chapters 8–10)

5.7. Ethical considerations (Chapter 11; reflections on ethics proposal)

5.8. Discussion

6 Discussion (1 A4)

6.1. Conclusion/key message

6.2. Self-reflection/limitations

6.3. Implications/recommendations/next research steps

F Research proposal

Frontpage

Abstract

1 Introduction (1–2 A4)

1.1. Appealing opening

1.2. Essay aims or key message (e.g., summarise research aims/methodology)

1.3. Personal background/motivation (e.g., critical-theoretical framework)

1.4. Definitions/criteria of central concepts

1.5. Chapter overview

2 Research background (1–2 A4)

(Chapter 3; sketch conceptual framework, cf. literature review; focus on the field's main problem or gap in literature)

2.1. Introduction

2.2. Review aims and method

2.3. Findings

2.4. Discussion

3 Literature review (1–2 A4)

(Chapter 3; systematic major-review of studies similar to your research project)

3.1. Introduction

3.2. Review aims and method

3.3. Findings
3.4. Discussion

4 Research aims (1–2 A4)

(Chapter 6)
4.1. Introduction
4.2. Summary of problem in field and gap in literature
4.3. Aim
4.4. Objectives/questions
4.5. Hypotheses
4.6. Contributions to field
4.7. Discussion

5 Methodology (1–6 A4)

(Chapters 7–10; explain, justify, and specify)
5.1. Introduction
5.2. Ontological and epistemological position
5.3. Study design
5.4. Sample
5.5. Recruitment
5.6. Data-collection tools
5.7. Analysis preparation (e.g., transcription, coding, preparatory statistical analysis)
5.8. Data analysis
5.9. Organisation and timeline
5.10. Ethical reflections (Chapter 11; summary of ethics proposal)
5.11. Discussion

6 Self-reflection

(Chapter 4)
6.1. Introduction
6.2. Self-reflection methods
6.3. Validity and reliability and/or trustworthiness
6.4. Discussion

7 Discussion (1 A4)

7.1. Conclusion/key message
7.2. Self-reflection/limitations
7.3. Implications/recommendations/next research steps

Appendices

- Recruitment material
- Questionnaires/interview schedule
- Treatment manual/experiment protocol

- Scoring/coding schemes
- Timetable

G Ethics proposal

Frontpage

Abstract

1 Introduction (1 A4)

1.1. Appealing opening
1.2. Essay aims or key message
1.3. Definitions/criteria of central concepts
1.4. Chapter overview

2 Theoretical background (1 A4)

(Chapter 11)
2.1. Definitions and relevance of ethics in research
2.2. Relevant ethical frameworks and principles
2.3. Relevant laws and professional guidelines
2.4. Discussion

3 Research rationale (1–2 A4)

(Explain and justify need for this study; summarise research proposal)
3.1. Introduction
3.2. Rationale (e.g., gap in literature, problem in field)
3.3. Research aim, objectives, questions, hypotheses
3.4. Contributions to field (e.g., participants, field, society)
3.5. Methodology
3.6. Specification of research material (e.g., what will participants receive)
3.7. Role of funding and personal conflicts of interest
3.8. Self-reflection
3.9. Discussion

4 Ethical reflection on sample

(Chapters 7, 11)
4.1. Introduction
4.2. Inclusion/exclusion criteria
4.3. Voluntary participation (e.g., no coercion, withdrawal right)
4.4. Recruitment procedures (e.g., no deception)
4.5. Possible advantages of participation
4.6. Possible disadvantages of participation
4.7. Data protection

4.8. Privacy protection

4.9. Informed-consent procedures

5 Risk assessment and risk management

(Chapter 11; discuss likelihood, prevention and management of risks)

5.1. Introduction

5.2. Physical risks

5.3. Interpersonal risks

5.4. Vulnerable individuals

5.5. Distress protocol

5.6. Suicidal-risk protocol

5.7. Other risks

5.8. Insurance

5.9. Discussion

6 Discussion (1 A4)

6.1. Conclusion/key message

6.2. Self-reflection/limitations

6.3. Implications/recommendations/next research steps

Appendices

- Participant information form
- Recruitment material
- Informed consent
- Participant debrief form
- Research material (e.g., questionnaire/interview schedule)
- Other forms (e.g., research proposal, risk assessment, distress protocol, suicidal-risk protocol, data protection)

H. Final thesis

Option I: Thesis based on a research monograph

Frontpage

Abstract

1 Introduction

1.1. Appealing opening

1.2. Key message (e.g., summary of key findings/contributions)

1.3. Personal background

1.4. Definitions/criteria of central concepts

1.5. Chapter overview

2 Research background (1–4 A4)

(Chapter 3; sketch conceptual framework via non-systematic mini-reviews, cf. literature review)

2.1. Introduction

2.2. Critical-theoretical framework (if relevant)

2.3. Literature review aims and method

2.4. Findings (present multiple sections/sub-sections with headings/sub-headings)

2.5. Gaps in literature and problems in field

2.6. Discussion

3 Literature review (1–4 A4)

(Chapter 5; systematic major-review of studies similar to your research project)

3.1. Introduction

3.2. Review aims and method

3.3. Findings (present multiple sections/sub-sections with headings/sub-headings)

3.4. Discussion

4 Research aims (1–2 A4)

(Chapter 6)

4.1. Introduction

4.2. Summary of the main problems in the field and gaps in the literature

4.3. Aim

4.4. Objectives/questions

4.5. Hypotheses

4.6. Contributions to field

4.7. Discussion

5 Methodology

(Chapters 7–10)

5.1. Introduction

5.2. Ontological and epistemological position

5.3. Study design

5.4. Sample and recruitment

5.5. Data collection

5.6. Data analysis

5.7. Self-reflection methods (Chapter 4)

5.8. Ethics (Chapter 11)

6 Findings

(Chapters 7–10; present multiple sections/sub-sections with headings/sub-headings)

6.1. Introduction

6.2. Preliminary analysis

6.3. Sample

6.4. Findings objective 1/theme 1

6.x. Findings objective x/theme x

6.y. Synthesis and self-reflection (if applicable)

7 Discussion

(Chapter 12)

7.1. Conclusion/key message

7.2. Contextualise key findings

7.3. Interpret and conceptualise key findings

7.4. Self-reflection/limitations

7.5. Implications/recommendations/next research steps

Option II: Thesis based on articles

Frontpage

Abstract

1 Introduction

1.1. Appealing opening

1.2. Research aim/objectives/questions/hypotheses

1.3. Personal background (e.g., critical-theoretical framework; Chapter 4)

1.4. Definitions/criteria of central concepts

1.5. Overview of chapters

2 Literature review

(Chapter 5; may be integrated in chapters on specific articles/studies)

2.1. Introduction

2.2. Review aims and findings

2.3. Review of research background (sketch conceptual framework via non-systematic mini-reviews; Chapter 3)

2.4. Review of similar studies (systematic major-review of similar studies; Chapter 3)

2.5. Findings (present multiple sections/sub-sections with headings/sub-headings)

2.6. Discussion

3 Methodology

(Chapters 7–10; may be integrated in chapters on specific articles/studies)

3.1. Introduction

3.2. Ontological and epistemological position

3.3. Study design

3.4. Sample and recruitment

3.5. Data collection

3.6. Data analysis

3.7. Self-reflection methods

3.8. Ethics (Chapter 11)

4 Article/study 1 (repeat for next articles/studies)

(Present multiple sections/sub-sections with headings/sub-headings)
4.1. Introduction
4.2. Methods
4.3. Findings
4.4. Discussion

5 Discussion

(Synthesise findings, go beyond individual articles/studies; Chapter 12)
5.1. Conclusions
5.2. Contextualisation of key findings
5.3. Interpretation and conceptualising of key findings
5.4. Validity and reliability, and/or trustworthiness
5.5. Other self-reflection/limitations
5.6. Implications and recommendations

Appendices (see research/ethics proposals)

I Article

1 Introduction

1.1. Introduction/appealing opening
1.2. Key problem in field
1.3. Review of research background (e.g., critical-theoretical framework; conceptual framework via non-systematic mini-reviews)
1.4. Review of similar studies (systematic major-review of similar studies)
1.5. Research aim, questions, objectives, hypotheses

2 Methods

(Chapters 7–10)
2.1. Introduction
2.2. Study design
2.3. Sample and recruitment
2.4. Data collection
2.5. Data analysis
2.6. Ethics (Chapter 11; including ethics committee approval, disclosure of conflicts of interest, pre-registration, available data access)
2.7. Discussion

3 Findings

3.1. Preparatory analyses (if relevant)
3.2. Sample characteristics
3.3. Findings objective 1 or theme 1

3.x. Findings objective x or theme x

3.y. Synthesis and self-reflection (if applicable)

4   Discussion

(Chapter 12)

4.1. Conclusions

4.2. Contextualisation of key findings

4.3. Interpretation and conceptualisation of key findings

4.4. Validity and reliability, and/or trustworthiness

4.5. Other self-reflection/limitations

4.6. Implications and recommendations

REFERENCES

Abbas, R.K. (2022). Insider-outsider Research in Qualitative Inquiry. Routledge.

Aggarwal, C.C. (2017). *Outlier analysis*. Springer.

Ahn, H.N., & Wampold, B E. (2001). Where oh where are the specific ingredients? A meta-analysis of component studies in counseling and psychotherapy. *Journal of Counseling Psychology*, 48(3), 251.

Alaszewski, A. (2006). *Using diaries for social research*. Sage.

American Psychological Association. (2020). *Publication manual*. APA.

Amin, M.E.K., Nørgaard, L.S., Cavaco, A.M., Witry, M.J., Hillman, L., Cernasev, A., & Desselle, S.P. (2020). Establishing trustworthiness and authenticity in qualitative pharmacy research. *Research in Social and Administrative Pharmacy*, 16(10), 1472-1482.

Andresen, R., Oades, L.G., & Caputi, P. (2011). *Psychological recovery*. Wiley.

APA Presidential Task Force on Evidence-Based Practice. (2006). Evidence-based practice in psychology. *American Psychologist*, 61(4), 271–285.

Archer, M., Bhaskar, R., Collier, A., Lawson, T., & Norrie, A. (2013). *Critical realism*. Routledge.

Ashworth, P. (2003). An approach to phenomenological psychology. *Journal of Phenomenological Psychology*, 34(2), 145–156.

Atkins, D.C., & Christensen, A. (2001). Is professional training worth the bother? *Australian Psychologist*, 36(2), 122–130.

Atkinson, P. (2007). *Ethnography*. Routledge.

Avdi, E., & Georgaca, E. (2007). Narrative research in psychotherapy. *Psychology and Psychotherapy: Theory, Research and Practice*, 80(3), 407–419.

Azevedo, V., Carvalho, M., Fernandes-Costa, F., Mesquita, S., Soares, J., Teixeira, F., & Maia, A. (2017). Interview transcription. *Revista de Enfermagem Referência*, 4(14), 159–167.

Baer, A.R., Zon, R., Devine, S., & Lyss, A.P. (2011). The clinical research team. *Journal of Oncology Practice*, 7(3), 188.

Bager-Charleson, S., & McBeath, A.G. (2021). What support do therapists need to do research? *Counselling and Psychotherapy Research*, 21(3), 555–569.

Bager-Charleson, S., McBeath, A., & Vostanis, P. (2021). Building bridges with mixed methods research? *Counselling and Psychotherapy Research*, 21(1), 48–51.

Bagnoli, A. (2009). Beyond the standard interview. *Qualitative Research*, 9(5), 547–570.

Baldwin, S.A., & Imel, Z.E. (2020). Studying specificity in psychotherapy with meta-analysis is hard. *Psychotherapy Research*, 30(3), 294–296.

Bandelow, B., Reitt, M., Röver, C., Michaelis, S., Görlich, Y., & Wedekind, D. (2015). Efficacy of treatments for anxiety disorders. *International Clinical Psychopharmacology*, 30(4), 183–192.

Bargar, R.R., & Duncan, J.K. (1982). Cultivating creative endeavour in doctoral research. *Journal of Higher Education*, 53(1), 1–31.

Barker, C., Pistrang, N., & Elliott, R. (2015). *Research methods in clinical psychology*. Wiley.

Barkham, M., & Lambert, M.J. (2021). The efficacy and effectiveness of psychological therapies. In M. Barkham, W. Lutz, & L.G. Castonguay (2021), *Bergin and Garfield's Handbook of Psychotherapy and Behavior Change* (pp. 135 189). Wiley.

Barkham, M., & Mellor-Clark, J. (2003). Bridging evidence-based practice and practice-based evidence. *Clinical Psychology & Psychotherapy, 10*(6), 319–327.

Barkham, M., Connell, J., Stiles, W.B., Miles, J.N.V., Margison, F., Evans, C., & Mellor-Clark, J. (2006). Dose-effect relations and responsive regulation of treatment duration. *Journal of Consulting and Clinical Psychology, 74*(1), 160–167.

Barkham, M., Stiles, W.B., Connell, J, et al. (2008). Effects of psychological therapies in randomized trials and practice-based studies. *British Journal of Clinical Psychology, 47*(4), 397–415.

Barkham, M., Hardy, G.E., & Mellor-Clark, J. (2010). *Developing and delivering practice-based evidence*. Wiley.

Barkham, M., Lutz, W., & Castonguay, L.G. (2021). *Bergin and Garfield's handbook of psychotherapy and behaviour change*. Wiley.

Barlow, D.H., Nock, M., & Hersen, M. (2008). *Single case research designs*. Allyn.

Baron, R.M., & Kenny, D.A. (1986). The moderator–mediator variable distinction in social psychological research. *Journal of Personality and Social Psychology, 51*(6), 1173.

Beck, A.P., & Lewis, C.M. (2000). *The process of group psychotherapy*. APA.

Billig, M. (2009). *Discursive psychology, rhetoric and the issue of agency*. Semen.

Birkenstein, C., & Graff, G. (2018). *They say/I say: The moves that matter in academic writing*. Norton.

Birks, M., Chapman, Y., & Francis, K. (2008). Memoing in qualitative research. *Journal of Research in Nursing, 13*(1), 68–75.

Blair, J., Czaja, R.F., & Blair, E.A. (2013). *Designing surveys*. Sage.

Blanca, M.J., Arnau, J., López-Montiel, D., Bono, R., & Bendayan, R. (2013). Skewness and kurtosis in real data samples. *Methodology, 9*(2), 78–90.

Boddy, C.R. (2016). Sample size for qualitative research. *Qualitative Market Research, 19*(4), 426–432.

Bohart, A.C., & Tallman, K. (1998). The person as active agent in experiential therapy. In L.S. Greenberg, J.C. Watson, & G. Lietaer (Eds.), *Handbook of experiential psychotherapy*. Guildford.

Böhnke, J.R., Lutz, W., & Delgadillo, J. (2014). Negative affectivity as a transdiagnostic factor in patients with common mental disorders. *Journal of Affective Disorders, 166*, 270–278.

Bolstad, W.M., & Curran, J.M. (2016). *Introduction to Bayesian statistics*. Wiley.

Bond, T. (2015). *Standards and Ethics for Counselling in Action*. Sage.

Borenstein, M., Hedges, L.V., Higgins, J.P., & Rothstein, H.R. (2021). *Introduction to meta-analysis*. Wiley.

Bornstein, R.F. (2017). Evidence-based psychological assessment. *Journal of Personality Assessment, 99*(4), 435–445.

Boréus, K., & Bergström, G. (2017). *Analyzing text and discourse*. Sage.

Borgatti, S. (2023). Introduction to grounded theory. http://www.analytictech.com/mb870/introtoGT.htm

Boswell, J.F., Bentley, K.H., & Barlow, D.H. (2015). Motivation facilitation in the unified protocol for transdiagnostic treatment of emotional disorder. *Counselling and Psychotherapy Research, 21*(3), 555–569.

Bowen, N.K., & Guo, S. (2011). *Structural equation modelling*. Oxford University Press.

Bradford-Hill, A. (1965). President's address. *Proceedings Royal Society of Medicine, 58*(5), 295–300.

Braun, V., & Clarke, V. (2021). *Thematic analysis: a practical guide*. Sage.

Bretag, T. (2016). *Handbook of academic integrity*. Springer.

Brinkmann, S. (2013). *Qualitative interviewing*. Oxford University Press.

Bruner, J. (1985). Narrative and paradigmatic modes of thought. *Teachers College Record, 86*(6), 97–115.

Bryman, A. (2006). Integrating quantitative and qualitative research: how is it done?. *Qualitative Research, 6*(1), 97–113.

Burgess, R., & Moorhead, J. (2011). *New principles of best practice in clinical audit*. Radcliffe.

Butcher, J.N. (2002). Clinical personality assessment: Practical approaches. Oxford University Press.

Butler, J. (2011). *Bodies that matter*. Routledge.

Butlin, H. (2016). *Searching for wisdom*. Thesis. University of Western Ontario.

Cahill, J., Barkham, M., & Stiles, W.B. (2010). Systematic review of practice-based research on psychological therapies in routine clinic settings. *British Journal of Clinical Psychology, 49*(4), 421–453.

Campbell, M., McKenzie, J.E., Sowden, A., et al. (2020). Synthesis without meta-analysis (SWiM) in systematic reviews. *British Medical Journal, 368,* 16890.

Carey, M.A., & Asbury, J.E. (2016). *Focus group research.* Routledge.

Carroll, K.M., & Nuro, K.F. (2002). One size cannot fit all: A stage model for psychotherapy manual development. *Clinical Psychology: Science and Practice, 9*(4), 396–406.

Carroll, M., & Shaw, E. (2013). *Ethical maturity in the helping professions.* Kingsley.

Carpenter, S. (2018). Ten steps in scale development and reporting. *Communication methods and measures, 12*(1), 25–44.

Carrozzino, D., Patierno, C., Guidi, J., et al. (2021). Clinimetric criteria for patient-reported outcome measures. *Psychotherapy and Psychosomatics, 90*(4), 222–232.

Carter, D., & Gradin, S. (2001). *Writing as Reflective Action.* Addison-Wesley.

Castonguay, L.G., & Beutler, L.E. (2005). *Principles of therapeutic change that work.* Oxford University Press.

Castonguay, L.G., & Hill, C.E. (2017). *How and why are some therapists better than others?* APA.

Chambless, D.L. (2002). Beware the dodo bird. *Clinical Psychology, 9*(1), 13–16.

Chambless, D.L., & Ollendick, T.H. (2001). Empirically supported psychological interventions. *Annual Review Psychology, 52,* 685–716.

Chan, A.W., Tetzlaff, J.M., Altman, D.G., et al. (2013). SPIRIT 2013 statement. *Annals of Internal Medicine, 158*(3), 200–207.

Chapman, S., & Schwartz, J.P. (2012). Rejecting the null. *Counselling and Values, 57*(1), 24–30.

Charmaz, K. (2015). *Constructing grounded theory.* Sage.

Clark, V.L.P., & Ivankova, N.V. (2015). *Mixed methods research.* Sage.

Clarke, V., & Braun, V. (2018). Using thematic analysis in counselling and psychotherapy research. *Counselling and Psychotherapy Research, 18*(2), 107–110.

Cleophas, T.J., & Zwinderman, A.H. (2018). *Modern Bayesian statistics in clinical research.* Springer.

Colaizzi, P.F. (1978). Psychological research as the phenomenologist views it. In R.S. Valle & M. King (Eds.), *Existential-phenomenological alternatives for psychology.* Oxford University Press.

Coley, S.M., Scheinberg, C.A., & Strekalova, Y.A.L. (2021). *Proposal writing.* Sage.

Collins, P.H., & Bilge, S. (2020). *Intersectionality.* Wiley.

Cooper, A.A., & Conklin, L.R. (2015). Dropout from individual psychotherapy for major depression. *Clinical Psychology Review, 40,* 57–65.

Cooper, M. (2013). *Essential research findings in counselling and psychotherapy.* Sage.

Cooper, M., McLeod, J., & Ogden, G.S. (2015). Client helpfulness interview studies. Unpublished manuscript retrieved 24 February 2023 from www.researchgate.net/profile/Mick_Cooper.

Cooper, M., Norcross, J.C., Raymond-Barker, B., & Hogan, T.P. (2019). Psychotherapy preferences of laypersons and mental health professionals. *Psychotherapy, 56*(2), 205.

Copp, D. (2005). *The Oxford handbook of ethical theory.* Oxford University Press.

Corbin, J., & Strauss, A. (2014). *Basics of qualitative research.* Sage.

Creswell, J.W. (2021). *A concise introduction to mixed methods research.* Sage.

Creswell, J.W., & Clark, V.L.P. (2017). *Designing and conducting mixed methods research.* Sage.

Creswell, J.W., & Tashakkori, A. (2007). *Developing publishable mixed methods manuscripts.* APA.

Creswell, J.W., Klassen, A.C., Clark, V.L.P., & Smith, K.C. (2011). Best practices for mixed methods research in the health sciences. *National Institutes of Health, 2013,* 541–545.

Cronbach, L.J. (1951). Coefficient alpha and the internal structure of tests. *Psychometrika, 16*(3), 297–334.

Crotty, M. (1996). *Phenomenology and nursing research.* Saunders.

Cuijpers, P. (2016). Are all psychotherapies equally effective in the treatment of adult depression? The lack of statistical power of comparative outcome studies. *BMJ Mental Health, 19*(2), 39–42.

Cuijpers, P., & Cristea, I.A. (2016). How to prove that your therapy is effective, even when it is not. *Epidemiology and Psychiatric Sciences, 25*(5), 428–435.

Cuijpers, P., Van Straten, A., Andersson, G., & Van Oppen, P. (2008). Psychotherapy for depression in adults. *Journal of Consulting and Clinical Psychology, 76*(6), 909–920.

Cuijpers, P., Donker, T., van Straten, A., Li, J., & Andersson, G. (2010). Is guided self-help as effective as face-to-face psychotherapy for depression and anxiety disorders? *Psychological Medicine*, *40*(12), 1943–1957.

Cuijpers, P., Driessen, E., Hollon, S.D., van Oppen, P., Barth, J., & Andersson, G. (2012). The efficacy of non-directive supportive therapy for adult depression. *Clinical Psychology Review*, *32*(4), 280–291.

Cuijpers, P., Hollon, S.D., van Straten, A., Bockting, C., Berking, M., & Andersson, G. (2013). Does cognitive behaviour therapy have an enduring effect that is superior to keeping patients on continuation pharmacotherapy? *British Medical Journal*, *3*(4), e002542.

Cuijpers, P., Weitz, E., Cristea, I.A., & Twisk, J. (2017). Pre-post effect sizes should be avoided in meta-analyses. *Epidemiology and Psychiatric Sciences*, *26*(4), 364–368.

Cuijpers, P., Reijnders, M., & Huibers, M.J. (2019). The role of common factors in psychotherapy outcomes. *Annual Review of Clinical Psychology*, *15*(1), 207–231.

Das, K.R., & Imon, A.H.M.R. (2016). A brief review of tests for normality. *American Journal of Theoretical and Applied Statistics*, *5*(1), 5–12.

De Beurs, E., Boehnke, J.R., & Fried, E.I. (2022). Common measures or common metrics? *Clinical Psychology & Psychotherapy*, *29*(5), 1755-1767.

Dechartres, A., Altman, D.G., Trinquart, L., Boutron, I., & Ravaud, P. (2014). Association between analytic strategy and estimates of treatment outcomes in meta-analyses. *JAMA*, *312*(6), 623–630.

Delaney, K.J. (2007). Methodological dilemmas and opportunities in interviewing organizational elites. *Sociology Compass*, *1*(1), 208–221.

Denzin, N.K. (1978). *The research act*. McGraw-Hill.

Denzin, N.K., & Lincoln, Y.S. (2021). *The Sage handbook of qualitative research*. Sage.

Devellis, R.F., & Thorpe, C.T. (2021). *Scale development*. Sage.

Dilthey, W. (2010). *Hermeneutics and the study of history*. Princeton University Press.

Dixon-Woods, M., Agarwal, S., Jones, D., Young, B., & Sutton, A. (2005). Synthesising qualitative and quantitative evidence. *Journal of Health Services Research & Policy*, *10*(1), 45–53.

Donohoe, G. (2022). How adverse childhood experiences shape our brains. *The Psychologist*, *37*(9), 19–25.

Dowling, M. (2007). From Husserl to van Manen. *International Journal of Nursing Studies*, *44*(1), 131–142.

Duffy, R.D., & Dik, B.J. (2013). Research on calling: What have we learned and where are we going? *Journal of Vocational Behavior*, *83*(3), 428-436.

Duffy, R.D., Torrey, C.L., Bott, E.M., Allan, B.A., & Schlosser, LZ. (2013). Time management, passion, and collaboration. *The Counseling Psychologist*, *41*(6), 881-917.

Duncan, B.L., Miller, S.D., & Sparks, J.A. (2011). *The heroic client*. Wiley.

Easton, K.L., McComish, J.F., & Greenberg, R. (2000). Avoiding common pitfalls in qualitative data collection and transcription. *Qualitative Health Research*, *10*(5), 703–707.

Ellingson, L.L. (2009). *Engaging crystallization in qualitative research*. Sage.

Elliott, R. (1986). Interpersonal Process Recall as a psychotherapy process research method. In L.S. Greenberg & W.M. Pinsof (Eds.), *The psychotherapeutic process*. Guilford.

Elliott, R. (1989). Comprehensive Process Analysis. In M.J. Packer & R.B. Addison (Eds.), *Entering the circle*. State University of New York Press.

Elliott, R. (1998). A guide to the empirically supported treatments controversy. *Psychotherapy Research*, *8*(2), 115–125.

Elliott, R. (2010). Psychotherapy change process research. *Psychotherapy research*, *20*(2), 123–135.

Elliott, R., & Rodgers, B. (2008). Client change interview schedule. Unpublished research instrument, University of Strathclyde.

Elliott, R., & Shapiro, D.A. (1988). Brief structured recall. *British Journal of Medical Psychology*, *61*(2), 141–153.

Elliott, R., Fischer, C.T., & Rennie, D.L. (1999). Evolving guidelines for publication of qualitative research studies in psychology and related fields. *British Journal of Clinical Psychology*, *38*(3), 215–229.

Emanuel, E.J., Grady, C.C., Crouch, R.A., Lie, R.K., Miller, F.G., & Wendler, D.D. (2008). *The Oxford textbook of clinical research ethics*. Oxford University Press.

Emmel, N. (2013). Sampling and choosing cases in qualitative research. Sage.

England, K.V. (1994). Getting personal: Reflexivity, positionality, and feminist research. *The Professional Geographer, 46*(1), 80–89.

Erford, B.T., Savin-Murphy, J.A., & Butler, C. (2010). Conducting a meta-analysis of counselling outcome research. *Counselling Outcome Research and Evaluation, 1*(1), 19–43.

Etherington, K. (2004). *Becoming a reflexive researcher*. Kingsley.

Eurelings-Bontekoe, E.H.M., & Snellen, W.M. (2010). *Dynamische persoonlijkheidsdiagnostiek*. Harcourt.

Eysenck, H.J. (1952). The effects of psychotherapy. *Journal of Consulting Psychology, 16*(5), 319.

Farber, B.A. (2003). Patient self-disclosure. *Journal of Clinical Psychology, 59*(5), 589–600.

Fern, E.F., & Fern, E.E. (2001). *Advanced focus group research*. Sage.

Fetterman, D.M. (2019). *Ethnography*. Sage.

Field, A. (2013). *Discovering statistics using IBM SPSS statistics*. Sage.

Finlay, L. (2006). The body's disclosure in phenomenological research. *Qualitative Research in Psychology, 3*(1), 19–30.

Finlay, L., & Gough, B. (Eds.) (2008). *Reflexivity: A practical guide*. Wiley.

Firth, N., Barkham, M., & Kellett, S. (2015). The clinical effectiveness of stepped care systems for depression in working age adults. *Journal of Affective Disorders, 170*, 119–130.

Fisher, J.E., & O'Donohue, W.T. (2006). *Practitioner's guide to evidence-based psychotherapy*. Springer.

Fisher, M. (2017). *Qualitative computing*. Routledge.

Fonseca-Pedrero, E. (2018). Network analysis in psychology. *Psychologist Papers, 39*(1), 1–12.

Fontana, A., & Frey, J. (1994). The art of science. In Y.L. Denzin (Ed.), *The handbook of qualitative research*. Sage.

Fonteyn, M.E., Kuipers, B., & Grobe, S.J. (1993). A description of think-aloud method and protocol analysis. *Qualitative Health Research, 3*(4), 430–441.

Fraser, K.D., & Al Sayah, F. (2011). Arts-based methods in health research. *Arts & Health, 3*(2), 110–145.

Friese, S. (2019). *Qualitative data analysis with ATLAS*. Sage.

Furukawa, T.A., Noma, H., Caldwell, D.M., et al. (2014). Waiting list may be a nocebo condition in psychotherapy trials. *Acta Psychiatrica Scandinavica, 130*(3), 181–192.

Gadamer, H.G. (2013). *Truth and method*. A&C Black.

Galletta, A. (2013). *Mastering the semi-structured interview and beyond*. NYU Press.

Garber, J., & Hollon, S.D. (1991). What can specificity designs say about causality in psychopathology research? *Psychological Bulletin, 110*(1), 129–140.

Gelso, C.J., Baumann, E.C., Chui, H.T., & Savela, A.E. (2013). The making of a scientist–psychotherapist. *Psychotherapy, 50*(2), 139–145.

Gergen, K.J., & Gergen, M.M. (1988). Narrative and the self as relationship. *Advances in Experimental Social Psychology, 21*(1), 17–56.

Gibbs, G. (1988). *Learning by doing*. FEU.

Giorgi, A.P. (2009). *The descriptive phenomenological method in psychology*. Duquesne University Press.

Giorgi, A.P., & Giorgi, B.M. (2003). The descriptive phenomenological psychological method. In P.M. Camic, J.E. Rhodes, & L. Yardley (Eds.), *Qualitative Research in Psychology*. APA.

Girden, E.R., & Kabacoff, R.I. (2010). *Evaluating research articles from start to finish*. Sage.

Glaser, B.G. (1978). *Theoretical sensitivity*. The Sociology Press.

Glaser, B.G., & Strauss, A.L. (2017). *The discovery of grounded theory*. Routledge.

Glesne, C. (2007). Research as solidarity. In N.K. Denzin & M.D. Giardina (Eds.), *Ethical futures in qualitative research*. Left Coast Press.

Gobo, G. (2008). *Doing ethnography*. Sage.

Goertz, G., & Mahoney, J. (2012). Concepts and measurement: Ontology and epistemology. *Social Science Information, 51*(2), 205–216.

Goldberg, S.B., Tucker, R.P., Greene, P.A., et al. (2018). Mindfulness-based interventions for psychiatric disorders. *Clinical Psychology Review, 59*, 52–60.

Goodheart, C.D., Kazdin, A.E., & Sternberg, R.J. (2006). *Evidence-based psychotherapy*. APA.

Gøtzsche, P. C. (2000). Why we need a broad perspective on meta-analysis. *BMJ, 321*(7261), 585–586.

Gough, D., Oliver, S., & Thomas, J. (2012). *An Introduction to systematic reviews*. Sage.

Goss, S., & Mearns, D. (1997). A call for a pluralist epistemological understanding in the assessment and evaluation of counselling. *British Journal of Guidance and Counselling, 25*(2), 189–198.

Grawe, K.(1997). Research-informed psychotherapy. *Psychotherapy research, 7*(1), 1–19.

Greenberg, L.S. (1986). Change process research. *Journal of Consulting and Clinical Psychology, 54*(1), 4.

Greenberg, L.S. (2007). A guide to conducting a task analysis of psychotherapeutic change. *Psychotherapy Research, 17*(1), 15–30.

Greenberg, L.S., & Pinsof, W.M. (1986). *The psychotherapeutic process: A research handbook.* Guilford.

Greetham, B. (2020). How to write your literature review. Bloomsbury

Gregory, R.J. (2014). *Psychological testing.* Pearson.

Groth-Marnat, G. (2003). Handbook of psychological assessment. Wiley.

Guest, G., MacQueen, K.M., & Namey, E.E. (2011). *Applied thematic analysis.* Sage.

Gyani, A., Shafran, R., Layard, R., & Clark, D.M. (2013). Enhancing recovery rates. *Behaviour Research and Therapy, 51*(9), 597–606.

Hak, T., Van der Veer, K., & Jansen, H. (2004). *The three-step test-interview.* SSRN: 636782.

Hamera, J.A. (2006). *The Sage handbook of performance studies.* Sage.

Hansen, N.B., Lambert, M.J., & Forman, E.M. (2002). The psychotherapy dose-response effect and its implications for treatment delivery services. *Clinical Psychology, 9*(3), 329.

Hanson, W.E., Creswell, J.W., Clark, V.L.P., Petska, K.S., & Creswell, J.D. (2005). Mixed methods research designs in counselling psychology. *Journal of Counselling Psychology, 52*(2), 224.

Harkin, B., Webb, T.L., Chang, B.P., et al. (2016). Does monitoring goal progress promote goal attainment? *Psychological Bulletin, 142*(2), 198.

Harkness, J., Pennell, B.E., & Schoua-Glusberg, A. (2004). Survey questionnaire translation and assessment. In L. Presser (Ed.), *Methods for testing and evaluating survey questionnaires.* Wiley.

Haynes, C.A., & Shelton, K. (2018). *Handbook of research on innovative techniques.* IGI.

Heidegger, M. (1927). *Sein und Zeit.* Niemeyer Verlag.

Henrich, J., Heine, S.J., & Norenzayan, A. (2010). Most people are not WEIRD. *Nature, 466*(7302), 29–39.

Herman, L., & Vervaeck, B. (2019). *Handbook of narrative analysis.* University of Nebraska Press.

Herr, K., & Anderson, G.L. (2014). *The action research dissertation.* Sage.

Hesse-Biber, S. (2015). Mixed methods research. *Qualitative Health Research, 25*(6), 775–788.

Higgins, J.P., Thomas, J., Chandler, J., Cumpston, M., Li, T., Page, M.J., & Welch, V.A. (2019). *Cochrane handbook for systematic reviews of interventions.* Wiley.

Hill, C.E., Knox, S., Thompson, B.J., Williams, E.N., Hess, S.A., & Ladany, N. (2005). Consensual qualitative research. *Journal of Counselling Psychology, 52*(2), 196.

Höfler, M. (2005). The Bradford-Hill considerations on causality. *Emerging Themes in Epidemiology, 2*(1), 1–9.

Hoyle, R.H. (2012). *Handbook of structural equation modelling.* Guilford Press.

Hsu, C.C., & Sandford, B.A. (2007). The Delphi-technique. *Practical Assessment, Research, and Evaluation, 12*(1), 10.

Hullinger, A.M., DiGirolamo, J.A., & Tkach, J.T. (2019). Reflective practice for coaches and clients. *Philosophy of Coaching, 4*(2), 5–34.

Hunt, B. (2011). Publishing qualitative research in counselling journals. *Journal of Counselling & Development, 89*(3), 296–300.

Husserl, E. (1999). *The essential Husserl.* Indiana University Press.

Hutchby, I., & Wooffitt, R. (2008). *Conversation analysis.* Polity.

Imenda, S. (2014). Is there a conceptual difference between theoretical and conceptual frameworks. *Journal of Social Sciences, 38*(2), 185–195.

Ioannidis, J.P., Evans, S.J., Gøtzsche, P.C., & CONSORT. (2004). Better reporting of harms in randomized trials. *Annals of Internal Medicine, 141*(10), 781–788.

Jabareen, Y. (2009). Building conceptual frameworks. *International Journal of Qualitative Methods, 8*(4), 25–40.

Jackson, K., & Bazeley, P. (2019). *Qualitative data analysis with NVivo.* Sage.

Jacobson, N.S., & Truax, P. (1991). Clinical significance. *Journal of Consulting and Clinical Psychology, 59*, 12–19.

Jasper, M.A. (2005). Using reflective writing within research. *Journal of Research in Nursing*, 10(3), 247–260.

Jesson, J., Matheson, L., & Lacey, F.M. (2011). *Doing your literature review*. Sage.

Jinha, A. (2010). Article 50 million. *Learned Publishing*, 23(3), 258–263.

Johnson, P., & Duberley, J. (2003). Reflexivity in management research. *Journal of Management Studies*, 40(5), 1279-1303.

Jones, S.H., Adams, T.E., & Ellis, C. (2016). *Handbook of autoethnography*. Routledge.

Jørgensen, M.W., & Phillips, L.J. (2002). *Discourse analysis as theory and method*. Sage.

Jovanović, G. (2011). Toward a social history of qualitative research. *History of the Human Sciences*, 24(2), 1–27.

Jung, T., & Wickrama, K.A. (2008). An introduction to latent class growth analysis and growth mixture modelling. *Social and Personality Psychology Compass*, 2(1), 302–317.

Jussim, L., Krosnick, J.A., & Stevens, S.T. (2022). *Research integrity*. Oxford University Press.

Kahn, J.H., & Schneider, W.J. (2013). It's the destination and it's the journey. *Journal of Clinical Psychology*, 69(6), 543–570.

Kaplan, R.M., & Saccuzzo, D.P. (2017). Psychological testing: Principles, applications, and issues. Cengage.

Kasket, E. (2012). The counselling psychologist researcher. *Counselling Psychology Review*, 27(2), 64–73.

Kasket, E., & Gil-Rodriguez, E. (2011). The identity crisis in trainee counselling psychology research. *Counselling Psychology Review*, 26(4), 20–30.

Kazdin, A.E. (2007). Mediators and mechanisms of change in psychotherapy research. *Annual Review of Clinical Psychology*, 3, 1–27.

Kazdin, A.E. (2009). Understanding how and why psychotherapy leads to change. *Psychotherapy Research*, 19(4–5), 418–428.

Kazdin, A.E. (2011). Evidence-based treatment research. *American Psychologist*, 66(8), 685.

Kazdin, A.E. (2015). Evidence-based psychotherapies. *South African Journal of Psychology*, 45(1), 3–21.

Kazdin, A.E. (2021). *Research design in clinical psychology*. Cambridge University Press.

Keeney, S., McKenna, H., & Hasson, F. (2011). *The Delphi-technique*. Wiley.

Keightley, E., Pickering, M., & Allett, N. (2012). The self-interview. *International Journal of Social Research Methodology*, 15(6), 507–521.

Kendall, G., & Wickham, G. (2004). The Foucauldian framework. *Qualitative Research Practice*, 141–150.

Kenny, D.A., & Hoyt, W.T. (2014). Multiple levels of analysis in psychotherapy research. In W.E. Lutz & S.E. Knox (Eds.), *Quantitative and qualitative methods in psychotherapy research*. Routledge.

Killen, M., & Smetana, J.G. (2013). *Handbook of moral development*. Psychology Press.

Knapp, M., McDaid, D., & Mossialos, E. (2006). *Mental health policy and practice across Europe*. McGraw-Hill.

Knapp, S.J., Gottlieb, M.C., Handelsman, M.M., & VandeCreek, L.D. (2012). *APA handbook of ethics in psychology*. APA.

Kopta, S.M., Howard, K.I., Lowry, J.L., & Beutler, L.E. (1994). Patterns of symptomatic recovery in psychotherapy. *Journal of Consulting and Clinical Psychology*, 62(5), 1009.

Kraemer, H.C., & Kupfer, D.J. (2006). Size of treatment effects and their importance to clinical research and practice. *Biological Psychiatry*, 59(11), 990–996

Kraemer, H.C., Stice, E., Kazdin, A., Offord, D., & Kupfer, D. (2001). How do risk factors work together? *American Journal of Psychiatry*, 158(6), 848–856.

Kraemer, H.C., Frank, E., & Kupfer, D.J. (2011). How to assess the clinical impact of treatments on patients, rather than the statistical impact of treatments on measures. *International Journal of Methods in Psychiatric Research*, 20(2), 63–72.

Kuhn, T.S. (1970). *The structure of scientific revolutions*. University of Chicago Press.

Kühne, F., Maas, J., Wiesenthal, S., & Weck, F. (2019). Empirical research in clinical supervision. *BMC Psychology*, 7(1), 1–11.

Kumar, R. (2018). *Research methodology*. Sage.

Labov, W. & Waletzky, J. (1967). Narrative analysis. In J. Helm (ed.), *Essays on the Verbal and Visual Arts*. University of Washington Press.

Ladmanová, M., Řiháček, T., & Timulak, L. (2022). Client-identified impacts of helpful and hindering events in psychotherapy. *Psychotherapy Research, 32*(6), 723–735.

Lambert, M. (2007). What we have learned from a decade of research aimed at improving psychotherapy outcome in routine care. *Psychotherapy research, 17*(1), 1–14.

Lambert, M.J. (2011). Psychotherapy research and its achievements. In J.C. Norcross, G.R. VandenBos, & D.K. Freedheim (Eds.), *History of psychotherapy*. APA.

Lambert, M.J., & Hill, C.E. (1994). Assessing psychotherapy outcomes and processes. In A.E. Bergin & S.L. Garfield (Eds.), *Handbook of psychotherapy and behaviour change*. Wiley.

Landrum, B., & Garza, G. (2015). Mending fences. *Qualitative Psychology, 2*(2), 199.

Lane, D.A., & Corrie, S. (2007). *The modern scientist-practitioner*. Routledge.

Langridge, D. (2007). *Phenomenological psychology: Theory, research and method*. Pearson.

Langridge, D., & Hagger-Johnson, G. (2009). Introduction to research methods and data analysis in psychology. Pearson.

Lauer, G. (1999). Concepts of quality of life in mental health care. In S. Priebe, J.P.J. Oliver & W. Kaiser (Eds.), *Quality of Life and Mental Health Care*. Wrightson.

Leavy, P. (2020). *Method meets art*. Guilford.

Lefebvre, C., Glanville, J., Briscoe, S., & Cochrane (2019). Searching for and selecting studies. In J.P. Higgins, J. Thomas, J. Chandler, M. Cumpston, T. Li, M.J. Page, & V.A. Welch (Eds.), *Cochrane handbook for systematic reviews of interventions*. Wiley.

Lempert, L.B. (2007). Asking questions of the data. In A. Bryant & K. Charmaz (Eds.), *Sage handbook of grounded theory*. Sage.

Leon, A.C., Davis, L.L., & Kraemer, H.C. (2011). The role and interpretation of pilot studies in clinical research. *Journal of Psychiatric Research, 45*(5), 626–629.

Lerum, K. (2001). Subjects of desire. *Qualitative Inquiry, 7*(4), 466–483.

Levitt, H.M., Motulsky, S.L., Wertz, F.J., Morrow, S.L., & Ponterotto, J.G. (2017). Recommendations for designing and reviewing qualitative research in psychology. *Qualitative Psychology, 4*(1), 2.

Liamputtong, P. (2011). *Focus group methodology*. Sage.

Lilienfeld, S.O. (2007). Psychological treatments that cause harm. *Perspectives on Psychological Science, 2*(1), 53–70.

Lilienfeld, S.O., Ritschel, L.A., Lynn, S.J., Cautin, R.L., & Latzman, R.D. (2013). Why many clinical psychologists are resistant to evidence-based practice. *Clinical Psychology Review, 33*(7), 883–900.

Lincoln, Y.S., & Guba, E.G. (1985). *Naturalistic inquiry*. Sage.

Linden, M., & Schermuly-Haupt, M.L. (2014). Definition, assessment and rate of psychotherapy side effects. *World Psychiatry, 13*(3), 306.

Linstone, H.A. & Turoff, M.. (2002). *The Delphi method: Techniques and applications*. Addison-Wesley.

Little, T.D. (Ed.) (2013). *The Oxford handbook of quantitative methods*. Oxford University Press.

Locke, L.F., Spirduso, W.W., & Silverman, S.J. (2013). *Proposals that work*. Sage.

Lopez, S.J., & Snyder, C.R. (2003). Positive psychological assessment: A handbook of models and measures. APA.

Luborsky, L., Diguer, L., Seligman, D.A., et al. (1999). The researcher's own therapy allegiances. *Clinical Psychology, 6*(1), 95–106.

Luborsky, L., Rosenthal, R., Diguer, L., Andrusyna, T.P., Berman, J.S., Levitt, J.T., Seligman, D.A., & Krause, E.D. (2002). The dodo bird verdict is alive and well – mostly. *Clinical Psychology, 9*(1), 2–12.

Lynn, M.R. (1986). Determination and quantification of content validity. *Nursing Research, 35*, 382–385.

Machi, L.A., & McEvoy, B.T. (2016). *The literature review*. Sage.

MacLean, L.M., Meyer, M., & Estable, A. (2004). Improving accuracy of transcripts in qualitative research. *Qualitative Health Research, 14*(1), 113–123.

Madill, A., Jordan, A., & Shirley, C. (2000). Objectivity and reliability in qualitative analysis. *British Journal of Psychology, 91*(1), 1–20.

Madison, D.S. (2011). *Critical ethnography*. Sage.

Malterud, K., Siersma, V.D., & Guassora, A.D. (2016). Sample size in qualitative interview studies. *Qualitative Health Research, 26*(13), 1753–1760.

Margison, F.R., Barkham, M., Evans, C., McGrath, G., Clark, J.M., Audin, K., & Connell, J. (2000). Measurement and psychotherapy. *The British Journal of Psychiatry, 177*(2), 123–130.

Marshall, B., Cardon, P., Poddar, A., & Fontenot, R. (2013). Does sample size matter in qualitative research? *Journal of Computer Information Systems, 54*(1), 11–22.

Marshall, C., Gerstl-Pepin, C., & Johnson, M. (2020). *Educational Politics for Social Justice*. Teachers College Press.

Marshall, C., & Rossman, G.B. (2014). *Designing qualitative research*. Sage.

Mason, M. (2010). Sample size and saturation in PhD studies using qualitative interviews. *Forum: Qualitative Social Research, 11*(3), 1–15.

Maxwell, J. (2012). *Qualitative research design*. Sage.

McKay, M.T., Cannon, M., Chambers, D., et al. (2021). Childhood trauma and adult mental disorder. *Acta Psychiatrica Scandinavica, 143*(3), 189–205.

McLeod, J. (1997). *Narrative and Psychotherapy*. Sage.

McLeod, J. (2010). *Case study research in counselling and psychotherapy*. Sage.

McLeod, J. (2011). *Qualitative research in counselling and psychotherapy*. Sage.

McLeod, J. (2022). *Doing research in counselling and psychotherapy*. Sage.

McNiff, J. (2016). *You and your action research project*. Routledge.

Mearns, D., & Cooper, M. (2017). *Working at relational depth in counselling and psychotherapy*. Sage.

Mellor-Clark, J., Cross, S., Macdonald, J., & Skjulsvik, T. (2016). Leading horses to water. *Administration and Policy in Mental Health and Mental Health Services Research, 43*(3), 279–285.

Merleau-Ponty, M. (1964). *Sense and non-sense*. Northwestern University Press.

Merleau-Ponty, M. (1996). *Phenomenology of perception*. Motilal Banarsidass.

Meyer, G.J., Finn, S.E., Eyde, L.D., et al. (2001). Psychological testing and psychological assessment. *American Psychologist, 56*(2), 128.

Midgley, N., Hayes, J., & Cooper, M. (2017). *Essential research findings in child and adolescent counselling and psychotherapy*. Sage.

Miles, M.B., Huberman, A.M. & saldana, J. (2019). *Qualitative data analysis*. Sage.

Miller, N.E., Luborsky, L.E., Barber, J.P., & Docherty, J.P. (1993). *Psychodynamic treatment research*. Basic Books.

Miller, S.J., & Binder, J.L. (2002). The effects of manual-based training on treatment fidelity and outcome. *Psychotherapy, 39*(2), 184.

Milosevic, I., & McCabe, R.E. (Eds.). (2015). Phobias: The psychology of irrational fear: The psychology of irrational fear. Abc-Clio.

Minami, T., Wampold, B.E., Serlin, R.C., Kircher, J.C., & Brown, G.S.J. (2007). Benchmarks for psychotherapy efficacy in adult major depression. *Journal of Consulting and Clinical Psychology, 75*(2), 232.

Minami, T., Brown, G.S., McCulloch, J., & Bolstrom, B.J. (2012). Benchmarking therapists. *Quality & Quantity, 46*(6), 1699–1708.

Moher, D., Liberati, A., Tetzlaff, J., Altman, D.G., & PRISMA. (2009). Preferred reporting items for systematic reviews and meta-analyses. *PLoS Medicine, 6*(7), e1000097.

Mohlman, J., Deckersbach, T., & Weissman, A. (2015). *From symptom to synapse*. Routledge.

Moran, D. (2002). *Introduction to phenomenology*. Routledge.

Morrow, S.L. (2005). Quality and trustworthiness in qualitative research in counselling psychology. *Journal of Counselling Psychology, 52*(2), 250.

Morrow-Bradley, C., & Elliott, R. (1986). Utilization of psychotherapy research by practicing psychotherapists. *American Psychologist, 41*(2), 188.

Morse, J.M. (2016). *Mixed method design*. Routledge.

Morse, J.M., Barrett, M., Mayan, M., Olson, K., & Spiers, J. (2002). Verification strategies for establishing reliability and validity in qualitative research. *International Journal of Qualitative Methods, 1*(2), 13-22.

Moser, P.K., Mulder, D.J., & Trout, J.D. (1998). *The theory of knowledge*. Oxford University Press.

Moustakas, C. (1990). *Heuristic research*. Sage.

Moyn, S. (2018). *Not enough*. Harvard University Press.

Mulrow, C.D. (1994). Systematic reviews. *British Medical Journal, 309*(6954), 597–599.

Munder, T. (2013). Researcher allegiance in psychotherapy outcome research. *Clinical Psychology Review, 33*(4), 501–511.

Murphy, D., Irfan, N., Barnett, H., Castledine, E., & Enescu, L. (2018). A systematic review and meta-synthesis of qualitative research into mandatory personal psychotherapy during training. *Counselling Psychotherapy Research, 18*(2), 199–214.

Naji, B., & Ekhtiari, H. (2016). New generation of psychotherapies inspired by cognitive neuroscience development. *Basic and Clinical Neuroscience, 7*(3), 179.

Nathan, P.E., & Gorman, J.M. (2015). *A guide to treatments that work*. Oxford University Press.

Nathan, P.E., Stuart, S.P., & Dolan, S.L. (2000). Research on psychotherapy efficacy and effectiveness. *Psychological Bulletin, 126*(6), 964.

Nicol, A.A., & Pexman, P.M. (2003). *Displaying your findings*. APA.

Noblit, G.W., & Hare, R.D. (1988). *Meta-ethnography*. Sage.

Norcross, J.C., & Karpiak, C.P. (2017). Our best selves. *The Counselling Psychologist, 45*(1), 66–75.

Norcross, J.C., & Lambert, M.J. (Eds.) (2019). *Psychotherapy relationships that work*. Oxford University Press.

Norcross, J.C., Beutler, L.E., & Levant, R.F. (2006). *Evidence-based practices in mental health*. APA.

O'Donohue, W., Buchanan, J.A., & Fisher, J.E. (2000). Characteristics of empirically supported treatments. *Journal of Psychotherapy Practice and Research, 9*(2), 69.

O'Reilly, M., & Dogra, N. (2016). *Interviewing children and young people for research*. Sage.

Orlinsky, D.E. (2022). *How Psychotherapists Live*. Routledge.

Orlinsky, D.E. (2009). The 'Generic Model of Psychotherapy' after 25 years. *Journal of Psychotherapy Integration, 19*(4), 319.

Orlinsky, D.E., & Rønnestad, M.H. (2005). *How psychotherapists develop*. APA.

Orlinsky, D.E., Grawe, K., & Parks, B.K. (1994). Process and outcome in psychotherapy. In A.E. Bergin & S.L. Garfield (Eds.), *Handbook of psychotherapy and behaviour change*. Wiley & Sons.

Orlinsky, D.E., & Howard, K.I. (1986). The psychological interior of psychotherapy. In L.S. Greenberg & W.M. Pinsof (Eds.), *The psychotherapeutic process*: A research handbook (pp. 477–501). Guilford.

Parent, M.C. (2013). Handling item-level missing data. *The Counselling Psychologist, 41*(4), 568–600.

Parker, I. (2014). *Discourse dynamics*. Routledge.

Paterson, B.L. (2011). 'It looks great but how do I know if it fits?' In K. Hannes & C. Lockwood (Eds.), *Synthesizing qualitative research*. Wiley & Sons.

Paterson, B.L., Thorne, S.E., Canam, C., & Jillings, C. (2001). *Meta-study of qualitative health research*. Sage.

Peirce, C.S. (1965). *Pragmatism and pragmaticism*. Belknap.

Pek, J., Wong, O., & Wong, A.C. (2018). How to address non-normality. *Frontiers in Psychology, 9*, 2104.

Pennington, B.F. (2002). *The development of psychopathology*. Guilford Press.

Pequegnat, W., Stover, E., & Boyce, C.A. (2011). *How to write a successful research grant application*. Routledge.

Pernecky, T. (2016). *Epistemology and metaphysics for qualitative research*. Sage.

Pilgrim, D. (2019). *Critical realism for psychologists*. Routledge.

Polkinghorne, D.E. (1989). Phenomenological research methods. In R.S. Valle & S. Halling (Eds.) *Existential-phenomenological perspectives in psychology*. Springer.

Pontcrotto, J.G. (2005). Qualitative research in counseling psychology. *Journal of Counseling Psychology, 52*(2), 126.

Ponterotto, J.G., & Grieger, I. (2007). Effectively communicating qualitative research. *The Counselling Psychologist, 35*(3), 404–430.

Pope, K.S., & Vasquez, M.J. (2016). *Ethics in psychotherapy and counselling*. Wiley & Sons.

Popper, K. (2005). *The logic of scientific discovery*. Routledge.

Potter, J. (2013). Discursive psychology and discourse analysis. In J.P. Gee & M. Handford (Eds.), *Routledge handbook of discourse analysis*. Routledge.

Prell, C. (2012). *Social network analysis*. Sage.

Prochaska, J.O., & Norcross, J.C. (2001). Stages of change. *Psychotherapy, 38*(4), 443.

Prochaska, J.O., & Norcross, J.C. (2018). *Systems of psychotherapy*. Oxford University Press.

Purtle, J., Nelson, K.L., Bruns, E.J., & Hoagwood, K.E. (2020). Dissemination strategies to accelerate the policy impact of children's mental health services research. *Psychiatric Services, 71*(11), 1170–1178.

Randolph, J. (2009). A guide to writing the dissertation literature review. *Practical Assessment, Research, and Evaluation, 14*(1), 13.

Raskin, J.D. (2002). Constructivism in psychology. *American Communication Journal, 5*(3), 1–25.

Ravitch, S.M., & Riggan, M. (2016). *Reason & rigor.* Sage.

Reason, P., & Bradbury, H. (Eds.) (2001). *Handbook of action research.* Sage.

Reeves, A. (2015). *Working with risk in counselling and psychotherapy.* Sage.

Reicher, S. (2000). Against methodolatry. *British Journal of Clinical Psychology, 39,* 1.

Reif-Lehrer, L. (2005). *Grant application writer's handbook.* Jones & Bartlett.

Rennie, D.L. (2007). Methodical hermeneutics and humanistic psychology. *Humanistic Psychologist, 35*(1), 1–14.

Rhodes, R.H., Hill, C.E., Thompson, B.J., & Elliott, R. (1994). Client retrospective recall of resolved and unresolved misunderstanding events. *Journal of Counselling Psychology, 41*(4), 473.

Ricoeur, P. (1986). Life. In M.C. Doeser & J.N. Kraay (Eds.), *Facts and values.* Springer.

Riding, N., & Lepper, G. (2005). *Researching the psychotherapy process.* Bloomsbury.

Riessman, C.K. (2008). *Narrative methods for the human sciences.* Sage.

Rivera, J. (2006). Conceptual encounter. In C.T. Fisher (Ed.), *Qualitative research methods for psychologists.* Academic Press.

Roberts, R. (2018). *Capitalism on campus.* Hunt.

Robinson, L., Delgadillo, J., & Kellett, S. (2020). The dose-response effect in routinely delivered psychological therapies. *Psychotherapy Research, 30*(1), 79–96.

Romanyshyn, R.D. (2020). *The wounded researcher.* Routledge.

Ronk, F.R., Hooke, G.R. & Page, A.C. (2012). How consistent are clinical significance classifications when calculation methods and outcome measures differ? *Clinical Psychology, 19,* 167–179.

Roos, J., & Werbart, A. (2013). Therapist and relationship factors influencing dropout from individual psychotherapy. *Psychotherapy Research, 23*(4), 394–418.

Rose, G. (2016). *Visual methodologies.* Sage.

Rossman, G.B., & Wilson, B.L. (1985). Numbers and words. *Evaluation Review, 9*(5), 627–643.

Rossi, P.H., Lipsey, M.W., & Freeman, H.E. (2004). *Assessing program impact.* Sage.

Roth, A. (2015). Are competence frameworks fit for practice? *Psychotherapy Research, 25*(4), 460–472.

Roth, A., & Fonagy, P. (2006). *What works for whom?* Guildford.

Roulston, K. (2010). *Reflective interviewing.* Sage.

Rounsaville B.J., Carroll K.M., Onken L.S.. (2008). A stage model of behavioral therapies research: Getting started and moving on from stage I. *Clinical Psychology: Science and Practice.* 8(2), 133–142.

Saaty, T.L., & Ozdemir, M.S. (2003). Why the magic number seven plus or minus two. *Mathematical and computer modelling, 38*(3-4), 233–244.

Safran, J.D., Abreu, I., Ogilvie, J., & DeMaria, A. (2011). Does psychotherapy research influence the clinical practice of researcher–clinicians? *Clinical Psychology, 18*(4), 357.

Salmons, J. (2009). *Online interviews in real time.* Sage.

Sartre, J.P. (2021). *Existentialism is a humanism.* Yale University Press.

Saxon, D., Firth, N., & Barkham, M. (2017). The relationship between therapist effects and therapy delivery factors. *Administration and Policy in Mental Health and Mental Health Services Research, 44*(5), 705–715.

Scheffer, J. (2002). Dealing with missing data. *Res. Lett. Inf. Math. Sci, 3*(1), 153-160.

Schiefele, A.K., Lutz, W., Barkham, M., et al. (2017). Reliability of therapist effects in practice-based psychotherapy research. *Administration and Policy in Mental Health and Mental Health Services Research, 44*(5), 598–613.

Schram, S. (2006). *Making political science matter.* NYU Press.

Schumacker, R.E., & Lomax, R.G. (2004). *A beginner's guide to structural equation modelling.* Lawrence Erlbaum.

Schwarzer, R., & Luszczynska, A. (2015). Health action process approach. In M. Conner & P. Norman (Eds.), *Predicting health behaviours.* Open University Press.

Seligman, M.E. (1995). The effectiveness of psychotherapy: The Consumer Reports study. *American psychologist*, 50(12), 965.

Sexton, T.L., Robbins, M.S., Hollimon, A.S., Mease, A.L., & Mayorga, C.C. (2004). Efficacy, effectiveness, and change mechanisms in couple and family therapy. In T.L. Sexton (Ed.), *Handbook of family therapy*. Routledge.

Shadish, W.R., Cook, T.D., & Leviton, L.C. (1991). *Foundations of program evaluation*. Sage.

Shalom, J.G., & Aderka, I.M. (2020). A meta-analysis of sudden gains in psychotherapy. *Clinical Psychology Review*, 76, 101827.

Shenton, A.K. (2004). Strategies for ensuring trustworthiness in qualitative research projects. *Education for Information*, 22(2), 63–75.

Shinebourne, P. (2011). The theoretical underpinnings of Interpretative Phenomenological Analysis. *Existential Analysis*, 22(1), 25–43.

Siddique, S. (2011). Being in-between: The relevance of ethnography and auto-ethnography for psychotherapy research. *Counselling and Psychotherapy Research*, 11(4), 310-316.

Sieber, J.E. (Ed.) (2012). *The ethics of social research*. Springer.

Silverman, D. (2021). *Doing qualitative research*. Sage.

Silvia, P.J. (2015). *Write it up*. APA.

Singer, P. (2011). *Practical ethics*. Cambridge University Press.

Smith, J.A. (2015). *Qualitative psychology*. Sage.

Smith, J.A., & Fieldsend, M. (2021). *Interpretative Phenomenological Analysis*. APA.

Smith, M.L., & Glass, G.V. (1977). Meta-analysis of psychotherapy outcome studies. *American Psychologist*, 32, 752–760.

Smyth, R. (2004). Exploring the usefulness of a conceptual framework as a research tool. *Issues in Educational Research*, 14(2), 167–180.

Snow, R.E. (1991). Aptitude-treatment interaction as a framework for research on individual differences in psychotherapy. *Journal of Consulting and Clinical Psychology*, 59(2), 205–216.

Sousa, F.J. (2010). Metatheories in research. In A.G. Woodside (Ed.), *Organizational culture*. Emerald.

Speer, D.C. (1992). Clinically significant change: Jacobson and Truax revisited. *Journal of Consulting and Clinical Psychology*, 60(3), 402.

Speer, D.C., & Greenbaum, P.E. (1995). Five methods for computing significant individual client change and improvement rates. *Journal of Consulting and Clinical Psychology*, 63(6), 1044–1048.

Spielmans, G.I., Berman, M.I., & Usitalo, A.N. (2011). Psychotherapy versus second-generation antidepressants in the treatment of depression. *Journal of Nervous and Mental Disease*, 199(3), 142–149.

Spinelli, E. (2005). *The interpreted world*. Sage.

Spradley, J.P. (2016). *The ethnographic interview*. Waveland.

Sprangers, M.A., & Schwartz, C.E. (1999). Integrating response shift into health-related quality of life research. *Social Science & Medicine*, 48(11), 1507–1515.

Sprangers, M.A., Sawatzky, R., Vanier, A., et al. (2023). Implications of the syntheses on definition, theory, and methods conducted by the Response Shift–in Sync Working Group. *Quality of Life Research*, 1(1), 1–14.

Stanghellini, G., Broome, M., Raballo, A., Fernandez, A.V., Fusar-Poli, P., & Rosfort, R. (2019). *The Oxford handbook of phenomenological psychopathology*. Oxford University Press.

Stanley, L., & Wise, S. (2002). *Breaking out again: Feminist ontology and epistemology*. Routledge.

Steinert, C., Hofmann, M., Kruse, J., & Leichsenring, F. (2014). Relapse rates after psychotherapy for depression–stable long-term effects? A meta-analysis. *Journal of Affective Disorders*, 168, 107-118.

Steinman, R.B. (2009). Projective techniques in consumer research. *International Bulletin of Business Administration*, 5(1), 37–45.

Stevens, A., & Gabbay, J. (1991). Needs assessment. *Health Trends*, 23(1), 20–23.

Stevens, J.P. (2012). *Applied multivariate statistics for the social sciences*. Routledge.

Stevens, S.E., Hynan, M.T., & Allen, M. (2000). A meta-analysis of common factor and specific treatment effects. *Clinical Psychology*, 7(3), 273–290.

Stiles, W.B. (2001). Assimilation of problematic experiences. *Psychotherapy*, 38(4), 462.

Stiles, W.B. (2007). Theory-building case studies of counselling and psychotherapy. *Counselling and Psychotherapy Research*, 7(2), 122–127.

Stivers, T., & Sidnell, J. (2012). *The handbook of conversation analysis*. Wiley & Sons.

Strupp, H.H., & Howard, K.I. (1992). A brief history of psychotherapy research. In D.K. Freedheim, H.J. Freudenberger, J.W. Kessler, S.B. Messer, D.R. Peterson, H.H. Strupp, & P.L. Wachtel (Eds.), *History of psychotherapy*. APA.

Sultan, N. (2018). *Heuristic inquiry*. Sage.

Swales, J.M., & Feak, C.B. (2019). *Academic writing for graduate students*. University of Michigan Press.

Swift, J.K., Callahan, J.L., Cooper, M., & Parkin, S.R. (2018). The impact of accommodating client preference in psychotherapy. *Journal of Clinical Psychology, 74*(11), 1924–1937.

Swift, J.K., & Greenberg, R.P. (2012). Premature discontinuation in adult psychotherapy: a meta-analysis. *Journal of Consulting and Clinical Psychology, 80*(4), 547.

Tao, K.W., Owen, J., Pace, B.T., & Imel, Z.E. (2015). A meta-analysis of multicultural competencies and psychotherapy process and outcome. *Journal of Counselling Psychology, 62*(3), 337.

Tashakkori, A., & Teddlie, C. (2021). *Sage handbook of mixed methods in social & behavioural research*. Sage.

Teddlie, C., & Tashakkori, A. (2006). A general typology of research designs featuring mixed methods. *Research in Schools, 13*(1), 12–28.

Timulak, L. (2008). *Research in psychotherapy and counselling*. Sage.

Timulak, L. (2009). Meta-analysis of qualitative studies. *Psychotherapy Research, 19*(4–5), 591–600.

Timulak, L. (2010). Significant events in psychotherapy. *Psychology and Psychotherapy, 83*(4), 421–447.

Tingey, R., Lambert, M., Burlingame, G., & Hansen, N. (1996). Assessing clinical significance. *Psychotherapy Research, 6*(2), 109–123.

Toukmanian, S.G., & Rennie, D.L. (1992). *Psychotherapy process research*. Sage.

Truijens, F. (2022, 22-24 September). *"In hindsight, I was more depressed than I thought". Response shifts in psychotherapy research*. [Conference workshop]. Society of Psychotherapy Research, Rome, Italy.

Tryon, G.S. (2002). *Counselling based on process research*. Allyn & Bacon.

Tschacher, W., & Ramseyer, F. (2009). Modelling psychotherapy process by time-series panel analysis. *Psychotherapy Research, 19*(4–5), 469–481.

UCL Comeptence Frameworks. (2023). *UCL competence frameworks for the delivery of effective psychological interventions*. https://www.ucl.ac.uk/pals/research/clinical-educational-and-health-psychology/research-groups/competence-frameworks

Van der Linden, W.J. (2017). *Handbook of item response theory*. CRC.

Van Deurzen, E. (2014). Structural existential analysis. *Counselling Psychology Review, 29*(2), 70–83.

van Manen, M. (2016). *Phenomenology of practice*. Routledge.

van Rijn, B. (2014). *Assessment and case formulation in counselling and psychotherapy*. Sage.

Vanier, A., Oort, F.J., McClimans, L., et al. (2021). Response shift in patient-reported outcomes. *Quality of Life Research, 30*(12), 3309–3322.

Visser, G. (1998). *De Druk van de Believing*. SUN.

Vos, J. (2014). *The conceptual components model: How to build the conceptual model of your research or thesis*. British Psychology Society Research Conference, May, London.

Vos, J. (2017). *Meaning in life: An evidence-based handbook for practitioners*. Bloomsbury.

Vos, J. (2018). Death in existential psychotherapies. In R.E. Menzies, R.G. Menzies & L. Iverach. *Curing the dread of death*. Australian Academic Press Group.

Vos, J. (2019). Phenomenological-existential therapies: A review of its empirical evidence. In E. Van Deurzen (Ed.), *World Handbook of Existential Therapies*. Wiley.

Vos, J. (2020). *The economics of meaning in life*. University Professors Press.

Vos, J. (2021a). Systematic pragmatic phenomenological analysis. *Counselling and Psychotherapy Research, 21*(1), 77–97.

Vos, J. (2021b). The existential competences framework. *International Journal of Psychotherapy, 25*(1), 9–58

Vos, J. (2021). The Psychology of Covid-19. Sage.

Vos, J. (2022a). The Meaning Sextet: A Systematic Literature Review and Further Validation of a Universal Typology of Meaning in Life. *Journal of Constructivist Psychology*. [Epub ahead of print].

Vos, J. (2022b, 30 April-1 May). How to Create a Meaningful Society for All: Breaking the Cycles of Structural Injustice. [Keynote lecture]. *Advancing humanistic, existential & transpersonal psychology and scholarship*. Online.

Vos, J. (2023). Systematic Meaning in Life Psychotherapy: From systematic literature reviews to a systematic treatment manual. [Prepublication on Psyarxiv.com].

Vos, J., & Van Rijn, B. (2021). The evidence-based conceptual model of transactional analysis. *Transactional Analysis Journal*, 51(2), 160–201.

Vos, J. & Van Rijn, B. (2023). Brief Transactional Analysis Psychotherapy for Depression: The systematic development of a treatment manual. *Psychotherapy Integration*. [Epub ahead of print].

Vos, J., & Vitali, D. (2018). The effects of psychological meaning-centred therapies on quality of life and psychological stress: A meta-analysis. *Palliative & Supportive Care*, 16(5), 608–632.

Vos, J., Roberts, R., & Davis, J. (2019). *Mental health in crisis*. Sage.

Vos, J., Van Deurzen, E., & Tantam, D. (2020). The forgotten Brexistential crisis. *Psychologist*, 33(10), 10.

Vos, J., Chryssafidou, E., van Rijn, B., & Stiles, W.B. (2022). Outcomes of beginning trainee therapists in an outpatient community clinic. *Counselling and Psychotherapy Research*, 22(2), 471–479.

Vossler, A., & Moller, N. (2014). *The counselling and psychotherapy research handbook*. Sage.

Walsh, D., & Downe, S. (2005). Meta-synthesis method for qualitative research. *Journal of Advanced Nursing*, 50(2), 204–211.

Wampold, B.E., & Bhati, K.S. (2004). Attending to the omissions. *Professional Psychology*, 35(6), 563.

Wampold, B.E., & Imel, Z.E. (2015). *The great psychotherapy debate*. Routledge.

Wampold, B.E., Minami, T., Tierney, S.C., Baskin, T.W., & Bhati, K.S. (2005). The placebo is powerful: estimating placebo effects in medicine and psychotherapy from randomized clinical trials. Journal of clinical psychology, 61(7), 835-854.

Wampold, B.E., Mondin, G.W., Moody, M., Stich, F., Benson, K., & Ahn, H.N. (1997). A meta-analysis of outcome studies comparing bona fide psychotherapies. *Psychological Bulletin*, 122(3), 203.

Wampold, B.E., Lichtenberg, J.W., & Waehler, C.A. (2002). Principles of empirically supported interventions in counselling psychology. *The Counselling Psychologist*, 30(2), 197–217.

Wampold, B.E., Minami, T., Baskin, T.W., & Tierney, S.C. (2002). A meta-(re)analysis of the effects of cognitive therapy versus 'other therapies' for depression. *Journal of Affective Disorders, 68* (2–3), 159–165.

Ward, A.C. (2009). The role of causal criteria in causal inferences. *Epidemiologic Perspectives & Innovations*, 6(1), 1–22.

Watson, J.C., & Rennie, D.L. (1994). Qualitative analysis of clients' subjective experience of significant moments during the exploration of problematic reactions. *Journal of Counselling Psychology*, 41(4), 500.

Watson, J.C., & Wiseman, H. (2021). *The responsive psychotherapist*. APA.

Weisz, J.R., & Kazdin, A.E. (2010). *Evidence-based psychotherapies for children and adolescents*. Guilford.

Wempen, F. (2010). *PowerPoint bible*. Wiley.

Wertz, F.J. (1984). Procedures in phenomenological research and the question of validity. *Studies in the Social Sciences*, 23, 29–48.

Westen, D., & Morrison, K. (2001). A multidimensional meta-analysis of treatments. *Journal of Consulting and Clinical Psychology*, 69(6), 875–895.

Wicks, D. (2017). *The coding manual for qualitative researchers*. Sage.

Wiles, R. (2012). *What are qualitative research ethics?* A&C Black.

Willig, C. (2019). Ontological and epistemological reflexivity. *Counselling and Psychotherapy Research*, 19(3), 186–194.

Willig, C. (2012). Qualitative Interpretation and Analysis in Psychology. McGraw-Hill.

Willig, C. (2022). *Introducing Qualitative Research in Psychology*. McGraw-Hill.

Winter, D.A. (2003). Repertory grid technique as a psychotherapy research measure. *Psychotherapy Research, 13*(1), 25–42.

Wodak, R., & Meyer, M. (2015). *Methods of critical discourse studies*. Sage.

Wolitzky-Taylor, K.B., Horowitz, J.D., Powers, M.B., & Telch, M.J. (2008). Psychological approaches in the treatment of specific phobias. *Clinical Psychology Review, 28*(6), 1021–1037.

Wong, G., Greenhalgh, T., Westhorp, G., Buckingham, J., & Pawson, R. (2013). RAMESES publication standards. *Journal of Advanced Nursing, 69*(5), 987–1004.

Wrathall, M.A. (2010). *Heidegger and unconcealment*. Cambridge University Press.

Wright, J., & Bolton, G. (2012). *Reflective writing in counselling and psychotherapy*. Sage.

Xiao, H., Hayes, J.A., Castonguay, L.G., McAleavey, A.A., & Locke, B.D. (2017). Therapist effects and the impacts of therapy nonattendance. *Psychotherapy, 54*(1), 58.

Yardley, L. (2015). Demonstrating validity in qualitative psychology. In J.A. Smith (Ed.), *Qualitative psychology: A practical guide to research methods*. Sage.

Young, G. (2017). *Revising the APA ethics code*. Springer.

Zahavi, D. (Ed.) (2018). *The Oxford handbook of the history of phenomenology*. Oxford University Press.

INDEX

Note: Page numbers followed by "*f*" indicate figure and "*t*" indicate table in the text.

www.ingramcontent.com/pod-product-compliance
Ingram Content Group UK Ltd.
Pitfield, Milton Keynes, MK11 3LW, UK
UKHW050858130225
454838UK00004B/45